T0371821

Emerging Technologies for Combatting Pandemics

The COVID-19 pandemic has significantly affected the healthcare sector across the globe. Artificial Intelligence (AI) and the Internet of Medical Things (IoMT) play important roles when dealing with emerging challenges. These technologies are being applied to problems involving the early detection of infections, fast contact tracing, decision-making models, risk profiling of cohorts, and remote treatment. Applying these technologies runs against challenges including interoperability, lack of unified structure for eHealth, and data privacy and security. *Emerging Technologies for Combatting Pandemics: AI, IoMT, and Analytics* examines multiple models and solutions for various settings including individual, home, work, and society. The world's healthcare systems are battling the novel coronavirus, and government authorities, scientists, medical practitioners, and medical services are striving hard to surmount these challenges.

This book focuses on the design and implementation of AI-based approaches in the proposed COVID-19 solutions that are enabled and supported by the IoMT, sensor networks, cloud and edge computing, robotics, and analytics. It covers technologies under the umbrella of AI that includes data science, big data, machine learning (ML), semantic technologies, analytics, and cyber security.

Highlights of the book include:

- Epidemic forecasting models
- Surveillance and tracking systems
- IoMT and Internet of Healthcare Things-based integrated systems for COVID-19
- Social network analysis systems
- Radiological image-based diagnosis systems
- Computational intelligence methods

This reference work is beneficial for interdisciplinary students, researchers, and healthcare and technology professionals who need to know how computational intelligence could be used for surveillance, control, prevention, prediction, diagnosis, and potential treatment of the disease.

Emerging Technologies for Combatting Pandemics
AI, IoMT, and Analytics

Edited by
M. Rubaiyat Hossain Mondal, Utku Kose,
V. B. Surya Prasath, Prajoy Podder, Subrato Bharati,
and Joarder Kamruzzaman

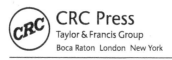

CRC Press
Taylor & Francis Group
Boca Raton London New York

CRC Press is an imprint of the
Taylor & Francis Group, an **informa** business
AN AUERBACH BOOK

Cover Image Credit: Shutterstock.com

First edition published 2023
by CRC Press
6000 Broken Sound Parkway NW, Suite 300, Boca Raton, FL 33487-2742

and by CRC Press
4 Park Square, Milton Park, Abingdon, Oxon, OX14 4RN

CRC Press is an imprint of Taylor & Francis Group, LLC

© 2023 M. Rubaiyat Hossain Mondal, Utku Kose, V. B. Surya Prasath, Prajoy Podder, Subrato Bharati, and Joarder Kamruzzaman

ISBN: 978-1-032-32828-7 (hbk)
ISBN: 978-1-032-34917-6 (pbk)
ISBN: 978-1-003-32444-7 (ebk)

DOI: 10.1201/9781003324447

Typeset in Garamond
by Newgen Publishing UK

Contents

Foreword

AI plays a significant part in today's technological progress. It has become more acceptable for computational solutions to participate actively in daily life as a result of the advances in computer and communication technology. As a result, AI-assisted smart technologies have become indispensable components in the twenty-first century. Before we began to see smart daily life technologies, AI-based solutions were viable options for resolving crucial challenges in a variety of disciplines. As a result, smart instruments have piqued interest in numerous areas including medicine, finance, and education. Healthcare is one of the industries where smart instruments play a significant part in enhancing efficacy and efficiency, because it relates to the wellbeing of the planet and humans. Because of the technological challenges that AI has produced in the healthcare area, it has become more important to apply AI to provide optimal smart healthcare applications.

This edited volume, *Emerging Technologies for Combatting Pandemics: AI, IoMT, and Analytics,* compiles the most recent research efforts for developing effective smart tools for healthcare applications. Many research projects today require multidisciplinary and interdisciplinary cooperation to build alternative solutions, as the lines between technology components from many disciplines are blurring. Hardware components to run physically equipped solutions are now included in today's innovations, in addition to AI and software-oriented touches. This edited book contains various chapters that provide readers with up-to-date information on universal healthcare breakthroughs. As a result, I would like to express my gratitude to the editors for including chapters on the application of popular ML, deep learning (DL), the Internet of Things (IoT), and smart tools in healthcare challenges. The book also includes specific research works to ensure remedies against pandemics, such as COVID-19's big data analysis and detection. As a result, from a relatively recent perspective, the technological side of smart healthcare applications has been well captured, resulting in significant information synergy for interested academics. In this context, I feel that academics, graduate students, and even experts from the public and private sectors who are involved in this field will benefit from this volume. As the world has been more concerned about pandemics in recent years, this book will provide essential insights into how to create effective smart technologies for healthcare tasks while avoiding detrimental repercussions on the climate.

Finally, I would like to express my gratitude to all the editors for their invaluable contributions to the related literature. This book could be effective in filling the knowledge gap between AI and healthcare, because there is a big need for fresh reference books on smart tools for current and future world advances. This book includes all the required information for further study activities, because new generations require the most up-to-date knowledge and capacity to employ the most up-to-date technology components. I would like to extend an invitation to all the readers to enjoy the pages that follow and to begin working for a better future world with a sustainable healthcare infrastructure!

Dr Aditya Khamparia
Assistant Professor, Department of Computer Science,
Babasaheb Bhimrao Ambedkar University, India

Preface

AI was initially described in the literature as a technology tool to increase the speed and success rate when solving critical real-world problems. As a result, it was a branch of research that focused on the technological background of doors. However, as a result of changing cultures and a growing need for digital tools to improve the standards in daily life, AI has been rapidly accepted across a wide range of businesses, ushering in a new 'brave world' equipped with technologically superior tools. As a result, smart applications have become one of the most popular areas of study in the modern era. Smart tools have been developed in conjunction with related research efforts to enable the development of smart applications for buildings, surroundings, campuses, and even cities. In this context, it is critical to apply critical touches to specific issue areas in order to establish the framework for technological solutions. This makes more sense when it comes to key concerns that affect humanity's future.

Agriculture is one of the most significant determinants of humanity's fate. Because the sustainability of human demands (e.g., eating, drinking, and living) is contingent on the sustainability of all agricultural regions in the world, technological advances must always be adapted to dynamically evolving issues. For example, for a lengthy period, the climate crisis and newly emerging environmental concerns have had a sizable impact on the agricultural components.

Therefore, as technological components become increasingly common in agricultural applications, it is critical to conduct a thorough analysis of the balanced instruments that do not have an adverse effect on the climate or environment. The concerns caused by biological processes, such as plant diseases, should be handled through the use of intelligent instruments that are more aware of the specific problem triggers. Additionally, developing self-contained intelligent solutions capable of regulating pandemics and massive amounts of data in healthcare has long been a favored study strategy. Based on the previous information, this edited book was created with the objective of educating a global audience on the most recent technological advances in pandemic prevention. Because AI plays such a critical role in this, the majority of chapters focus on the role of AI and data analytics components when enhancing healthcare applications.

The first chapter introduces an IoMT paradigm for pandemic preparedness. The influence of COVID-19 on the economy is then assessed in the second chapter, with a focus on mining, agricultural, manufacturing, textile, pharmaceutical, and service industries. The third chapter examines the influence of IoT adoption on the long-term viability of small and medium-sized businesses (SMEs) that are affected by the pandemic. The fourth chapter examines India's situation, assessing the negative impact of COVID-19 on key sectors and recommending actions to alleviate the situation. In chapter five, multiple AI models for identifying COVID-19 from computed tomography (CT) or X-ray images are described, as well as AI's involvement in medication research and development. The chapter also discusses the use of AI and blockchain to address security and privacy concerns. The long-term implications of COVID-19 on human health, as well as patient recovery and tracing, and the repercussions for discharged patients are discussed in chapter six. The seventh chapter discusses regression models to investigate the impact of COVID-19 on Bangladesh's seaborne trade. In chapter eight, the readers will discover how to use intelligent optimization and computational learning techniques to combat pandemics. A range of DL techniques for diagnosing and treating coronavirus are examined in chapter nine. The chapter also discusses AI-based DL approaches, as well as available datasets, methods, and performance in the COVID-19 campaign. In Chapter 10, decision tree-based methods (ensembles) for COVID-19 pandemic prediction are implemented and deployed on the global COVID-19 dataset. Using ML techniques, chapter eleven shows how to predict whether a COVID patient needs to stay in an intensive care unit. A long short-term memory (LSTM), which is a type of artificial recurrent neural network (RNN) model, is proposed in chapter twelve for the prediction of COVID-19 distribution in several regions of India. Finally, chapter 13 examines dengue in the presence of COVID-19 and assesses tree-based classifiers on a dengue dataset using stratified K-Fold.

As editors, we feel that this book offers academics, scientists, degree students who will be the future of science, and industrial practitioners who will work closely with academics, a valuable viewpoint on the technological knowledge and capability state. All the authors' efforts are much appreciated. Suggestions from readers are appreciated. We desire a better, more sustainable world with precise technical touches that yield effective and efficient outcomes.

Editors

Acknowledgments

The editors would like to thank and congratulate everyone who helped make this book a reality. We would like to convey our sincere gratitude to all the chapter authors for their contributions, the book would not have been possible without them. Our sincere gratitude and appreciation also go to the subject matter specialists who worked as reviewers and took the time to examine the chapters and provide them on time; therefore, boosting the book's quality, prominence, and consistent layout. We would like to express our gratitude to the entire CRC Press Release team for their constant support and assistance in the publication of this edited book. Finally, we would like to express our gratitude to the Institute of Information and Communication Technology (IICT) at the Bangladesh University of Engineering and Technology for providing technical assistance.

About the Editors

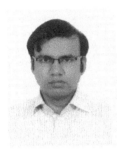

M. Rubaiyat Hossain Mondal received his BSc and MSc degrees in electrical and electronic engineering from the Bangladesh University of Engineering and Technology (BUET), Dhaka, Bangladesh. He obtained a PhD degree in 2014 from the Department of Electrical and Computer Systems Engineering, Monash University, Melbourne, Australia. From 2005 to 2010, and from 2014 to date he has been working as a Faculty Member at the IICT in BUET, Bangladesh. He has published a number of papers in journals of IEEE, IET, Elsevier, Springer, Wiley, De Gruyter, PLOS, and MDPI. He has published several conference papers and book chapters and edited a book published by DeGruyter in 2021. He has successfully supervised 10 students to complete their Masters' Thesis in Information and Communication Technology at BUET, Bangladesh. His research interests include AI, image processing, bioinformatics, wireless communications, and cryptography.

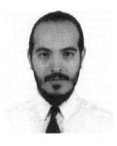

Utku Kose received his BSc degree in 2008 in computer education at Gazi University, Turkey, as a faculty valedictorian. He received his MS degree in 2010 from Afyon Kocatepe University, Turkey, in the field of computers and a DS/PhD degree in 2017 from Selcuk University, Turkey, in computer engineering. Between 2009 and 2011, he worked as a Research Assistant at Afyon Kocatepe University. Following, he has also worked as Lecturer and Vocational School Vice Director at Afyon Kocatepe University between 2011 and 2012, as a Lecturer and Research Center Director at Usak University between 2012 and 2017, and as an Assistant Professor at Suleyman Demirel University between 2017 and 2019. Currently, he is an Associate Professor at Suleyman Demirel University, Turkey. He has more than 100 publications including articles, authored and edited books, proceedings, and reports. He is also on the editorial boards of many scientific journals and serves as one of the editors of the Biomedical and Robotics Healthcare book series by CRC Press. His research interest includes AI, machine ethics, AI safety, optimization, chaos theory, distance education, e-learning, computer education, and computer science.

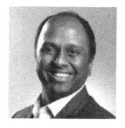

V.B. Surya Prasath graduated from the Indian Institute of Technology Madras, India, in 2009 with a PhD in Mathematics. He is currently an Assistant Professor in the Division of Biomedical Informatics at the Cincinnati Children's Hospital Medical Center, and in the Departments of Biomedical Informatics and Electrical Engineering and Computer Science at the University of Cincinnati from 2018. He has been a postdoctoral fellow at the Department of Mathematics, University of Coimbra, Portugal, for two years from 2010 to 2011. From 2012 to 2015 he was with the Computational Imaging and VisAnalysis Lab at the University of Missouri, USA, as a postdoctoral fellow, and from 2016 to 2017 as an assistant research professor. He had summer fellowships/visits at Kitware Inc. New York, USA; The Fields Institute, Canada; and IPAM, University of California Los Angeles, USA. His main research interests include nonlinear PDEs, regularization methods, inverse, and ill-posed problems, variational, PDE-based image processing, and computer vision with applications in remote sensing, and biomedical imaging domains. His current research focuses on data science and bioimage informatics with ML techniques.

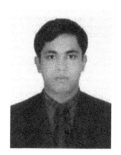

Prajoy Podder is currently a researcher at the IICT, BUET. He worked as a lecturer in the Department of Electrical and Electronic Engineering, Ranada Prasad Shaha University, Narayanganj, Bangladesh. Prajoy Podder received the BSc (Eng) degree in Electronics and Communication Engineering from Khulna University of Engineering and Technology, Khulna, Bangladesh, in 2014. He has recently completed his MSc in Information and Communication Technology from BUET, Dhaka, Bangladesh. Prajoy has authored or co-authored over 45 journal articles, conference proceedings, and book chapters published by IEEE, Elsevier, Springer, Wiley, Degruyter, and others. His research interests include wireless sensor networks, digital image processing, data mining, smart cities, IoT, ML, big data, digital signal processing, wireless communication, and VLSI.

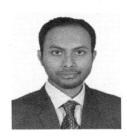

Subrato Bharati received his BSc degree in Electrical and Electronic Engineering from Ranada Prasad Shaha University, Bangladesh. He is currently working as a researcher at the IICT, BUET, Dhaka, Bangladesh. He is a regular reviewer for a number of international journals including those by Elsevier, Springer, Wiley, and other reputed publishers. He is an associate editor of the *Journal of the International Academy for Case Studies* and a guest editor of a special issue in the *Journal of Internet Technology* (SCI Index Journal). He is a member of the scientific and technical program committee for some conferences, such as CECNet 2021, ICONCS, ICCRDA 2020, ICICCR 2021, and CECIT 2021. His research interests include bioinformatics, medical image processing, pattern recognition, DL, wireless communications, data analytics, ML, neural networks, and feature selection. He has published a number of papers in journals by Elsevier, Springer, PLOS, and IOS Press and has also published several IEEE and Springer reputed conference papers. He has published Springer, Elsevier, De Gruyter, CRC Press, and Wiley book chapters as well.

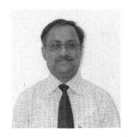

Joarder Kamruzzaman is currently Professor at the School of Science, Engineering and Information Technology, Federation University, Australia. Previously, he served as the Director of the Centre for Multimedia Computing, Communications and AI Research hosted first by Monash University and later by the Federation University. His interests include the IoT, ML, and cybersecurity. He has published over 250 peer-reviewed publications and received a Best Paper award at four international conferences. He has received nearly 2.4 million (AUD) in research funding, including prestigious Australian Research Council and large Collaborative Research Centre grants.

Contributors

Moruf Adeagbo
Mathematics and Computer Sciences
  Department
First Technical University
Ibadan, Nigeria

O. O. Adebowale
Veterinary Public Health and
  Preventive Medicine Department
Federal University of Agriculture
Abeokuta, Nigeria

Samuel Ayomikun Akinseinde
The Amateur Polymath
Lagos, Nigeria

Jide Ebenezer Taiwo Akinsola
Mathematics and Computer Sciences
  Department
First Technical University
Ibadan, Nigeria

A. A. Awoseyi
Mathematics and Computer Sciences
  Department
First Technical University
Ibadan, Nigeria

Mohammad Tameem Hossain Azmi
Department of Shipping and Maritime
  Science
Canadian University of Bangladesh
Dhaka, Bangladesh

Chitharanjan Billa
22nd Century Technologies Inc.
Washington, D.C., USA

M. Bohara
Computer Engineering
Devang Patel Institute of Advance
  Technology and Research,
  CHARUSAT
Gujarat, India

Jagadeesh Chandra Bose K.
Chandigarh University
Gharuan, India

Murthy Chavali
Faculty of Science and Technology
Alliance University
Bengaluru, India
NTRC-MCETRC
Tenali, India

J. Desai
Computer Science and Engineering
Devang Patel Institute of Advance
  Technology and Research,
  CHARUSAT
Gujarat, India

V. Aruna Devi
MIT Campus
Anna University
Chennai, India

A. Ganatra
Devang Patel Institute of Advance
  Technology and Research,
  CHARUSAT
Gujarat, India

Jyotsna Garikipati
Department of Information Technology
V R Siddhartha Engineering College
Kanurau, India

E. A. Gopalakrishnan
Center for Computational Engineering
  and Networking
Amrita School of Engineering
Coimbatore, India

Anshi Gupta
Chandigarh University
Gharuan, India

Jakir Hosain
Department of Shipping and Maritime
  Science
Canadian University of Bangladesh
Dhaka, Bangladesh

Supreet Kaur
Department of Computer Engineering
  and Technology
Guru Nanak Dev University
Amritsar, India

Reena Malik
Chitkara Business School
Chitkara University
Punjab, India

W. K. Mooi
Infrastructure University
Kuala Lumpur, Malaysia

Kayode Abiodun Oladapo
Babcock University
Ilisan-Remo, Nigeria

O. M. Oladoja
Mathematics and Computer Sciences
  Department
First Technical University
Ibadan, Nigeria

Fathia Onipede
First Technical University
Ibadan, Nigeria

Mredulraj S. Pandianchery
Center for Computational Engineering
  and Networking
Amrita School of Engineering
Coimbatore, India

B. Patel
Computer Science and Engineering
Devang Patel Institute of Advance
  Technology and Research,
  CHARUSAT
Gujarat, India

D. Patel
Computer Engineering
Chandubhai S Patel Institute of
  Technology, CHARUSAT
Gujarat, India

K. Patel
Computer Science and Engineering
Devang Patel Institute of Advance
    Technology and Research,
    CHARUSAT
Gujarat, India

Varalakshmi Perumal
MIT Campus
Anna University
Chennai, India

Bornali Rahman
Department of Shipping and Maritime
    Science
Canadian University of Bangladesh
Dhaka, Bangladesh

Sakthi Jaya Sundar Rajasekar
Melmaruvathur Adhiparasakthi
    Institute of Medical Sciences and
    Research
Melmaruvathur, India

Sandeep Sharma
Department of Computer Engineering
    and Technology
Guru Nanak Dev University
Amritsar, India

Sonia Sharma
Chandigarh University
Gharuan, India

R. Abd Shukor
Infrastructure University
Kuala Lumpur, Malaysia

K. P. Soman
Center for Computational Engineering
    and Networking
Amrita School of Engineering
Coimbatore, India

V. Sowmya
Center for Computational Engineering
    and Networking
Amrita School of Engineering
Coimbatore, India

Manas Kumar Yogi
Department of Computer Science and
    Engineering
Pragati Engineering College
Surampalem, India

Adebola Abdulwaheed Yusuf
Federal University of Petroleum
    Resources
Effurun, Nigeria

Chapter 1

Artificial Intelligence Leveraged Internet of Medical Things and Continuous Health Monitoring and Combating Pandemics within the Internet of Medical Things Framework

Chitharanjan Billa
22nd Century Technologies Inc., Washington, D.C., USA

Murthy Chavali
*Department of Science, Faculty of Science & Technology,
Alliance University, Karnataka, India*
NTRC-MCETRC, Tienali, India

DOI: 10.1201/9781003324447-1

Contents

1.1 Introduction

A flu-like outbreak in Wuhan, China in late 2019 spread rapidly to other parts of the world and the World Health Organization (WHO) declared it a pandemic (1) due to the large number of deaths that were associated with this outbreak. WHO also named this pandemic coronavirus disease or COVID-19 (2,3). Johns Hopkins University, Baltimore, MD, US calculated the case fatality rate at 2.15% as of July 2021 (4,5). The international committee on virus taxonomy named this virus SARS-Cov-2 on February 11, 2020. It was thought that this virus is transmitted via bats. Pangolins were initially thought to be the source but after several examinations, these were exonerated. There could be other direct or intermediate bird or animal hosts; however, they are yet to be identified and proved. Owing to its crown-like spiky appearance via microscopy this virus was named coronavirus. There were several fatal and adverse effects on humanity due to this virus. The Congressional Research Service (US) estimated the adverse effects of the virus and stated that the global economic growth in 2020 was reduced from -3.4% to -7.6% (annualized rate) and the recovery rate was projected from 4.2% to 5.6% for 2021. Trading at the global level was estimated to have tumbled by 5.3% in 2020; it is also poised to rise by 8.0% in 2021.

The need to mitigate and end this pandemic was severely felt not only to save lives but also to revive the economy; therefore, preventing other cascading adverse effects on humanity. Technology became the centerpiece for every solution, be it medical, financial, economic, or from any other solution standpoint. The race for an effective vaccination, finding the COVID-19 clusters in the countries to reduce transmission and helping the patients who are critically ill as well as who needs routine or emergency care for COVID, and non-COVID-related illness becomes a top priority to governments, scientific communities, and medical communities.

By setting up robust information technology (IT) infrastructure with the available cloud solutions and by leveraging artificial intelligence (AI), this pandemic could be successfully eradicated. With the use of the Internet of Medical Things (IoMT) from an AI perspective, the ongoing cybersecurity challenges and infrastructure challenges will be discussed at a deeper level.

This chapter mainly discusses how to scale the software when there is a surge in patient admissions to hospitals, perform quick genome-based diagnostic tests and share the results with the research and scientific community for effective treatments and vaccinations. AI-based analytics could help the government and medical agencies to determine the surge in trends and quantify the virus mutations in different clusters; it could help the administration to take decisions on border control and the procurement of emergency devices, such as PPE equipment. This chapter also proposes the latest Kubernetes technologies, edge computing, and genome-based rapid testing to quickly diagnose, track and trace infected patients and treat them rapidly using machine language and AI.

1.2 Defining the Role of AI from an IoMT Perspective

The term AI was first described by Pamela McCorduck in her book *Machines Who Think* (6). The author tried to portray AI as more of a possibility with human imagination in contrast to a standard scientific way of describing things, such as theorems that include hypotheses and conclusions. There is often confusion between machine learning (ML) and AI and it's imperative to understand that AI has more applications and comprehensiveness than machine language.

Although there are several important AI applications from the IoMT perspective, diagnosis stands on top of the list. Before the advent of the Internet of Things (IoT) or IoMT, most patient–doctor collaborations used to be via in-person clinical visits and the next popular option was teledoctor, where the patient interacts with a physician mostly over the telephone and explains the problem. This type of diagnosis is often error-prone and is not an absolute diagnosis. As the technology progressed, telediagnosis moved from teledoctor to agent-based dialogue where trained clinical agents used to note and store the patient's symptoms and other vital statistics, such as weight, hypertension, and blood glucose values in a notepad type of locally stored computer artifact and relay them the physician via email and other electronic means. Physicians used to review these records and then suggest appropriate medical regimens. This program worked for several years but this was constrained because it could only support a minor diagnosis. If the patient was suffering from a life-threatening disease, such as heart failure, the patient still had to be rushed to the clinic or emergency room for diagnosis and treatment.

One important role AI plays in the medical field is to provide an evaluation of previously stored data immediately in cases of emergencies and routine procedures. This is possible only by deploying IoMT devices, such as glucose, heartbeat, blood pressure monitors, and other devices that continually send patient data to the required parties, for example, emergency rooms, physicians, and pharmacies. IoMT devices also can simultaneously send the required data to insurance companies for appropriate analysis so that patient benefits are calculated and paid promptly. It is preferred to have almost near real time data and monitoring, particularly in case of emergencies where IoMT, which is powered by AI, will give a definite advantage to patients and physicians. These connected IoMT devices could significantly reduce hospital visits and avoid the spread of the virus during pandemics. Simple methods and IoMT devices to detect vital parameters and alert the hospitals could be achieved by the merger of AI with IoMT.

1.3 Relevance of AI During a Pandemic

Without a doubt, AI was well used during the COVID-19 pandemic. In particular, physicians, patients, and clinics were able to harness the advantages and power of AI. This pandemic generated an urgency for modernizing and enhancing the current AI systems and practices that are in place.

1.3.1 Predictive Analytics

AI could be successfully used in COVID-19 outbreak predictions and tracking. A successful initiative that was started by John Hopkins University, Baltimore, MD, US is being used widely across the public and medical communities. There is a variety of information including zip codes, number of cases, and number of deaths on a daily, weekly, and monthly basis. A few other companies, such as HealthMap, a lot of scientists, epidemiologists, and software engineers at Boston Children's Hospital, Boston, MA, US [founded in 2006 (7)] developed (content is aggregated from freely available information from several sources); www.diseasedaily.org/about) and BlueDot (2013), a Canadian software company with insights, used to plot the extent of infectious diseases, its software received substantial attention during the COVID-19 pandemic and is being used to trail outbursts of COVID-19 (8). HealthMap and BlueDot are very effective in harnessing publicly available data and providing valuable insights for government agencies, medical communities, and the public in general. Technical companies can provide effective forecasting methods leveraging multimodal data methods. Contact tracing is another very crucial function to alleviate the spread of rapidly communicable diseases, such as COVID-19.

China was the first country to experience the outbreak and it was the first country to apply AI to combat the pandemic. China also started using the IoMT during the peak pandemic situation. Its first application was the use of infrared thermometers, cameras, and AI-based face recognition systems. The deployment of AI-capable robots in critical crowded places helped the health authorities to avoid contact with the subjects and monitor temperatures at a very rapid rate. South Korea also demonstrated similar capability using AI to Test, Track, and Trace (famously called the 3-Ts) (9). Using these techniques, quick dashboards were set up to find the new cases and report the daily progress. Next-generation communication technology (5G) was also used to prevent the spread of this disease. China also used ML methods for genome studies, clustered regularly interspaced short palindromic repeats (CRISPR) assay was used to generate potential drug candidates against COVID-19.

1.3.2 Current Challenges

After several reviews across the globe, health auditors flagged errors in the recorded data; therefore, skewing patients' electronic health records (EHRs) (10). It was found that the clinical staff that entered the data were responsible for these unintentional human errors. Of interest, when the nurses or clinical staff entered data directly into the computers, there were several unforeseen errors. However, fewer errors or no errors were found when the data were directly read from radio frequency identification (radio) devices, barcoded, or when entered via a mobile application. The challenge when getting rid of paper records and moving to computers or mobile applications is there is a huge shortage of these special devices and hospitals must spend a lot of money on these devices when they are constrained by limited budgets.

Another critical challenge is computers or mobile devices may have to undergo regular maintenance, sometimes daily maintenance, for antivirus and patch updates that include Apple, Android, Windows, and Linux upgrades. The US government mandates every company in the health industry to comply with Health Information Technology (HITECH) (Health IT act) which requires quality health records (such as EHRs) in clinical settings in emergency rooms. This mandate helps insurance and government health care agencies, such as Medicaid and Medicare to send the payments to the beneficiaries quickly. The National Institute of Health is encouraging health-related IT vendors with grants and incentives to modernize their equipment, therefore, helping to adopt AI rapidly.

1.4 Proposed Technology Framework for IoMT Mobile Apps

Having a standardized framework across the health industry is the need of the hour. Considering the ongoing COVID-19 situation, It would be an efficient and effective decision to create an AI-based mobile application for COVID-related treatments, routine treatments, and emergency treatments. Emphasis should be given to easy-use devices, such as mobile tablets for use at check-in counters and hospital wards. For example, receptionists, physician assistants, nurses, and doctors should be provided with tablets instead of using common PCs.

Systems should have all the patients' available EHRs, which should include the latest doctor's visit, recent medication use, recent, and archived lab results. All available image data, such as X-rays and CT scans also should be available. It takes a lot of time to collect this data if the patient has medical records in different places.

Furthermore, it will encourage a new way of engaging patients and their families as physicians and staff can pull up a patient's record in real time to show them detailed X-ray images, and lab results. as part of the dialogue regarding the best course of treatment for the patient; therefore, creating a more intimate connection between patients and staff, and a better overall patient experience. The various stakeholders in the enterprise health model are shown in Figure 1.1.

Factors to be accounted for when designing the IoMT-related mobile applications.

1. As security is important, the framework should consider security with utmost importance. It should comply with all US regulatory frameworks, such as Health Insurance Portability and Accountability Act (HIPPA) and other health-related frameworks. If an authorization token (OAuth) protocol is being used for authentication, appropriate federated identity management services should be factored in during the design phase

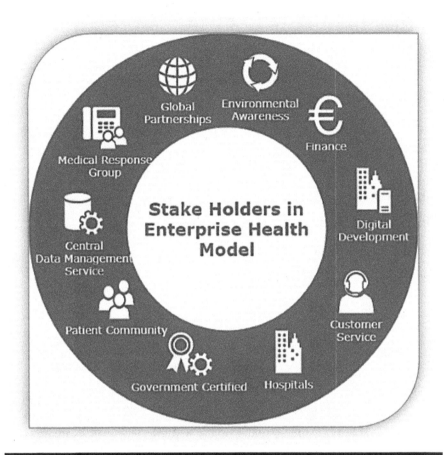

Figure 1.1   Various stakeholders in the enterprise health model

2. AI-based mobile applications should be able to interact with a variety of systems. The application should be open-ended and should not limit itself to a particular technology, database, or operating system commonly accepted data exchange protocols should be widely used, for example, JSON format
3. It is preferable to have a widely used and accepted technology stack so that the mobile application gains popular use and demand
4. Enough care should be taken about where the data would be stored to comply with local country regulations
5. Systems should have modern architecture, preferably service-oriented architecture. Proprietary application programming interfaces (APIs) should be included so that the mobile applications would be able to use huge historical data for rapid diagnosis and prescription management

6. Failover should be well thought out across the geographical locations so that emergency services would not be interrupted and there would be continuity for inpatient services
7. Load factor of >10,000 concurrent users should be considered and approximately 1,000,000 patient encounters should be considered from a sizing perspective

The proposed set of mobile applications and generic medical applications portal is given in Table 1.1.

Table 1.1 Proposed Mobile Applications and Generic Medical Applications Portal

Mobile Apps and Applications Portal	Description
EHR (IoMT) App	Mobile that has a capability that allows a person's EHR to be automatically updated by remote IoMT devices with a medical/emergency alerting capability (e.g., temperature, blood glucose, hypertension monitors, pacemakers, and EKG sensors)
Total Wellness App	This is a generic mobile application available for public consumption and available for download on iTunes/Google-Store
Care App	This is a generic mobile bedside application for clinical usage (e.g., receptionist, nurses, and physicians) and directly update the EHR of the patient during treatment, surgery, and pharmacy visits Information such as real time heartbeat, blood glucose, and blood pressure is gathered from other IoMT devices, such as Fitbit, Apple-watch, and medically approved wearables
Patient Portal	This is a generic portal to schedule hospital visits, manage repeat prescriptions, change scheduled visits, and print previous lab reports
Physician Social App	A secured social media app for connecting with registered doctors and seeking advice on treatment and getting a correct diagnosis
Genetic App	Allows physicians to enter the profile of a cancer patient (e.g., demographics, health, cancer diagnosis, medical history, hematology, drugs, and treatments) to find pattern matches against multiple data warehouses storing clinical cancer cases to compare and influence treatments and achieve better outcomes

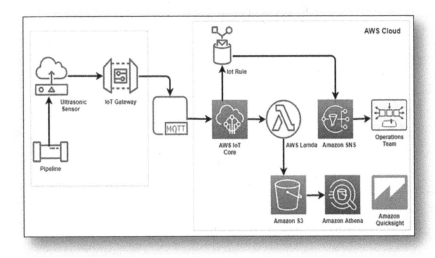

Figure 1.2   Typical IoMT architecture if Amazon Web Services are being used

The Food and Drug Administration (FDA) issued several emergency usage authorizations for IoMT devices during the SARS-COV-2 situation. These devices helped patients and the clinical staff community a lot to avoid physical contact with infected patients and helped when collecting vital parameters for treatment and continuous monitoring. These devices are noninvasive and do not need education to use. The approved wearables from the FDA are shown in Figure 1.2.

1.4.1 Example eHealth Standards for EHRs

EHRs are considered the base for any health application. Architecture and strategies for system integration and interoperability should be designed and developed for any health care service provider. EHealth Standards will continue to lead in planning a protected, interoperable, and scalable EHR system. This could be achieved by thoroughly applying a range of industry best practices to ensure a strong EHR. Mostly, the EHRs (Figure 1.3) are web and client-server-based as they use interactive databases and data access. A few EHRs were developed between 1971 and 1992, which were based on hierarchical or relational databases, and used systems that were established as clinical systems and used to advance medical research (11).

Avoiding duplication and promoting the accessibility of data require the privacy and security of personally identifiable information (PII) are required. This would be key to building a patient-centric EHR. The application will make use of the following parameters.

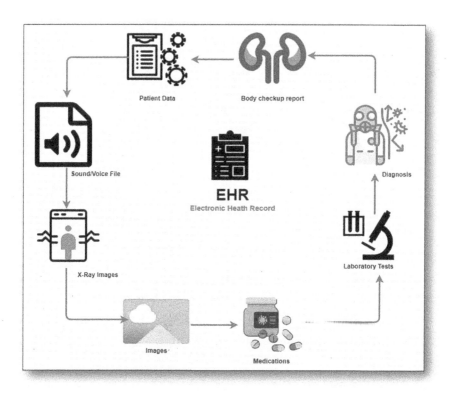

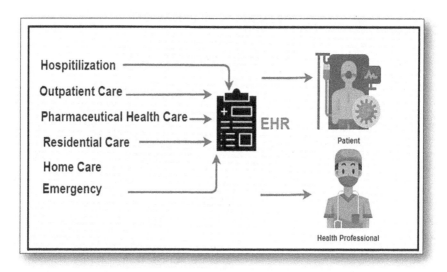

Figure 1.3 Showing: (Top) EHR; (Bottom) EHR, an integrated model of care. (Continued)

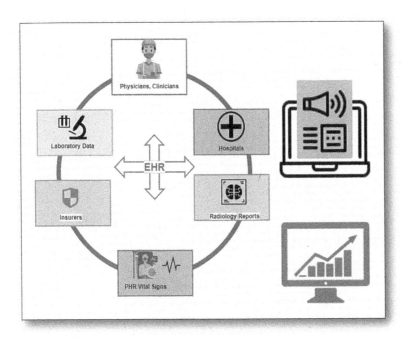

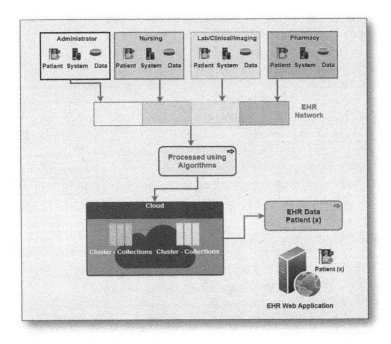

Figure 1.3 (Continued) Showing: (Top) EHR augmenting healthcare delivery system; and (Bottom) typical EHR framework for the healthcare system

1. Clinical file specification
2. Approval directives
3. Discharge summary standard
4. e-Referral standard
5. Health care audit standard
6. Provincial/state client registry standard (Canada/US)
7. Provincial/state clinical document architecture header standard (Canada/US)
8. Single sign-on/patient context sharing standard
9. Connect applications
10. Service-oriented architecture policies and principles (draft, which is important for overall system architecture)

1.4.2 EHRs in Developed Countries

In Europe, 19 out of 33 countries are at the stage of the planning and implementation of a patient summary and EHR-like system. A few countries including Sweden, Denmark, Finland, the UK, Austria, Germany, Norway, the Netherlands, and Switzerland are leading in EHRs (12). Countries like Canada and Australia are in the most advanced stage of nationwide EHR policies (13). Denmark leads where eHealth integration and daily services in healthcare are concerned (14). In England, the approach will introduce Summary Care Records with limited storage of data for the patients except for patients who do not want one (15). EHRs were initiated in Austria in 2005 with a health reorganization law. A single information exchange platform for health providers and authorities was developed by the government as the National Health Network in Norway. The health quality of Switzerland is high quality and costly.

In 2010, New Zealand introduced the National Health IT plan. In mid-1990, Israel was the first country that introduced a Health IT Information Exchange System with primary care doctors using EHRs. Among Asian countries, a health information exchange project was started that supported healthcare information by integrating wired and wireless networking with a healthcare information and communication technology infrastructure.

The EHR is of high priority in developed countries due to public funding while EHRs are still in a nascent stage in low to medium-income countries. In Canada, EHRs are interoperable nationwide through the Canada Health Info way initiative. Further, there is literature from countries, such as Australia and Hong Kong where EHRs were implemented based on the consumer's needs and patient's healthcare.

An EHR is a select e-record of a person's health over time that covers patient demographics, notes on clinical problems, treatment, medicines, previous health accounts, and clinical data and can be retrieved immediately and easily by certified personnel. This makes access instantaneous and secure to certified users about the information required on the patient in real time, treatment-centered records contain the therapeutic and medical management history of patients. The users are expanding order sets, mobile devices, voice recognition, barcodes, and documents system to transfer the data into EHRs.

EHRs are widely used in nursing homes, home health, and various organizations caring for homeless populations. There can be interfacing of personal health records within EHRs, which can be used largely for large facilities and vendors. The DNA can be used for clinical decision key support features for practitioners and a large amount of information can be used as a source of phenotypic information for analytical purposes. The data are the data sources for phenotypic and genomic information research, which can be stored in the records of EHRs. EHRs, in one way help to build an improved healthy future for a nation; they contain more information on the patient's complete wellbeing, which is broader than the electronic medical records of a patient.

1.4.2.1 Benefits

1. Electronic patient record files are easier to transfer; there is no confusion over illegible handwriting, possibly leading to cost savings for the patient and the medical provider
2. Electronic clinic management can reduce cancellations, missed appointments, and waiting times
3. The use of electronic prescriptions would help patients get their medications quicker
4. Surveillance of healthcare-associated infections (HAI)
5. Clinicians identify and classify chronically ill patients
6. EHRs can improve quality care by using data and analytics to prevent hospitalizations among high-risk patients
7. Facilitate the coordination of healthcare delivery in nonaffiliated healthcare facilities
8. Statistical reporting for quality enhancement, resource administration, and public health communicable disease surveillance
9. Can reduce the risk of data replication and the risk of lost paperwork
10. Digital information, for example, possible trends and long-term changes in a patient are searchable
11. Facilitate population-based studies

1.4.2.2 Limitations

1. Electronic medical records should only be stored on secure networks
2. Unauthorized access to records for illegitimate purposes is of major concern
3. During a natural disaster, a crisis with electricity would cause the proper network access to e-records will be difficult

4. Accessibility issues
5. It is important to realize that patient access to health data is an important component of patient engagement
6. Lack of uniform standards for national and international operations for electronic patient records. For the system to work seamlessly, the software must be uniform, or there must be a way to convert between different standards easily
7. Cost factor: a tool that was originally developed to increase communication and quality of care may create a riskier healthcare environment
8. Increased use of mobile technology may impact security measures and patient privacy rules
9. Health records long-term preservation and storage. There is a lack of consistent, well-regulated, and efficient standardized preservation infrastructures to support a wide variety of EHRs and data formats

1.4.3 EHR Resources for System Development

The potential value of EHRs lies in the transformation of the healthcare community. The creation of a database through an EHR system is a significant process due to spatial, complexity, interrelation, temporal, heterogeneous, and fast-evolving data. Nevertheless, data models are created through several processes.

An EHR is an integration process that involves a network of systems, databases, interfaces, physicians, entry orders, and electronic and clinical workstations. EHR systems consist of highly structured data, for example, medical, security, legal, and financial data. An EHR is an electronic record of the patient that keeps track of an individual's lifetime health. An EHR uses cloud computing for easy access as it reduces the cost of installation, hardware, and software. Software as a Service (SaaS) is applied to cloud computing with software-oriented architecture (SOA), which can access records from end to end web service. SOA can be accessible through web-portal and circumstantial services from the cloud, where stored HER data is present.

1.5 Kubernetes Advantages in AI-Based IoMT

Testing, decisions, and treatment should be carried out in a rapid phase during pandemic situations. The world has witnessed many deaths during the recent COVID-19 situation. Systems that are fragile and monolithic could not cope with the workload coming from patients and physicians. The best way to deal with these situations is to move away from on-premises or isolated server-based architecture to containers and run the applications on them. Emergency rooms or any other hospital and treatment centers would suffer many casualties if there was any downtime.

1.5.1 Kubernetes Example

In monolithic architecture, if one server goes down, bringing up another server will involve a lot of lead time. But containers can handle this transition seamlessly from one container to another. This is achieved automatically without any human intervention. Failover is handled seamlessly by Kubernetes and runs these distributed systems safely (Figure 1.4).

1.5.2 Distinctive Advantages of Kubernetes in the Medical Field

1.5.2.1 Password Management

Configuration and secrets management is very easy in Kubernetes and lets the owners and hospitals manage sensitive information, such as PII. Other information, such as secure shell (SSH) keys, and OAuth tokens could be stored well in Kubernetes. When a container has to be rebuilt, that can be done seamlessly without exposing any sensitive information.

1.5.2.2 Automated Deployment

The deployment of a medical-related mobile app can be done declaratively. Kubernetes eliminates the need for downtime and archives this immediately; therefore, helping with other processes.

1.5.2.3 Packaging Applications

There was a need to produce applications rapidly, in particular, during the COVID-19 pandemic situation. Automatic bin packing would be easier with Kubernetes and declaratively define how many central processing units and RAM should be provided for each container. Node or container design would be easy with Kubernetes compared with other orchestration tools.

1.5.2.4 Storage Management and Orchestration

Kubernetes provides different choices for storage and orchestration, such as On-Cloud and On-Prem. A hybrid solution also could be used in Kubernetes. As petabytes of data must be stored in servers, monolithic applications would not be able to store large data sets and retrieve them successfully.

1.5.2.5 Load-Balancing Mechanism

AI-based applications obtain data from various diverse sources. It must be load balanced properly so that the nodes that have high loads will be protected properly.

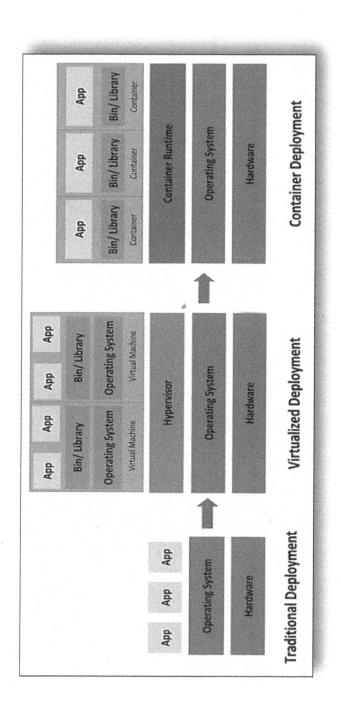

Figure 1.4 Typical deployments

Source: Google Inc.

1.6 Prescription and Medicine Administration using AI

We are used to visiting hospitals for routine and emergency care situations. This was thought to be the usual norm until COVID-19 was identified. After discovering the primary mode of disease transmission was via droplets and air to a certain extent, restrictions were introduced on physical movement. Virtual diagnosis using video calls and other technology applications became the new norm. Continuous monitoring while patients were at home and receiving treatments during homestays became a reality. In this section, how prescription administration using AI is discussed.

There are three essential areas from a prescription and administration viewpoint.

1. Routine care
2. Emergency care
3. Pandemic situation care

AI could be leveraged well in the previous three areas. AI would help in targeted medicine, customization, and diagnosis. Apart from the diagnosis, AI can priori-tize which patient should be investigated first when there are thousands of patients waiting for treatment at the same hospital. This will avoid a first-come-first-serve basis, which would be good under normal circumstances but not in pandemic situations.

Data is collected from the following sources, such as food habits, sleep and stress data, current prescription data, and other laboratory data and then sent to a cloud and used by all parties (e.g., hospitals, doctors, and ambulances) as shown in Figure 1.5.

We are on the brink of a new technological revolution in the medical field. How prescriptions are administered is going to change rapidly with the merger of the IoMT and AI.

1.7 Cybersecurity Challenges in AI-Based IoMT

Several reports suggest that the privacy of patients has been compromised. When AI systems have been deployed by hospitals and clinics, complex data is being transmitted on the pretext of improving the services. Service providers collect huge amounts of data from various sources to train their data models. Typical collections include heartbeat data, pregnancy progression, chronic kidney disease progression, and abnormal hypertension readings. Many big hospitals, such as the Mayo Clinic, Rochester, MIN, US, collect huge amounts of data from patients for their ongoing research purposes. The main concern is that patients are not aware of how their data is being used or if any products are being developed using their DNA profiles.

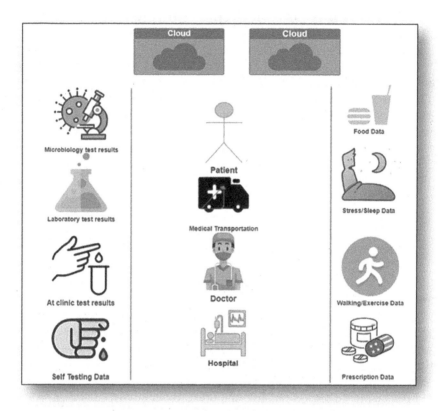

Figure 1.5 Various data sources from an IoMT perspective

AI companies should take all necessary steps to allay the fears of patients and communities and vouch for the ethical use of the data. A certain percentage of revenue generated from patients' data should be distributed back to the data owner, such as the copyright agreement.

1.7.1 Zero Trust Architecture for IoMT Devices

Data generated by IoMT devices are protected by law as they contain PII. The sensitive nature of the data and for the best interest of the enterprises and organizations must be taken into consideration in "zero trust" security architecture. In zero trust architecture, any IoMT device that cannot be verified is denied access to the dependent database and application servers. This principle applies regardless of the location of the device, which can be either located internally or externally to the security perimeter. All users, systems (including databases), devices, and wearables are considered suspect or threat vectors until they are verified by the connecting system or device. To implement this policy, security is applied at the following levels or access points: (1) OS Platforms; (2) network security; (3) data security; (4) Identity and access management security; and (5) device security (16).

1.7.2 Role-Based Authentication in AI-Based IoMT

Authentication and authorization are two critical factors in any identity management solution. Authentication confirms the identity of the users who are claiming access. Authorization gives the user permission to access or use certain or all applications. During the authentication process, user credentials are validated to confirm the authenticity. This is the primary or minimal function needed by any secure application. Applications connected to IoMT devices are recommended to have multifactor authentication (MFA).

1.7.3 Workflow of Authentication

The user enters a username and password and if both fields exactly match the identity data stored in the systems, access is granted. If MFA is used, a one-time pin is sent via an SMS and the user enters this pin to confirm authenticity. In addition to both validations, it is better to have authentication applications, such as the Google authentication app. Applications or devices are more secure these days using biometrics, such as fingerprints or iris scans to confirm their authenticity. After authentication, based on the approved roles, the user would have access to critical data. For example, a finance manager cannot access a medical image application, only physicians are allowed to access this information.

1.8 Scalability of IoMT

The world's data is expected to grow to 175 zettabytes by 2025 (an approximate increase of 61% as of 2021) (17). It was also projected that the storage industry would produce and ship 42 zettabytes of data by 2028. In total, 90 zettabytes of data would be generated by IoT devices, including IoMT devices. Overall, 90 zettabytes of data will be created on IoT devices by 2025. Almost 50% of the public data would be on the public cloud.

The majority of this data is generated by IoT devices including IoMT devices. The adoption of the cloud made data incorporation easy but as the data grew it became increasingly difficult to retrieve and use it on demand. A major problem is a latency between the source servers and destination servers or devices. The SaaS model, instant availability of the complex hardware, on demand setup of infrastructure using infrastructure as a code, and cost-effective operational costs are the major benefits of cloud computing. Although there are several benefits with cloud computing, it still lacks performance and scalability issues as described previously, in particular, with IoMT devices.

1.8.1 Introducing Edge Computing

Enterprises or organizations should consider latency and performance when designing their systems. Edge computing would be the best possible solution to address the major scalability and performance issues that are seen in the current cloud environments. Edge computing would be the preferred solution where IoMT devices are involved. It is imperative to distinguish between edge computing and IoMT. Although edge computing is not a one-fit solution for every latency problem, each case must be evaluated before spending any infrastructure budget on this architecture.

1.8.2 Components of Edge Computing

Generally, IoT sensors, cloud infrastructure, AI, ML, big data, and edge gateways are the major components involved in edge computing. These could vary depending on the use. The IoT or IoMT sensors collect the data and feed it to the cloud infrastructure and apply AI and ML algorithms. The previous processes are executed in different layers. The IoT and IoMT sensors are in device layers and these devices relate to the application layer where the AI and ML algorithms are applied for urgent or critical decisions. In the cloud servers, edge computing gateways are placed in a different layer that is in proximity to the devices. IoMT sensors play an important role in the diagnosis and treatment of patients in COVID-19 pandemic situations. Emphasis is placed on location in edge computing, which makes treatment and attending to patients easier compared with cloud computing, where there would be latency either in the transfer of data or in creating, inserting, updating, and deleting operations related to the patient's EHR.

1.8.3 Factors to Consider before the Adoption of Edge Computing

The following factors need to be considered when deciding if edge computing should be introduced to the new or existing architecture.

1. If there is an existing cloud infrastructure and the main problem is with bandwidth or latency, thorough and deep benchmarking statistics should be generated. Data load and the average data volumes and traffic should be taken into consideration. Target architecture should be in place with appropriate gateways
2. Faster implementation and results and safety are two important factors that need to be considered to adopt edge computing. In the current COVID-19

situation, where the infrastructure must be set up immediately in weeks, if not in days, anything that takes more time to set up or takes time to operate is considered negatively

3. Simplicity is another factor to be considered before implementing edge computing. Making current architecture as simple as possible without introducing complexities is another important factor

4. Government framework compliance, such as HIPPA and other country-related regulations to be incorporated helps to maintain the privacy and security of the individual health records and protects data from any cyber-attacks on the critical medical systems

5. Quick failover architecture is another important factor to be considered in IoMT devices as these would help critical diagnosis and procedures to be performed online.

Any interruptions during the patient consultation would result in a high number of adverse effects; therefore, failover architecture should be in place when considering edge computing.

1.8.4 Challenges in Implementing Edge Computing

As discussed previously, several advantages are associated with using or adopting edge computing. But edge computing has its limitations and challenges. The following challenges should be considered before deciding to adopt edge computing.

1. Expenses and costs are the most important challenges. This factor depends on the available infrastructure budget, including capital expenditures and operating expenses so this practice could be adopted for several years. Operational costs are huge to maintain this complex system as enterprises need to hire highly-skilled engineers and DevOps personnel. Edge computing costs are an addition to the ongoing cloud computing costs

2. Technical and operational challenges are the next main challenges to be addressed. From the IoMT perspective, we are dealing with millions of devices and in the current COVID-19 pandemic, these numbers could grow exponentially as the number of patients increases. As discussed earlier, edge computing mainly deals with access locations and communication with the medical sensors via several thousands of edge gateways. These gateways have their operating systems. If gateways are running on containerized and virtualized environments there are a lot of challenges in maintaining these containers, such as applying regular OS patches, security patches, or updates and monitoring the health of the containers regularly. These updates must be applied regularly and sometimes daily to keep the systems up and running. In addition to these, hardware upgrades would also be required

3. Cybersecurity challenges in edge computing are another area that must be noted. In edge computing, an additional layer (i.e., nodes or gateways) is introduced thus increasing the chance of cybersecurity issues or threats. These threats would be increased drastically as the number of connections with nodes or gateways increased. Cyber attackers can introduce malaise software to cause service disruption using denial-of-service methods.

1.9 Continuous Monitoring for the Availability of IoMT

After scalability, continuous availability is an important aspect of the IoMT. It is desirable to achieve 99.999% availability for all IoMT-related systems keeping the criticality of the application as these devices are vital for the diagnosis and treatment of patients during the COVID-19 pandemic. The 99.9% availability allows 8.76 h of downtime, 99.99% allows 1 h of downtime, and 99.999% availability allows 5 mins of downtime per year. There are two types of outages from an availability standpoint. The first one is a planned outage, where the users or customers are notified about the outage in advance, which is normal in any software enterprise. The second one is an unplanned outage, where unavailability occurs due to human, software, or hardware errors or failures. The unplanned outage is not desirable in the IoMT area. Hence, designing the systems for continuous availability is vital.

1.9.1 Designing IoMT Systems for High Availability

Cloud service providers or other technology providers who provide communication-related services generally state their availability between 99.9% and 99.999%. Enterprises need to adopt innovative measures to attain a high degree of availability, and these are the suggested guidelines.

1. The operations team should have a robust Standard Operating Procedure document that describes various scenarios to cover unplanned outages at various layers in the architecture, such as compute, network, and storage
2. A load balancer should be in place to mitigate single points of failure, which is commonly referred to as SPOF. Configurations generally use active–active or active–standby methods to avoid SPOF scenarios. Using a load-balancing mechanism and utilizing N+1 redundancy configuration SPOF could be mitigated or eliminated. N+1 configuration needs active–active nodes. A load-balancing cluster would help in achieving high availability configurations

3. Automated monitoring is critical to achieving high availability. Monitoring scripts, executing automated tests at regular intervals (i.e., checking the availability for every 30 s) and alerting the sysadmins and owners will help them to quickly bring back the systems after failover and even help avert a failure scenario

4. It is recommended to have a floating IP address always available so that distributed systems, databases, and application servers would be connected through this floating IP. Underlying systems may experience failure; however, the floating IP connects to the redundant or next available system automatically and for the end-user, this would be a seamless experience.

This concept is very important in IoMT-related apparatus, servers, and devices.

1.10 Practical uses of AI-Based IoMT in Pandemics

Current pandemics like COVID-19 presented humanity with unprecedented challenges. And many challenges are showing up simultaneously, throwing the physicians and scientific community with priority questions. Communities are struggling with the question of which task or action should be prioritized first.

1. Stop the massive number of deaths that occurred due to this pandemic
2. Diagnose accurately and treat the people who are admitted into intensive care units
3. Develop an effective vaccination for all age groups so that this pandemic can be softened
4. Administer the vaccine quickly across countries, including the unreachable areas keeping in mind the nonaffordability of the vaccination due to cost reasons.

AI-based IoMT devices and applications provide promising solutions to all these issues. One of the main features of AI applications or systems is that they manifest similar characteristics to a human mind or human thought processes. For example, facial recognition or learning once and repeating the same task several times. Some of the mathematical techniques would be randomization techniques and best or optimal solutions from a series of computational tests generated either by ML algorithms or other computer programs. The advantages of these AI systems are that they would be able to slow down the pandemic, identify and predict the clusters proactively, and alert the agencies for better preparedness. GAs play an important role in developing vaccines. There is an established approach known as formal concept analysis (18) where gene-disease identification is based on formal concepts known as biclusters7 or bicliques8. The mathematical structure could be produced using this data, which is hidden, and these structures are called lattices. Using these lattices, the relationships/dependencies among the diseases can be determined.

1.11 Predictive Analytics for Combating Pandemics

Big data analytics (19) would be best used for effective and speedy medical situations and other solutions to test, track, trace, prevent, and finally control the current COVID-19 pandemic. A robust analytics framework should be in place so that this technology could be rapidly used for the previous tasks. Today, public health institutions do not have a standardized analytics framework either to generate meaningful analytics for public consumption or scientific usage. Big data technology solutions are designed on volume, variety, velocity, and veracity (the 4Vs). With the advent of IoT and IoMT, there is an increased generation of data from social media and public cloud computing data sets. Big data technology is also used for good governance and rapid decision-making during pandemic situations. The data generated from the previously mentioned sources is stored in huge data warehouses, distributed systems, file systems, and large storage systems.

This data includes the real time generated data as well as historical data for analysis. Major data sources for generating big data analytics are.

1. Medical information or data generated by the IoMT, such as patient wearables, glucose and blood monitors, and thermometers. Geospatial data could also be collected to identify the patient location thus helping the government authorities with better tracking and to stop the spreading of the disease
2. Social media data generated helps the public and government to be better informed and helps both to make informed decisions. During lockdown situations, when no one was allowed to come out of their houses, social media played an important role in communication and collecting data. This collected data can be better used for generating analytics
3. The genome data bank is very useful to the scientific community that is working on producing vaccinations

Using the previous data and generating meaningful analytics, prevention, response, and recovery could be achieved at a rapid phase.

1.12 Conclusions

It is evident that by using the appropriate technologies, we can rapidly develop data models to prevent, respond to, and recover patients and economic situations (20–23).

Despite various issues, it is possible to improve the current situation involving the use of EHRs for research, which could improve awareness and motivation among professionals and patients, ease the legal obstacles to using EHRs for research, initiate actions by setting up tasks under strict guidance, help with technological innovations, improvements and security, cross-border cooperation, and the availability of resources at government and private levels to disseminate the benefits of research to everyone.

Since the IoMT is an amalgamation of medical devices and applications that can connect to healthcare, IT systems have revolutionized the healthcare system. As IoMT allows devices to securely communicate over the internet allowing the rapid and highly flexible analysis of medical data. For example, remote patient monitoring devices, telehealth devices, consumer wearables, logistics devices, sensors, and other tracking systems. In this chapter, various topics related to the IoMT, such as the need for a robust framework and merging IoMT with AI were thoroughly discussed. Speedy decisions with quality are the key to navigating successfully this pandemic, and AI and other branches of big data technologies could certainly help to over-come this situation and to provide a pathway for successful mitigations in any future pandemics. Certainly, COVID-19 taught us many technology lessons, tested IT infrastructures, and revealed the gaps that must be filled.

Five key factors that impact the performance of IoMT devices are: (1) IoMT platform sizing, which has an impact on all applications; (2) IoMT gateway sizing; (3) leveraging open source technology and standards, such as Apache Ignite and Kubernetes for IoMT devices provides several benefits from cost savings to easy access for enterprise versions of the relevant software; (4) observability and high availability; IoMT devices are part of a decentralized system and need the ability to connect rapidly to an enterprise network; and (5) communication protocol. The technological advances in healthcare information technologies have led to significant transformations in the healthcare sector. Even the reports predict that the global IoMT market is growing with a compound annual growth rate (CAGR) of 31% for the forecast period 2020–2026. Also, it is expected that the global IoMT market will grow from USD 30.79 billion in 2021 to USD 187.60 billion in 2028 at a CAGR of 29.5%. Thus, IoMT helps care providers will continue to harness the efficiency and cost benefits obtained from using connected medical devices, which provides access to better medical facilities across the world.

References

1. Munnangi AK , Sekaran R , Rajeyyagari S , Ramachandran M , Kannan S , Bharati S. Nonlinear Cosine Neighborhood Time Series-Based Deep Learning for the Prediction and Analysis of COVID-19 in India. Wirel Commun Mob Comput. 2022. doi.10.1155/2022/3180742.
2. Ma J. Coronavirus: China's first confirmed Covid-19 case traced back to November 17. South China Morning Post. 13. 2020.

3. Chaudhary V, Royal A, Chavali M. et al. Advancements in research and development to combat COVID-19 using nanotechnology. Nanotechnol Environ Eng. 2021; 6 (8).
4. CSSE. COVID-19 dashboard by the Center for Systems Science and Engineering at Johns Hopkins University. ArcGIS.
5. Johns Hopkins University & Medicine (2021). Coronavirus Resource Center. https://coronavirus.jhu.edu/
6. McCorduck P. Machines Who Think: A Personal Inquiry into the History and Prospects of Artificial Intelligence. New York: CRC Press. 2004
7. HealthMap (2021), Global Health and Local information. Available from: www.health map.org/en/
8. Niiler E. An AI epidemiologist sent the first warnings of the Wuhan virus. The BlueDot algorithm scours news reports and airline ticketing data to predict the spread of diseases like those linked to the flu outbreak in China. Science. Available from www.wired.com/story/ai-epidemiologist-wuhan-public-health-warnings
9. Hidayat R, Aini N, Ilmi A, Azzahroh F, Giantini A. Test, trace, and treatment strategy to control COVID-19 infection among hospital staff in a COVID-19 referral hospital in Indonesia. Acta medica Indonesiana. 2020; 52(3):206–13.
10. Evans RS. Electronic health records: Then, now, and in the future. Yearb med inform. 2016; (S1):S48–S61.
11. Barnett GO. The application of computer-based medical-record systems in ambulatory practice. New Engl J M. 1984; 310(25):1643–50.
12. Stroetmann KA, Artmann J, Stroetmann VN, Protti D, Dumortier J, Giest S, et al. European countries on their journey towards national eHealth infrastructures: Luxembourg. Office for Official Publications of the European Communities. 2011.
13. Thomson S, Osborn R, Squires D, Jun M. International profiles of health care systems 2012: Australia, Canada, Denmark, England, France, Germany, Iceland, Italy, Japan, the Netherlands, New Zealand, Norway, Sweden, Switzerland, and the United States. 2012; Available from: www.commonwealthfund.org/publications/fund-reports/2012/nov/international-profiles-health-care-systems-australia-canada
14. Kierkegaard P. eHealth in Denmark: a case study. J Med Syst. 2013; *37(6)*:1-10.
15. Cresswell KM, Robertson A, Sheikh A. Lessons learned from England's national electronic health record implementation: implications for the international community. 2nd ACM SIGHIT, Proceedings of the International Health Informatics Symposium; 2012; Miami (FLA) ACM: New York. pp. 685–90.
16. Robert D. Service recovery & availability disaster recovery and business continuity. 2010
17. Andy P. IDC: Expect 175 zettabytes of data worldwide by 2025. IDC Comm J. 2018; Available from: www.networkworld.com/article/3325397/idc-expect-175-zettabytes-of-data-worldwide-by-2025.html
18. Keller BJ, Eichinger F, Kretzler M. Formal concept analysis of disease similarity. AMIA Joint Summits on Translational Science proceedings. AMIA Joint Summits on Translational Science. Mar 19–22 San Francisco (CA). 2012; 42–51.
19. Jia Q, Guo Y, Wang G, Barnes SJ. Big data analytics in the fight against major public health incidents (Including COVID-19): A conceptual framework. Int J Environ Res Pub Health. 2020; 17(5):81–99.

20. James KJ, Martin AW, Andres BS, Rebecca MN, Karen MS, Michael DS. Global economic effects of COVID-19. Congressional Research Service (CRS). 2021; Available from: https://sgp.fas.org/crs/row/R46270.pdf
21. Mondal MRH, Subrato B, Prajoy P, Priya P. Data analytics for novel coronavirus disease. Inform Med Unlocked. 2020; 20:100374.
22. Bharati S, Mondal MRH. 12 Applications and challenges of AI-driven IoHT for combating pandemics: a review. In: Khamparia A, Mondal MRH, Podder P, Bhushan B, Albuquerque V, Kumar S. editors. Computational intelligence for managing pandemics. Berlin, Boston: De Gruyter; 2021. pp. 213–30. doi.10.1515/9783110712254-012
23. Paul P, Bharati, S, Podder P, Mondal, MHR. 10 The role of IoMT during pandemics. In Khamparia A, Mondal MRH, Podder P, Bhushan B, Albuquerque V, Kumar S. editors. Computational intelligence for managing pandemics Berlin, Boston: De Gruyter. 2021. pp. 169–86. doi.10.1515/9783110712254-010

Chapter 2

Assessing the Economic Impact of COVID-19

Sonia Sharma, Anshi Gupta, and
Jagadeesh Chandra Bose K.

Chandigarh University, Gharuan, Punjab, India

Contents

DOI: 10.1201/9781003324447-2

2.1 Introduction

Starting from Wuhan's crowded food market, the virus spread unpredictably, and then the governments of almost every country announced a complete lockdown that included social distancing, travel restrictions, quarantine, and no public events for the sake of human lives. In addition, the world experienced a huge economic crisis during this long pandemic (December 2019 to July 2021), which might take years to recover from, specifically in developing countries. Based on one report, which compared different countries, the UK faces the highest uncertainty level with an index of 128.36. The markets face huge financial losses of millions and trillions. The International Monetary Fund (IMF) and multilateral financial institutions are successfully working to improve the economy.

For social intervention programs (e.g., support labor markets, social assistance, and insurance) an economic response policy was used. The Organization for Economic Co-operation and Development (OCED) countries provided complete financial relaxation to local firms going through losses and start-ups, >95% of the population (self-employed) are receiving income support. Around 48%–68% of people who are COVID-19 positive and quarantined workers receive their income regularly (Mondal et al., 2020).

Moreover, for industries and factories, the budget of approximately EUR 39 billion was decided. The World Bank provides approximately TND 40 million to Tunisia for recovery from pandemics. In addition, USD 745 million (an emergency loan) was received by Tunisia and USD 32 million went to Saudi Arabia to support medical facilities and business. Fiscal debt shows an increment of 6%–9% of GDP is expected. A 30%–50% of GDP increment was observed in the debt ceiling. Different efforts have been initiated by the governments of different countries to maintain the balance between health and finance (Fund, 2020; Gautam & Trivedi, 2020; Gentilini et al., 2020; Sarkodie & Owusu, 2020, 2021; Stubbs et al., 2021; Wang & Su, 2020).

In this chapter special attention is given to economically affected sectors from pandemics, the impact on various start-ups business, the effect on the growth rate of Indian GDP (2017–2021), and the effect of the medical crisis have disturbed the entire system. In addition, comparisons between inflation and employment between India and UK, the decline in the stock market, effects on travel and tourism services, and actions taken by the governments, and the people are mentioned in detail.

2.2 Economically Affected Indian Sectors by Pandemics

As shown in Figure 2.1, almost every sector of the economy has been affected drastically, such as primary sectors (mining and agricultural sectors), secondary sectors, such as manufacturing industries (automobile, textile, chemical, electronic, and solar power industries), and industries in the service sectors (tourism, healthcare, IT, transportation, BFSI, entertainment, and retail).

The primary sector contributes to both employment and Indian GDP. Approximately 16% of GDP is due to the primary sector and approximately 43% of the population are working as employees and labor in the primary sectors. Secondary sectors get their materials from the primary sector. After lockdown, the labor force went back to their villages, and then public transport was completely banned and borders were sealed. Due to this, the agricultural industries must face the consequences, because without labor there is less production of crops which means less profit. Furthermore, bakeries, restaurants, tea stalls and many more food shops were closed due to the lack of raw materials, such as sugar, wheat, gram flour, rice, and bran. The damage caused by lockdown is listed in Table 2.1.

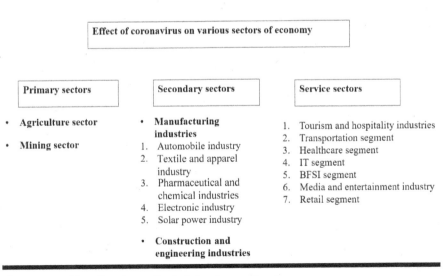

Figure 2.1   List of sectors affected due to pandemics

Source: Rakshit & Paul (2020)

Table 2.1 Damage Caused by Lockdown on Listed Sectors

Various Industries and Sectors	Effect Due to Pandemics
1. Mining sector	Share prices of mining entities drop down due to less demand for minerals and metals
2. Agricultural sector	Less production of crops as the movement of agricultural labor is prohibited
3. Automobile industry	All plants are closed, imports are being sealed up, and automobile companies go through losses
4. Textile and apparel industry	Export–import of yarn, fabric, and other materials is prohibited. The spinning mills in India financially suffer a lot
5. Pharmaceutical and chemical industries	Due to banned import–export of drugs and their raw material to China, this caused losses to this industry
6. Electronic industry	Production and sales of electronic goods are affected because every raw material and the fully working final product, was from China
7. Solar power industry	Around 79.99% of solar modules were purchased from Chinese manufacturers whereas Indian manufacturers have limited stock. Thus, the sector was also affected
8. Construction and engineering industries	Massive amounts of the labor force return to their villages and without labor, no industry can run
9. Tourism	No movement of tourists since March 2020. Huge loss to GDP, as tourism is the largest contributor to India's GDP
10. Transportation segment	Due to travel restrictions, sealed borders and prohibited mobility of tourists, this sector faces financial strain
11. Media and entertainment industries	Theaters cannot have movie shows whereas shooting of movies was also postponed
12. Retail segment	Malls and many shops were closed due to which their products expired, such as bakery shops. Only essential shops are permitted to open within given timings. Huge loss to the retail segment

Source: Rakshit & Paul (2020)

In the mining industries, share prices dropped due to less demand for metals. The contribution of the secondary sector to GDP is 29.6% whereas approximately 24.99% of the population gain employment from this sector. This pandemic also affected the manufacturing industries, because of the lack of a labor force, the production of goods could not proceed.

Industries are not preprepared for these conditions. The biggest industry is the textile industry, which provides employment to >45 million people but due to curfew and no labor force, these industries were shut down for a temporary basis affecting the economic conditions drastically. India used a partnership with China for the export and import of medical drugs, raw materials for manufacturing electronic goods, and solar panels. Since the Indian government has banned the import and export of anything with China, many sectors were affected economically, such as the pharmaceutical, solar power, and electronic industries.

The service sectors of India, which gives employment to approximately 32% of the population and contributes approximately 54.3% to the GDP, which travel, and tourism play a massive role in the Indian economy; however, due to curfew, this area of the sector came under huge financial strain. This pandemic condition affected the retail segment of the service sector because only necessary shops, such as confectionery and medical shops were allowed to open at fixed times. Furthermore, releasing new films and their filming was being delayed, due to which producers and makers of movies were at a loss (Rakshit & Paul, 2020).

2.3 Impact of Medical Crisis on Economic Conditions

Until medicine or vaccines were available, the lockdown was the only solution to eliminate this deadly virus. Coronavirus is spreading everywhere and causing deaths, due to which many people have no income source now. Due to this high illness rate and the nonworking population, the impact of this virus on economic conditions has been drastic. In the US, the employment loss was 24% and a 22% loss in GDP was reported (del Rio-Chanona et al., 2020; Podder et al., 2021). It is evident that in Pakistan, microfinance is facing a colossal financial crash in communities with less income. There was a 90% drop in household income and small enterprise owners and borrowers cannot pay back their loans. Various sectors are suffering economic losses.

Some interventions were taken by the government. In April 2020, these interventions were first measured by the IMF. In total, 10% of the world's GDP was the amount (USD 9 trillion) decided to be consumed to tackle this crisis. From which USD 4.6 trillion was for equity injections, quasi-fiscal operations, guarantees, and public sector loans. Overall. USD 4.4 trillion was the direct budgetary support (Battersby et al., 2020; IMF, 2020a; Malik et al., 2020; Sevilla & Smith, 2020). During the financial crisis (2007–2008) this was quite stable. Under a different scheme, such as the Job Retention Scheme (JRS), employees who are nonworking due to illness, receive 80% of their salary in the UK. It has been reported that all policies that were applied were not enough to recover all the problems, for instance, approximately 20% of the laborers were not covered, and we cannot rely on these figures (Giese & Haldane, 2020; Mayhew & Anand, 2020). The effects of this virus (economic and medical crisis) will remain with us for a few years. But if these consequences remain with us for a longer time, all the relief policies will need to be renewed again. Because unlocking starts in various places, new policies should be set up that contain relief from business property taxes, extension in the time of shops opening (restaurants, malls, and other confectionaries) and a reduction in VAT. Difficulties will occur because the structure of economics will never be the same as they were before the pandemics (Bharati et al., 2020; Devereux et al., 2020).

2.4 Start-Up Businesses

The corporate sector is having to take new risks after the implications of the new economic interventions. Loans are being given to different firms to start up their business again. Many firms are unaware of this; a survey should be conducted after some time to determine the default rate. A high default rate and its after-effects are possible. However, in 2007–2008, financial support was given to the commercial banks. They stopped showing the significant cost to society and their preference was to rebuild their balance sheets. This should be stopped to save society from bankruptcy. All these consequences threaten our economy. This time business and finance are not responsible for pandemics, such as in 2007–2008. Stress conditions are built-in for the financial sector due to its failing systems. A clear idea and strategy for what and how to recover and get profits is required (Mayer, 2013; Morris & Vines, 2014). This pandemic proved that governments and businesses were completely dependent on each other. Both need each other for good profits. It is very significant to form good relationships between the private and government sectors (Morris & Vines, 2014).

Data should be provided so that ideas and strategies for different experiments should be planned by the private sectors that cover all the problems arising among people and that plan should be executed under the supervision of the government. A high risk to enterprises (small and medium-size) in the developing areas, funding from the public sector is needed for financial support (Collier & Mayer, 2020). The hiring process has been frozen in 43% of European start-ups. From the previous decade, for the sake of economic growth start-ups are the only solution. COVID-19 has had a drastic effect on Europe's start-up companies. Relaxation packages offered by the governments have improved the situation to some context. In May 2021, a scheme of EUR 750 billion was declared. Many difficulties occur when starting up a business after and during pandemics; however, the execution of plans and policies as a remedy could speed up this process (Kalogiannidis & Chatzitheodoridis, 2021), as given in Table 2.2.

Table 2.2   Conclusions after Survey

Employment Issues are due to Collapsing Business among Europeans	Difficulties Occur in Reforming Business	Policies for Enhancing the Recovery Rate
It is concluded that massive unemployment occurs in each industry	Due to pandemics, constructing start-ups for industries and business is a challenge	It is observed that after the execution of the policies, the financial recovery of industries has been speeding up
Industries are not hiring an employee for a very long period	Industries are facing massive losses for more than a year. So, the industries going to start up will have great difficulties	Policies and plans by the government are not suitable for long-term relaxation of the business and industries
In start-up industries, employees are receiving a very low salary	Unstable economic conditions make industries start-up very risky	It limits the boundaries for encouragement and entrepreneurship

Source: Cunningham (2020); Kalogiannidis (2020b); Kalogiannidis & Chatzitheodoridis (2021); Morales-Narváez & Dincer (2020); Tromberg (2020)

2.5 Effects on Indian GDP (2017–2021)

The pandemic is ongoing, and we cannot predict the actual economic decrease in GDP in India. The decrease in the GDP of the nation shows that every country is suffering from financial losses in 2020. As there is an increase in the population every day, and therefore, a decrease in GDP results in a decrease in per capita income that affects the overall population of a country. The intensity of the economic crisis depends on the severity and duration of the lockdown. India was the fastest-growing economy during 2003–2008 having approximately an 8%–9% growth rate. Price stability, and bearable fiscal and payment deficit were the icing on the cake. But India's GDP growth rate decreased from 2017 onwards as shown in Figure 2.2. Many economists explained the reasons behind this major downfall of India's growth rate, such as the demonetization policy, the introduction of the Goods and Services Tax (GST), rising bad debts, rising fiscal deficit, and rising balance of payment deficit.

As India is fighting all the above challenges, the first case of COVID-19 was found in Kerala on January 27, 2020. The Reserve Bank of India's (RBI) estimates of growth rate showed that India grew by 4% in 2019–2020 compared with 6.5%

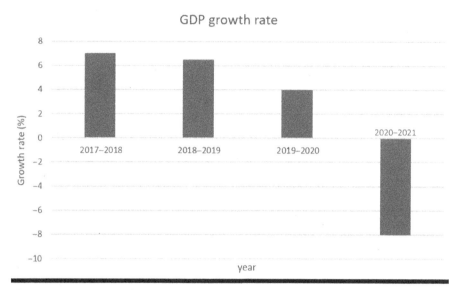

Figure 2.2   Decrease in GDP

Source: RIB (2021)

in 2018–2019. Approximately Rs. 3,397,049 crores were the gross value added in quarter four of 2019–2020 and the results of nationwide lockdown can be seen in the next quarter, estimated figure to be around INR 2,553,320 crores. The first wave had a massive impact and statisticians are still calculating the second wave's effect on growth rates, which is four times worse than in the previous wave. It is expected that India is going to experience the third wave around October–November, 2021 so the future still looks unclear. However, data from The National Council of Applied Economic Research predicted that the Indian economy would grow by 8.4%–10.1% in the present financial year (2020) (Andrews et al., 2020) (Chaudhary et al., 2020).

GDP's skid down is obvious because there is no employment in any sector. From 2017, there was a continuous fall in the GDP analyzed but after 2020, GDP growth became negative, which takes years and years to recover from (RBI, 2021).

2.6 Comparing Inflation and Employment between India and the UK

The after-effects of the pandemics on India and the UK are not the same because investments and trades are different. The economy of India was stable in 2009 whereas in 2016 it fell and in 2019 the economy of India slowed down. Demonetization and GST in India come with the belief that their after-effects will be for a short period; after that economy will rise in a few months. India was unable to recover as expected because of such schemes, and some informal sectors were affected negatively (Bhatt, 2011; Dasgupta, 2010; Ghosh, 2017; Kumar, 2009; Nataraj, 2018; RBI, 2017; Sharma, 2019; Victor, 2021). Starting with the GDP, growth was recorded in late 2020 at approximately 24% of India's GDP decrease. This decrease was recorded as the largest comparison with any other country (IMF, 2020b). The GDP fell 20.5% in the UK, for instance, the highest among developed countries. In 2020, between Europe and UK, there is an agreement, for instance, the Brexit Withdrawal Agreement. Until 2020, the UK had to remain as an isolated market and exit on January 1, 2021, if the British Parliament disagrees with this exit plan (Loayza & Pennings, 2020). The British Parliament's policy has had a huge impact on the UK's growth (Hantzsche et al., 2018)(2020a). It is evident that due to pandemics there is a massive negative impact on production, employment, supply, and demand (Loayza & Pennings, 2020).

In 2020, the sudden rise in unemployment in India was recorded due to the lower or lack of employment in every sector of the economy (Figure 2.3). Figure 2.4 shows the comparison of the unemployment and inflation rates in India (2016–2020).

It demonstrated that after 2017 unemployment rates rose. Because it is visible that both unemployment and inflation graphs rise and fall simultaneously, the economy shows unbelievable loss because of the extremely high level of unemployment. Sources of data used for plotting graphs are from the Centre for Monitoring Indian Economy (CMIE) and the Ministry of Statistics and Programme Implementation (Victor et al., 2021).

The JRS effectively gave relief to the laborer. As the lockdown was extended, the scheme tends to be useless (Mayhew & Anand, 2020). People that had no

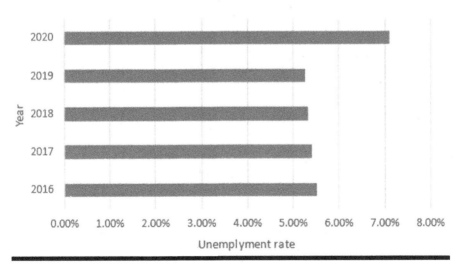

Figure 2.3   Unemployment rate in India

Source: CMIE Unemployment Rate in India

INDIA INFLATION AND UNEMPLOYMENT (2015–2020)

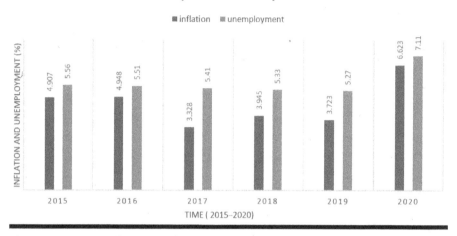

Figure 2.4 Comparing unemployment and the inflation rate in India (2016–2020)

Source: https://data.worldbank.org

income during the lockdown, after the limited unlocking in June–July, it was observed that they gave some relief to the economy. This crisis could soon be at its worst as the third wave is coming soon. Stability levels in unemployment were recorded; however, after 2019 there was an increase. It is obvious that due to a suppression of unemployment, there was an increment in the inflation level. It has been reported that the economy of the UK did not collapse similar to the Indian economy.

Figure 2.5 shows the comparison of the unemployment and inflation rates in the UK from 2015–2020. Unlike India, the UK does not have these situations. If the unemployment rate increase, the inflation rate is decrease for the convenience of the population.

From all previous and current studies, there is a horrible indication that if COVID-19 is not controlled and eradicated from India then it will collapse the whole system (Khanna, 2021; Perumal, 2020). Showing consistency with Phillip's theory, the inflation and unemployment relationship is negative in the UK whereas India shows a positive relationship. Due to the lack of supply in India, people are facing unemployment, the collapse of finances, and a high inflation rate. This condition became intense in India during the pandemic. After observing all the problems in different sectors, new policies (that give positive outcomes in a short period) must be implemented to give relief from this pandemic situation. For this, 15% of the GDP is utilized. This information will surely help to make recovery strategies. Some policies had disadvantages for industries (Victor et al., 2021).

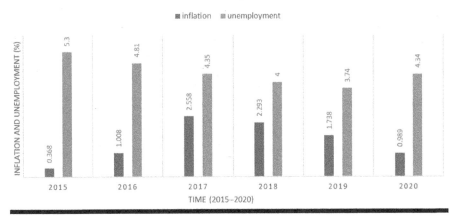

UK INFLATION AND UNEMPLOYMENT (2015–2020)

Figure 2.5   Comparing unemployment and inflation in the UK from 2015–2020

Source: https://data.worldbank.org/

2.7 Stock Market Crashes due to Pandemic

Not every industry and firm faced a financial crisis, but many sectors collapsed completely. Stimulus packages from the government failed to benefit many and the status of the stock markets after lockdowns is recorded in this section of the chapter. It was reported that negative returns were generated by 90% of the S&P 1500 stocks. The crude petroleum sector collapsed completely in a day, with a 60% decrease in market value.

However, the chemicals sectors gained benefits with a 10% of return. At the beginning of 2020, even the leading industries, such as software and technology, natural gas, food, and healthcare had massive losses. Some sectors, such as hospitality, real estate, and petroleum earned profits during the lockdown, which shows the dramatic fluctuations in the stock market by up to 70%. Most frequent changes are recorded in the petroleum sector whose prices skid the most. The selected firm's responses are mentioned because they were the most affected due to the collapse of the stock market during the pandemics (Table 2.3).

Many industries were shut during the lockdown period. Not only weaker economic foundations were the reason behind the stock market going into shock, but reduced earnings and spending by consumers are the big reasons. After firms that made crude oil experienced great losses in March 2020, they stopped giving compensation to the concerned authorities. Exceptions, such as Gulfport Energy gave increases in the salaries of senior management even when almost all organizations

Table 2.3 Responses of Firms to Pandemics

Firms	Monthly Return	Date	Responses
SM Energy	-81.43	April 9, 2020	A semi-annual cash dividend (USD 0.01 per share) was approved by directors
		April 17, 2020	Salary was reduced by 20%, which is given to the CEOs temporarily; if there was no improvement in business conditions, less salary was awarded to other departmental officers; compared with 2019, the reduction was observed in 2020. LTIP target grant values; reduction and cancellation of bonus and awards to executive officers and will be paid by the end of 2021
Gulfport Energy	-45.74	March 11, 2020	On March 16, 2021, cash awarded was approved to the officers (CFO, senior executives, and CEO)
Penn Virginia	-80.56	April 7, 2020	5% of increment in salary of CEO and 10% for engineering
Apache	-83.22	March 31, 2020	Immediately giving up position by the vice president, data analytics and practicable intelligence and energy technology. 90% reduction in dividend from USD 0.25
Oasis Petroleum	-78.59	March 30, 2020	No response from this firm

Source: Mieszko Mazur (2020)

were collapsing. In addition, Oasis Petroleum firm did not provide any compensation for the pandemic.

The question of why all firms in the same section did not share their response toward pandemics arose. The decision-making by these firms was controlled by corporate governance. An assessment of Gulfport Energy discovered that this company does not hold strategy-related meetings and that the remuneration committee works more actively than the nomination committee and corporate governance (Adams, 2007; Almazan, 2003).

2.7.1 Black Days of the Stock Market

It is very surprising, that even in early 2020 when industries and organizations with high performance had massive losses, there was a company called Natural Gas whose stock earnings were around +17% on Black Monday and Tuesday. As of March 2020, the prices of oil have decreased, after which the output of petroleum was reduced. When extracting crude petroleum, natural gas is the by-product. Therefore, the production of petroleum and natural gas decreased simultaneously. This must be the reason behind the increasing rates of natural gas. Furthermore, stocks of petroleum bounced up to 60%. Therefore, the sudden increase in prices of ≤20% of firms (Kraton and United Natural Foods) (Mieszko Mazur, 2020).

2.7.2 Effects on Travel and Tourism Services

Demand and supply issues are intensely affected globally due to pandemics. Due to the border's being closed, restricted traveling, quarantine time, and closed tourist places, this sector has suffered a lot. Some countries were dependent on consumption abroad. Restricting traveling was the only solution to regulate the increasing cases; however, it completely collapsed the tourism sector, because domestic and international travel were restricted until a vaccine was made (Barkas et al., 2020). Market shares of e-tourism have increased. Different aspects were examined and connected with the overall trade to demonstrate the disastrous effect of traveling and tourism on the country's economy.

It was reported in 2018, that travel and tourism services were the source of almost 319 million jobs and had a 10.4% contribution to total global GDP; in addition, international trading had a massive loss. Different measures are taken with respect to the advancement and expansion of countries to stabilize the economic conditions. In some countries, there are jobs where the income majorly depends upon tourism, and their economy has been massively affected (Barkas et al., 2020). The contribution of the Organization for Economic Co-operation and Development (OECD) is approximately 21.5% in exports (service-related),. 4.4% in GDP, and 7% in employment.

Before the economic crisis impacted, national tourism and traveling were the most important sector of the country's economy, it has increased the GDP level consistently. It not only contributes to GDP and employment and has a momentous role in various sectors, such as trade retailing, construction, real estate, and many more. International tourism spending is approximately 28.8%, which is less important than 71.3% of domestic spending (Poole, 2020).

Foreign tourist arrivals increased every year until 2020. However, no tourists arrived in India after March 2020 (Figure 2.6), which meant that this sector faced massive loss. Less than 3 million foreign tourists visited India in 2020 because of the restrictions imposed on international and national flights and transportation, to decrease the spread of COVID-19. In 2019, the greatest number of foreign tourists arrived in India (10.93 million), whereas in 2018, 10.56 million tourists arrived.

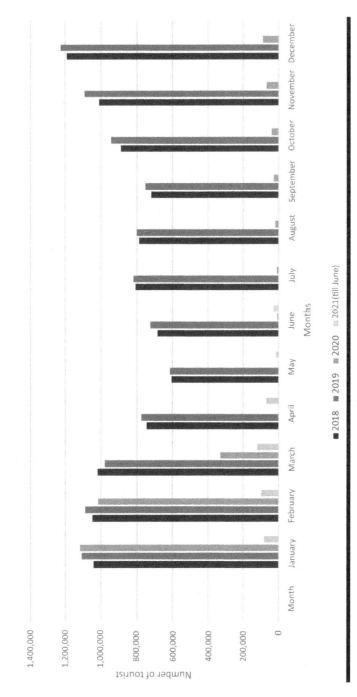

Figure 2.6 Month-wise FTA in India

However, after analyzing the graph mentioned previously it is very clear that the tourism sector of the economy faced massive losses, which has significantly harmed the GDP since 2020. In 2021 the graph rises again, but after March 2021 the situation becomes crucial. As the tourism ministry said, foreign tourist arrival (FTA) in the previous 9 months from April 2020 to December 2020 stood at 0.2 million.

2.7.9 Action Must Be Taken by the Government

A stimulus policy with a proper strategy should be executed to encourage and stabilize the companies that have real potential. This could benefit the employees who have no income. Some programs should be organized to counsel firms and employees. This could help the firms to earn profits. The measures taken by the government are specific to the sector. Different stimulus plans should be implemented for different sectors.

The government should also focus on a freeze in payments, tax cuts, insolvency prevention clauses, and liquidity injections. Service providers should also benefit by providing them soft loans, rearrangements of interest and tax payments, subsidies, and tax breaks. Except for firms and different businesses, special attention should be paid to employees who are working part-time, and to temporary and seasonal workers (Barkas et al., 2020).

2.7.10 Actions People Should Take

People who work in tourism should be flexible during the pandemic so that they can also apply for other jobs. They must be ready to move into those sectors that are still growing and giving wages to workers; therefore, they don't go bankrupt due to this extreme economic crisis.

Adaptability, multitasking, and flexibility are crucial to adjusting every niche of the division. In this crisis, the labor market should proceed by balancing diversification and specialization. Therefore, they should select different pieces of training; however, specialization leads to competition between employees to be selected (Figure 2.7) (Barkas et al., 2020).

Workers should be given new training, reskilling themselves so that they can apply for different and more convenient jobs to boost their income and survive this pandemic. In conclusion, digital skills are in demand in the market today, and employees should pay attention to this sector. Labor demand will automatically decrease due to digitalization. Nonskilled workers have been fired who worked as tourism service providers in the tourism sector because of digitalization (Kalogiannidis, 2020; OECD, 2020c). In this time of tough competition, to attract more clients, the tourism market should offer different schemes, which give benefit the client and market and tourists should be aware of these schemes and offers. After a long period of lockdown, people will want to travel. All actions must be completed within the boundaries of the rules and regulations of the COVID-19 norms.

Actions people should take
1. Maintaining flexibility of employment opportunities within the sector.
2. Upskilling and reskilling to adapt to evolving labour market needs.
3. Keeping an eye out for the tourism offers and destinations of the future.

Figure 2.7   Some actions that people can take during this economic crisis

Source: Barkas et al. (2020)

Recovery of the tourism and health sector should be simultaneous so that no further spread of the virus occurs (Barkas et al., 2020; Carty, 2020). In summary, if the cases of COVID-19 do not decrease, it will increase the economic shock, and thus, an economic collapse, if it is not controlled. The requirements of every sector should be discussed with the government. Therefore, new and revised policies should be applied to give the best possible outcomes. The world health organizations should analyze the economic conditions of every developed and underdeveloped country and take bold actions to stabilize their collapsing economy. Donations from the stakeholders should be collected after the pandemic for better recovery of the nation (Barkas et al., 2020; UNWTO, 2020a).

Different types of strategies and the graph of recovery rate due to these policies will help to decide the economic condition in post-COVID life. It was assessed that this economic crisis could increase the competition in the market. This virus has spread uncontrollably and globally, due to which flights are restricted, and there was zero mobility. These will be in place in 2020 until the vaccination is made. The tourism sector should collaborate and be coordinated to end the crisis. Globally, only 45% of 217 destinations were closed during the pandemic. In total, 18% of countries banned tourists and the area which was marked as the containment zone, 30% stopped flights partially or completely and the remaining 7% make it essential to be quarantined for a fixed period (Barkas et al., 2020; UNWTO, 2020b). All segments of the economy must come together for a speedy economic recovery. In addition, we should be prepared for post-COVID-19 life (Kalogiannidis, 2020a, b).

2.8 Challenges after Pandemics

2.8.1 Inflation

All countries globally have faced recession during the pandemic. Central bankers are pumping more currency into the system to deal with this economic shock. Most notable is in the US where >USD 5 trillion was created out of thin air. The world's biggest economy, the US, has already increased housing prices and crude oil is increasing. The New York Stock Exchange and cryptocurrency are breaking records and getting higher each day (IMF, 2021). Very likely by 2023, the US interest rate will increase again (due to hyper-inflation in the US), and the country that borrows in USD will all go to Holland. The countries that will be the worst hit will include India, because 52.1% of foreign debt is dominated by USD. Macroeconomic policymakers are making predictions to create mistakes as there is a lot of uncertainty in the system. The growth rate will be severely affected if the money supply is controlled, but inflation will raise if don't control it. So, policymakers are facing a trade-off.

2.8.2 Market Recovery

Due to the pandemic, major industries, such as travel, food, hotel, and tourism were hit. Consumer tastes and preferences changed, and more people were likely to have negativity and depression. So, given the rising unemployment and negative consumer sentiment, it is believed that the market will take some time to return to prepandemic levels. As we know, consumer expenditure is the major and the most significant component of total demand; therefore, it will drive down the national income.

2.8.3 Rise in Debt

Many governments across the world have introduced special relief packages to combat the crisis of COVID-19, such as the Indian Finance Minister introducing an INR 1.7 trillion package on March 26, 2021. These packages include extending loan guarantees, concessional credit for pandemic-hit sectors, and more investment to boost health care capacities. All these add up to a rising fiscal burden on the government. Analysts and economists are expecting higher taxes to be imposed by the government in the near future to deal with rising debt and fiscal burden.

2.8.4 Trade Impact

As we all know, all livelihoods and lives have been affected because of the pandemic. As corona and its spread increase, economical activities are also changing, resulting in the downfall in the trading business. Across the globe, the flow of trade fell by 7% in 2020. For various reasons, international trades were also affected, which was the impact of the economic crises due to the pandemic in the countries traded with, the impacts on health and changes associated with it, an increase in penalties and taxes by the management, and steps taken by the administration to decrease the spread of COVID-19. The spontaneous spread of viruses impacting trade is a well-known aspect. As Baldwin (2020) said, pandemics are creating an impact on demand and supply. As both have a damaging impact on trade, the result influences a country's import demand. This disease has a ripple effect on the imports and exports of each country and due to globalization, the entire supply chain was restricted. The consequences are still ambiguous.

2.8.5 Sustainable Development

Sustainable development goals include reducing poverty, and zero hunger, ensuring healthy lives, promoting well-being, quality education, and financial awareness. We are a long way from achieving these inspirational and ambitious goals and after COVID-19, these aims look difficult and tough to achieve. COVID-19 will lead to an increase in the world's hunger, poverty, and inequality, dampen the education system, and the funding of healthcare policies and welfare policies will become burdensome. Analysis by the OECD highlighted the significance of public spending to transition to a green economy; major investments for improvements in technology and research, and innovation through biotechnology to combat these kinds of viruses are required. Steps should be taken to provide financial assistance, provide funding to new entrepreneurs to get over the economic crises caused by the coronavirus pandemic and these are essential to speed up the achievement of the sustainable development goals (Shulla, 2021).

2.8.6 Social Issues

This pandemic is said to be the worst nightmare for all sectors of society, but it is particularly detrimental for poor people, the elderly, people with disabilities, and Indigenous tribes. People with no access to clean water, migrants, and refugees all stand to suffer disproportionately from the outbreak and they have fewer employment opportunities. Schools, universities, and offices were closed for quite a long time causing lower sectors like maids, servants, watchmen, and peons to lose their jobs (WEF, 2020). Because of the issues created because of the outbreak, we can expect rising crime rates as people have less money and an unstable source of income that will eventually lead them to criminal activities. If proper care is not taken, this could give rise to discrimination, inequality, long-term global unemployment, and exclusion.

2.9 Future Scope

2.9.1 Possible Scope of Data Analysis

All types of diseases that come in the near future will require proper data analysis techniques to follow the diseases and then further research can be carried out. Some points for data analytics could be applied to make the research easier.

1. We must know how the spread of the virus takes place. The regions that have the greatest number of clusters of the viruses must be recognized and restricted to decrease the spread of the virus. Also, people should know that these areas should be avoided
2. People should have full knowledge of the virus so that when a pandemic takes place they will know whether they are affected by the virus or are safe from it
3. A warning system should be applied for the affected patients so that the detection and classification become easy and fast. For example, if a person is going for a CT scan, the scanner should have an arrangement in which there's an image of the lung of a healthy patient and then there should be an image of the lung of the patient affected with coronavirus. By this method, if there are slight changes in the lungs the scanner will automatically give warning signals. This will save time and immediate action could be taken
4. Find the basic multiplicative number of viruses
5. To find if the virus that causes the disease affects patients that already have other diseases, like in the heart, lungs, cancer, diabetes, and kidneys
6. Predict if isolation and other modes of quarantine are affecting the outbreak of the virus or not
7. Find out if a baby born during a pandemic suffers from any type of disease
8. Continue monitoring the effect of vaccinations on the virus-infected patients and their treatments, so that it is not an alarming threat to the community
9. Those countries that have poor health care systems need to be more careful in the future as these types of pandemics could occur at any time. Healthcare systems must be improved and properly managed (Mondal, 2020)

2.9.2 Change in Economic Structure

Due to the December 2019 outbreak, the traditional ways of doing business changed. Now, people are using technology in every way possible to reduce personal interactions, decreasing the number of visits to the shops and traveling to other places due to stringent lockdown norms. Online businesses are expanding, and educational organizations must shift to online classes, even doctors are giving online appointments to patients. So, some of the trades experienced a positive impact while others experienced a negative impact.

2.9.3 Self-Sufficiency

2.9.3.1 Atmanirbhar Bharat Rozgar Yojana

This special economic package was announced to make India immune to the tough global supply chain competition and help empower the laborers, poor, and migrants who have been badly exaggerated by the COVID-19 outbreak. This scheme was launched in India on November 12, 2020, so that employment could be increased in various sectors of society with the assistance of production-linked incentives. Over USD 360 billion has been invested for the benefit of employees and employers. To boost the competitive manufacturing of goods, 10 sectors have been acknowledged under the production-linked incentives. This yojana also supports the real estate and construction sectors to enhance employment. This initiative has been applied to rural development and the agricultural sector. Boosting exports for the country and industrial sectors have been taken care of under the Atmanirbhar yojana. For research and development of the country over INR 9 billion has been given to biotechnology departments for the initiation of vaccine making and marketing and to make India covid free. This initiative, if properly implemented, will help to strengthen of GDP of India and we will not have to rely on other nations for goods and development; therefore, giving more power to local goods.

2.9.4 Digital Changes after COVID-19

Enhancement of digital technologies for medical purposes by boosting the practice of artificial intelligence must be a great initiative, which we could see in the near future (Figure 2.8). After this pandemic, peer pressure on the management should give the nation all the amenities but with social spacing. Through artificial intelligence and robotics, this issue can be resolved. Chaos has been created by parents whose children can afford the technology to gain educational benefits. Not everyone can afford a good mobile and laptop for education. Various IT companies are providing different tools for social interaction and commercial interactions like video

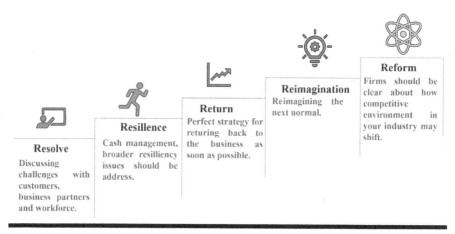

Figure 2.8 Steps should be taken by the companies and firms for a speedy recovery

Source: Co. (2020)

conferencing. From this initiative, people understood that one can work when sitting at home, which saves acres of office space and that space could be used to make more hospitals and quarantine sectors. The rapid increase in digitization during COVID-19 has enhanced the work from the home initiative, video conferencing across the globe, working without offices, and the development of businesses with fewer amenities, in a short time, which could take longer without the pandemic situation. To transfer cash and do digital payments for indispensable goods during a pandemic was possible because of India's digital ID system. Various technologies like three-dimensional (3D) printing of ventilators were initiated during the pandemic and 3D printing is money-making and could be widely used in the future. Digitization will help the economy in the long run as financial innovation could reduce black money, make governance efficient, and reduce the recurring cost of businesses, such as rent for offices and buildings. So, digitization will be a positive step toward development.

2.10 Conclusions

This chapter concluded that various sectors, such as manufacturing industries (automobile industry, textile industry, pharmaceutical industries, electronic industry, and solar equipment industries) and service sectors (tourism and hospitality industries, healthcare, IT, BFSI, retail, and entertainment industries) were irreversibly affected by the pandemic caused by COVID-19 since early 2020. Various countries had severe crises that showed a significant negative impact on the economic statistics. There was about a 70% of stock market loss, and decreased production of fossil fuel with an increment in the prices of crude and petroleum was observed. The tourism industry was one of the most affected sectors. The growth levels of Indian GDP went into minus after 2020. Many policies and stimulus packages were executed by the government for business start-ups, but it was found that these policies were still not efficient enough to stabilize the economic crash, which has been seen in the responses of different companies and business firms after March 2020 via surveys. Challenges prevented the economic recovery, for example, the country's worst hit included India as 52.1% of foreign debt is dominated by USD. Market recovery was very tough after the pandemics, as consumer tastes and preferences changed, and people were prone to negativity and depression. Analysts and economists are expecting higher taxes to be imposed by the government in the future to deal with rising debt and fiscal burden. The pandemic has had a ripple effect on the exports and imports of each country and due to globalization, the entire supply chain was restricted. Rising cybercrimes rates are expected as people have less money and an unstable source of income that will eventually lead them to cybercriminal activities. The future scope to recover from all these challenges, such as prepreparation of health facilities, funding, and proper data analysis should be done to avoid future pandemics. The traditional ways of doing business should be changed (more technology-based and contactless). Countries must become self-sufficient in every aspect like trading and manufacturing so, that import–export expenses will be saved and could be used in the economic recovery. Digitalization will decrease black money in the country. By following all these points, the economic conditions will surely recover.

References

Adams, R. B. A. F., D., (2007). A theory of friendly boards. *Journal of Finance, 62*(1) 217–250.

AIER. (2020). Retrieved from: www.aier.org/article/the-economy-after-covid-19/

Almazan, A. A. S., J. (2003). Entrenchment and severance pay in optimal governance structures. . *The Journal of Finance, 58*(2), 519–547.

Andrews, M., Areekal, B., Rajesh, K., Krishnan, J., Suryakala, R., Krishnan, B., … Santhosh, P. (2020). First confirmed case of COVID-19 infection in India: A case report, *The Indian journal of medical research, 151*(5), 490.

Baldwin, R. (2020). The greater trade collapse of 2020: Learnings from the 2008-09 great trade collapse. Retrieved from www.voxeu.org/article/greater-trade-collapse-2020

Barkas, P., Honeck, D., & Rubio, E. (2020). International trade in travel and tourism services: Economic impact and policy responses during the COVID-19 crisis. Retrieved from www.wto.org/english/res_e/reser_e/ersd202011_e.htm

Battersby, B., Lam, W. R., & Ture, E. (2020). Tracking the $9 trillion global fiscal support to fight COVID-19, *IMF Blog, 20.*

Bharati, S., & Mondal, M. R. H. (2021). Computational intelligence for managing pandemics. In K. Aditya, M. Rubaiyat Hossain, P. Prajoy, B. Bharat, C. D. A. Victor Hugo, & K. Sachin (Eds.) *12 Applications and challenges of AI-driven IoHT for combating pandemics: A review* (pp. 213–230). Berlin/Boston: De Gruyter. doi:10.1515/9783110712254-012

Bharati, S., Podder, P., & Mondal, M. R. H. (2020). Hybrid deep learning for detecting lung diseases from X-ray images. *Informatics in Medicine Unlocked, 20,* 100391.

Bharati, S., Podder, P., Mondal, M., & Prasath, V. (2021). Medical imaging with deep Learning for COVID-19 diagnosis: A comprehensive review. *arXiv preprint arXiv:210 7.09602.*doi.10.48550/arXiv.2107.09602

Bhatt, R. K. (2011). Recent global recession and Indian economy: An analysis. *International Journal of Trade, Economics and Finance, 2*(3), 212.

Carty, J. (2020). Tourism – How the business of happiness can emerge from the crisis, Galway International Hotel School. *GMIT Tourism Arts.* Retrieved from www.adv ertiser.ie/galway/article/114296/tourism-how-the-business-of-happiness-can-emerge-from-this-crisis

Chaudhary, M., Sodani, P., & Das, S. (2020). Effect of COVID-19 on economy in India: Some reflections for policy and programme, *Journal of Health Management, 22*(2), 169–180.

CMIE (2020). Unemployment Rate in India. Retrieved from https://unemploymentinindia.cmie.com/

Co., N. B. (2020). COVID-19 and its impact on Indian economy & business. *Taxguru:* Retrieved from www.taxguru.in/finance/covid-19-impact-indian-economy-business.html.

Collier, P., & Mayer, C. (2020). Reforming the UK financial system to promote regional development in post-COVID Britain, *Oxford Review of Economic Policy, 36*(1), S270–S280.

Cunningham, S. (2020). 3 tips for pharma startup success. *Drug Discovery Today, 25*(8), 1291.

del Rio-Chanona, R. M., Mealy, P., Pichler, A., Lafond, F., & Farmer, J. D. (2020). Supply and demand shocks in the COVID-19 pandemic: An industry and occupation perspective, *Oxford Review of Economic Policy, 36*(1), S94–S137.

Devereux, M. P., Güçeri, İ., Simmler, M., & Tam, E. H. (2020). Discretionary fiscal responses to the COVID-19 pandemic. *Oxford Review of Economic Policy, 36*(1), S225–S241.

Donthu, N., & Gustafsson, A. (2020). Effects of covid-19 on-business and research. *Journal of Business Research, 117,* 284–289.

Gentilini, U., Almenfi, M., Orton, I., & Dale, P. (2020). Social protection and jobs responses to COVID-19. Retrieved from https://openknowledge.worldbank.org/handle/10986/37186

Ghosh, A. N.(2017). Impact of demonetisation on India: A macro-theoretic analysis. *Trade and Development Review, 9*(1).

Giese, J., & Haldane, A. (2020). COVID-19 and the financial system: a tale of two crises. *Oxford Review of Economic Policy, 36*(1), S200-S214.

Gulf Today. (2020). Saudi Arabia announces $32b support to mitigate coronavirus impact on economy. Retrieved from www.gulftoday.ae/business/2020/03/20/saudi-arabia-announces-.

Hantzsche, A., Kara, A., & Young, G. (2018). The economic effects of the Government's proposed Brexit deal. *NIESR report, November.* Retrieved from www.imf.org/en/Publications/WEO

IMF. (2020a). Policy responses to COVID-19. Retrieved from www. imf. org/en/Topics/imf-and-covid19/Policy-Responses-to-COVID-19.

IMF. (2020b). World economic outlook update. Retrieved from www.imf.org/en/Publications/WEO/Issues/2020/06/24/WEOUpdateJune2020

IMF. (2021). Retrieved from www.imf.org/en/Topics/imf-and-covid19/Policy-Responses-to-COVID-19#V

Kalogiannidis, S. (2020a). Covid impact on small business. *International Journal of Social Science and Economics Invention, 6*(12), 387–391.

Kalogiannidis, S. (2020b). Impact of effective business communication on employee performance. *European Journal of Business and Management Research, 5*(6).

Kalogiannidis, S., & Chatzitheodoridis, F. (2021). Impact of Covid-19 in the European start-ups business and the idea to re-energise the economy. *International Journal of Financial Research, 12*(2), 56–61.

Knoema (2020). Retrieved from https://knoema.com

KPMG. (2020). Employment-related measures. Retrieved from https://home.kpmg/xx/en/home/insights/2020/04/india-government-and-institution-measures-in-response-to-covid.html

Kumar, R. Vashisht, P. (2009). The global economic crisis: Impact on India and policy responses. ADBI working paper 164. Retrieved from www.adbi.org/working-paper/2009/11/12/3367.global.economic.crisis.india/

Loayza, N., & Pennings, S. M. (2020). Macroeconomic policy in the time of COVID-19: A primer for developing countries. *World Bank Research and Policy Briefs.* Retrieved from https://openknowledge.worldbank.org/handle/10986/33540

Malik, K., Meki, M., Morduch, J., Ogden, T., Quinn, S., & Said, F. (2020). COVID-19 and the future of microfinance: Evidence and insights from Pakistan. *Oxford Review of Economic Policy, 36*(1), S138–S168.

Mayer, C. (2013). *Firm commitment: Why the corporation is failing us and how to restore trust in it.* Oxford. OUP.

Mayhew, K., & Anand, P. (2020). COVID-19 and the UK labour market. *Oxford Review of Economic Policy, 36*(1), S215–S224.

Mieszko Mazur, M. D., Miguel Vega. (2020). COVID-19 and the March 2020 stock market crash. Evidence from S&P1500. doi.10.1016/j.frl.2020.101690

Ministry of Tourism. India tourism statistics. Retrieved from https://tourism.gov.in/market-research-and-statistics

Mondal, M. R. H., Bharati, S., & Podder, P. (2020). Data analytics for novel coronavirus disease. *Informatics in Medicine Unlocked, 20*, 100374.

Mondal, M. R. H., Bharati, S., & Podder, P. (2021). Diagnosis of COVID-19 using machine learning and deep learning: A Review, *Current Medical Imaging, 17*(12), 1403–1418. doi.10.2174/1573405617666210713113439

Morales-Narváez, E., & Dincer, C. (2020). The impact of biosensing in a pandemic outbreak: COVID-19. *Biosensors and Bioelectronics, 163*, 112274.

Morris, N., & Vines, D. (2014). *Capital failure: Rebuilding trust in financial services.* Oxford: OUP

Nataraj, G. (2018.). Demonetisation in India: An impact assessment. *Journal of Business Thought, 9*, 11–23.

OECD. (2020c). Retrieved from www.oecd.org/daf/competition/competition-concerns-in-labour-markets.htm, Competition in Labour Markets,

Paul, P. K., Bharati, S., Podder, P., & Mondal, M. R. H. (2021). Computational Intelligence for Managing Pandemics. In K. Aditya, M. Rubaiyat Hossain, P. Prajoy, B. Bharat, C. d. A. Victor Hugo, & K. Sachin (Eds.) *10 The role of IoMT during pandemics* (pp. 169–186). Berlin/Boston: De Gruyter. doi.10.1515/9783110712254-010

Perumal, P. (2020). Is the Indian economy staring at stagflation. *The Hindu.* Retrieved from www.thehindu.com/business/Economy/is-the-indian-economy-staring-at-stagflation/article30595793.ece

Podder, P., Khamparia, A., Mondal, M. R. H., Rahman, M. A., & Bharati, S. (2021). Forecasting the Spread of COVID-19 and ICU Requirements. *International Journal of Online and Biomedical Engineering. 17*(5), 81–99

Poole, J. (2020). World Travel and Tourism Council (WTTC), Presentation on April 1st, 2020 at the OECD Tourism Committee.

Rakshit, D., & Paul, A. (2020). Impact of COVID-19 on sectors of Indian economy and business survival strategies. *Available at SSRN 3620727.*

RBI. (2021a). Retrieved from www.rbi.org.in/Scripts/BS_PressReleaseDisplay.aspx?prid=51819

RBI (2021b). Retrieved from www.rbi.org.in/Scripts/AnnualReportPublications.aspx?year=2021

RBII. (2017). Macroeconomic impact of demonetisation: A preliminary assessment. Retrieved from: https://rbidocs

Sarkodie, S. A., & Owusu, P. A. (2020). Impact of meteorological factors on COVID-19 pandemic: Evidence from top 20 countries with confirmed cases. *Environmental Research, 191*, 110101.

Sarkodie, S. A., & Owusu, P. A. (2021). Global assessment of environment, health and economic impact of the novel coronavirus (COVID-19). *Environment, Development and Sustainability, 23,* 5005–5015.

Sevilla, A., & Smith, S. (2020). Baby steps: the gender division of childcare during the COVID-19 pandemic. *Oxford Review of Economic Policy, 36*(S1), S169–S186.

Sharma, S. N. (2019). Severe slowdown: When will the Indian economy recover and how. *The Economic Times.* Retrieved from https://economictimes.indiatimes.com/news/econ omy/indicators/severe-slowdown-when-will-the-indian-economy-recover-and-how/ articleshow/72310684.cms?from=mdr

Shulla, K., Voigt, B.-F., Cibian, S., Scandone, G., Martinez, E., Nelkovski, F., & Salehi, P. (2021). Effects of COVID-19 on the Sustainable Development Goals (SDGs). *Discover Sustainability, 2*(1), 15. doi.10.1007/s43621-021-00026-x

Stubbs, T., Kring, W., Laskaridis, C., Kentikelenis, A., & Gallagher, K. (2021). Whatever it takes? The global financial safety net, Covid-19, and developing countries. *World Development, 137,* 105171.

Tromberg, B. J., Schwetz, T. A., Pérez-Stable, E. J., Hodes, R. J., Woychik, R. P., Bright, R. A., … Collins, F. S. (2020). Rapid scaling up of Covid-19 diagnostic testing in the United States—the NIH RADx initiative. *New England Journal of Medicine, 383*(11), 1071–1077.

United Nations. Everyone included: Social impact of COVID-19. Retrieved from www. un.org/development/desa/dspd/everyone-included-covid-19.html

UNWTO. (2020a). Calling on innovators and entrepreneurs to accelerate tourism recovery. Retrieved from www.unwto.org/calling-on-innovators-and-entrepreneurs-to-acceler ate-tourism-recovery

UNWTO. (2020b). 100% of Global Destinations Now Have COVID-19 Travel Restrictions. Retrieved from www.unwto.org/news/COVID-19-travel-restrictions

Victor, V., Karakunnel, J. J., Loganathan, S., & Meyer, D. F. (2021). From a recession to the COVID-19 pandemic: Inflation–unemployment comparison between the UK and India. *Economies, 9*(2), 73.

VoxEU. (2021). The 202 trade impact of the Covid-19 pandemic. Retrieved from www. voxeu.org/article/2020-trade-impact-covid-19-pandemic

Wang, Q., & Su, M. (2020). A preliminary assessment of the impact of COVID-19 on environment–A case study of China. *Science of the total environment, 728,* 138915.

WEF. (2020). Coronavirus: Over 20 million Americans have now applied for unemployment benefit. Retrieved from www.weforum.org/agenda/2020/04/united-states-unemploym ent-claimantscoronavirus-covid19/

Wolff, A. (2020). Time to start planning for the post-pandemic recovery. *WTO News.* Retrieved from www.wto.org/english/news_e/news20_e/ddgaw_09apr20_e.htm

Chapter 3

Assessing the Economic Impact of COVID-19 on the Implications of the Internet of Things Adoption on Small and Medium Enterprise Business's Sustainability

R. Abd Shukor and W. K. Mooi

Infrastructure University, Kuala Lumpur, Malaysia

Contents

DOI: 10.1201/9781003324447-3

3.1 Introduction

Current developments of the COVID-19 pandemic all around the world have increasingly impacted small and large businesses (Bharati, 2020). The conventional ways of doing business are making it harder to supplement the enterprises' continuity. Therefore, business owners and entrepreneurs are trying to sort out the best solution to overcome the situation since it was predicted that the pandemic will have a long-lasting effect on humans' daily routines (Podder et. al., 2021). The once-neglected solution before COVID-19, which is the Internet of Things (IoT) then came into mind wherein many situations help to overcome the problems that are faced by the majority of the enterprises all around the world (Karale, 2021). IoT was based on artificial intelligence (AI) that helps to eliminate security threats yet increases the level of accuracy; therefore, making it a very good basis in many sectors and industries (Paul et.al., 2021).

Small and medium enterprises (SMEs); however, must follow a more complicated route towards business sustainability, which involves technical involvement in their day-to-day operations. In reality, modern business relationships contain technological advances that require businesspeople to adapt to a unique analytical environment. Perhaps 30 years ago, businesses had to be imaginative and original to differentiate themselves from the rest of the pack without data. In fact, a new dimension of the whole industry was launched in Germany in the last 6 years, when the Industrial Revolution 4.0 was introduced (IR4.0). It develops a variety of components, which centralised data unification (Moore, 2019), encourages the development of operational flexibility, enhances productivity, and increases production capacity and precision, leading to cost savings and resource improvement when automating sales and marketing activities (Margherita & Braccini, 2020).

In IR4.0, the IoT is the most important component of integration, connection, compilation, and processing of data which can be found at any one moment and location in real-time. IoT fundamentally focuses on social information and the use of collective data to improve the present strategic methods and enhance machine-to-machine connectivity (Awan, Sroufe, & Shahbaz, 2021). Although a high-level management framework may be the main assumption for declining businesses, the fast return on investment and drastic cost savings suggest no extra expense for IoT frameworks. The IoT was characterised as "a theoretical structure that affects the availability of various gadgets and network interconnects, as well as an increasing number of actual objects that provide a common worldwide database that speculates about means of use including the two persons and portrayals at similar virtual levels" (Lea, 2020). Furthermore, technology, such as the cyber–physical system (CPS), consolidates the hypothesis of AI, mechatronics, planning, and interface science (Schranz, 2021). Implanted frames, in general place more emphasis on computational components and actual components for rotational control (Baumann, 2020). A CPS has a similar core architecture to the IoT. In all cases, a CPS offers a greater combination and coordination between the physical and computer components (Laarouchi, 2020). In fact, every tool helps individuals, and notably, entrepreneurs like SMEs, to know and predict the most precise road to be followed to continue to exist.

It is hoped that this chapter should contribute to all the stakeholders, readers, as well as enterprises around the world on the importance of enabling SMEs with innovative technologies, such as the IoT by shedding and highlighting additional knowledge and awareness as well as an understanding of the subject. The novelty of this chapter is that the past research outcomes, such as the theoretical aspects based on an applicable transformational concept, are adaptable to SMEs, especially with regard to the COVID-19 situation. This chapter will also introduce several knowhows about business resilience, a technology recently in the spotlight like IoT itself; and there will be more discussion about how the future will be with the consequences of the COVID-19 pandemic.

3.2 Methodology

This chapter was written based on collective secondary data that was gathered from various sources including journals, earlier research, blogs from reputable research organisations, and other well-known news providers that are easily accessible for use in this exploratory work (Johnston, 2014). The collected information will be used for the general research purpose (Donnellan & Lucas, 2013).

3.3 SMEs Business Sustainability

SME organisations have various types of employees. Numerous private associations, particularly single proprietors, and numerous other minuscule SMEs are involved in this classification (Ward, 2020). There are a large number of SMEs, which are sometimes considered a core part of most economies worldwide, SMEs are very opposed to their expansion. This is not how the term "small business" reflects the size of a company, can be appreciated, or anticipated for the internationalisation of companies. The direction of development, as well as internationalisation, are important aspects of SME internationalisation (Vanderstraeten et. al., 2020).

In general, what establishes an SME are as follows.

1. Resource limitation (Welsh & White, 1981). An SME by and large have restricted assets. Startups carry a significant risk of failure, but they may also be very interesting places to work with great benefits, an emphasis on innovation, and ample learning opportunities. Therefore, it is subject to the capacity of the proprietor to produce assets

2. Adhocracy (flexible) administration style (Bhargava, 2007). For SMEs, the administration is typically casual, proprietors are required to do nearly everything, and workers are typically expected to have the option to be generalists as there is no marked division of tasks

3. Adaptability (Ungureanu, 2020). The venture has greater adaptability to adjust to changes in the environment because of its size and casual design. For instance, any adjustments in government strategy or innovation may impact the organisations since these changes require extra assets or capital. This may turn into a requirement for the organisations to support themselves on the lookout

4. Reliance on singular decision makers (Feltham, Feltham & Barnett, 2005). The organisations are overseen, and the proprietor works in them. The business innovators of the business lead the organisation and assume a role as both workers and boss. The development of the organisations is dynamically controlled by the proprietor

Sustainable development demands agreements that solve the problems of the present without negotiating the capability of people in the future to address their challenges, particularly over time (Fukuda-Parr & Muchhala, 2020). To survive and sustain businesses, entrepreneurs have to manage their businesses in order to profit and provide a source of cash. Enterprises that do not supervise intertemporal companies damage the opportunity of the existing one. At a modest level, companies incur immediate risks by ignoring income streams and innovation (Tur-Porcar, Roig-Tierno, & Mestre, 2018).

Conventional business practices prevent SMEs from developing large supply chain operations that involve more demands and supplies from the market (Alkhoraif, Rashid & McLaughlin, 2019). Improved communication and innovation simplified the cooperation of SMEs in numerous fields. The globalisation of big enterprises and specialised organisations has granted SMEs more leeway to participate in different parts of their worthwhile supply chain (Romann, 2020). New and imaginative corporate approaches, including additional business models in the organisation, allow SMEs greater freedom to manage their business with larger businesses. The intensity and characteristics of organisations across the board have boosted the spread of executive education and business devices. The government of Malaysia is involved in promoting knowledge and awareness programmes for SME businesses in Malaysia via agencies and departments in the Ministry for Entrepreneur Development and Cooperatives (MEDAC), the Ministry of Finance (MOF), and the Ministry of Science Technology and Innovation (MOSTI). Financial aid is to help SMEs to cope with the hazards of the pandemic and to provide the know-how to enable SMEs to adopt the IoT more effectively. In total, MYR 95.7 billion of benefits indicate how serious the government is about uplifting the SMEs as the main gross domestic product contributors in Malaysia.

Knowledge and understanding of the necessity of technology, and its implementation in a business-wide operation are important to support SMEs in this highly linked world (Krüger & Meyer, 2021). Business sustainability indicates that the company must, in order to maintain its existence, cope with any radical change with great adaptability. How this can be achieved typically depends on the amount of flexibility of the SME businesses to accept change to improve the way SMEs operate (Hermawati & Gunawan, 2020). It was also asserted by Dobrovič, and Timková, (2017) that the way changes are arranged, changes are controlled, and the time to implement the changes was predicted to have an important role and substantial influence on an organization's progress achievement or disappointment. Procrastination will have a major role in the progress of an SME towards achieving sustainability as an ongoing concern.

3.4 The IoT

The IoT, as well as many innovative sectors, including sustainable company development and climate protection, will become crucial in the current scenario in years to come. The IoT has the potential to automate supply chain transactions when certain criteria are satisfied. The hypotheses of IoT agreements are high and reliable in order to alter business acumen by increasing the complex development of support equipment, such as medical and transport systems, clever urban regions, savvy energy management, and the cyclical economy (Nasiri, Tura & Ojanen, 2017).

IoT can dramatically transform organisations and society within a hyper-associated economy via increased straightforwardness, simplified creation methods, and reduced labour expenses. Future cyber–physical systems (CPCs) will rely on profoundly skilled, loaded, and related knowledge, such as smart urban communities, self-governing cars, or autonomous automobiles (Broo, Boman & Törngren, 2021). In general, the board has drawn up a six-part IoT research strategy, which covers IoT effects on IoT adaptation, society, businesses, and customer advantages. With greater accessibility, more efficient production methods, and lower overhead costs, IoT has the potential to profoundly alter the way businesses and society function in today's hyper-connected economy. IoT's impact on business and society, IoT monetization and end-user services, IoT as a distributed platform, the convergence of IoT and blockchain, security problems and solutions, and IoT and ethics were all listed as key areas for future IS research (Avital et. al., 2019). In general, adequate information will help organisations to track a subsidy and conduct an analysis on the utilization of husbandry, climate change, reducing outflows, and then again; where necessary, information has been collected, and organisations have been empowered to take account of that (Buntz, 2019).

Information sharing creates a knowledge base that allows a transition from the use of buyer profiles to the targeted promotion and evaluation of individualised offerings (Xu & Gao, 2021). The essential complexity of purchaser information as well as understanding the environment is needed to combine the efforts across organisations and remove the barriers between modern IoT apps and shoppers (Zhang & Chen, 2020). As businesses accumulate more and more information, including highly personal biometric data, they expose themselves to greater cyber security threats. Serious worries about discrimination, privacy, security, and consent come from the increased possibility of security breaches and the problems connected with obtaining meaningful consumer consent. Millions of customer records containing personal information like social security numbers, addresses, and credit card numbers have been compromised by large organizations like the credit scoring company Equifax, for example. Because features like your iris or fingerprint cannot be altered, biometric information poses even greater risks than regular credit card information. The exchange of personal health and biometric information is growing (Donner & Steep, 2021).

3.5 Contemporary Issues: A Malaysian's Scenario

3.5.1 SMEs Ecology

3.5.1.1 Digitalisation

Technical advancements, as in the digitalisation of enterprises by means of modern equipment, may help SMEs to reduce costs, standardise their companies, and automate the operation of their equipment, as well as help to optimise work (World Bank Group, 2018; Tong & Gong, 2020). As proven by Haseeb et. al. (2019), IR4.0 is the solution to preserve business efficiency for SMEs in this unpredictable market. The IR4.0 building blocks include the IoT, large-scale data systems, and smart production systems. This increases company sustainability and increases the progressive development of data innovation. In addition to organisational structures and processes, the interconnection of IR4.0 and IoT implementation will be strengthened (Haseeb et. al., 2019). As underlined, the digitisation of SMEs was important for sustainability and was pandemic-driven (COVID-19). SMEs during the pandemic in South-East

Asia were expected to reduce their sales by 2020 (Annuar, 2020), as early as the start of 2020, with eight in ten or more SME businesses in the area. Governments and financial institutions quickly make subsidies and programmes available to assist this vital sector to survive; however, there is historical evidence that technology and innovation are the keys to sustainable SMEs (SMECorp. 2021a).

Therefore, the COVID-19 epidemic has contributed to the use of IoT innovation in the daily lives of customers, and digitalisation was not just the driving force behind current businesses but also the driving force behind new enterprises. The use of digital applications is expanding and physically mobile; lifestyles were revitalised as a result of the COVID-19 pandemic. In fact, the epidemic has changed the way people do things. However, losing a brand name is truly damaging to ordinary customers or potential customers in terms of their trust. Internally, there has been a negative impact on staff morale in SMEs, which was to do with reducing compensation and resource diversion to others, and more vital tasks were required to survive the initial wave of the pandemic. When the crisis struck, the firm was affected by regulations and legal issues, which substantially influenced the value of the SME, in addition to the external and internal impact.

3.5.1.2 Cyber Security

Malaysia wanted to encourage SMEs to meet the needs of a growing digital environment before the COVID-19 pandemic, with the objective of becoming a globally digital economy by 2022. SME Corp has indicated that, if the firm is digitised, the cash-free transaction could provide SMEs benefits. Recent developments already provide around 5,634 SME government grants through SME Business Digitalisation (SMECorp., 2021b). In reality, they enable Malaysian SMEs to survive. In contrast, the growth in cybercrime activities is extremely worrying since digitalisation offers criminals and hackers the chance to take advantage of weak SMEs and customers (Wiggen, 2020). Hassan (2021) claimed that since firms increasingly employed work from home to deal with the pandemic, cybersecurity problems were caused. Threats, such as ransomware and email phishing, persuade internet users to visit malicious URLs that have downloaded unauthorised remote management tools (RATs). As asserted by Kaspersky Safety Network (KSN, n.d), in 2020, 767,000 Malaysian consumers were virtually infected by Internet-borne malware. In early 2020, phishing attempts were documented on about 269,533 incidents involving Malaysian SMEs, an increase of 56% in 2019. Crypto-mining efforts were reported to be 238,780; approximately twice as much as in 2019, compared with the first half of 2020 targeting SMEs (KSN, n.d.). The circumstances of single data theft to an SME in Southeast Asia can cost up to RM 400,000 on average (KSN, n.d.). However, Tiong (2020) said that cybersecurity will be on top, regardless of the size of the enterprise, as Malaysian SMEs continue to embrace digitisation. SMEs need to integrate cyber security digitalisation so that they do not become the victims of cybercrime SMEs (Tiong, 2020). When the economy is turbulent, it is smart to invest, but not after recovery.

3.5.2 Establishing a High-Level Tasks Force to Promote IoT/IR4.0

Tong & Gong (2020) proposed government and policy interventions to facilitate the IoT digitisation process for SMEs in Malaysia, as well as some other actions to help these SMEs. Indeed, the Malaysian government already established (since March 2017) a team known as the High-Level Task Force (HLTF), which is chaired by the MITI with representatives from many ministries involved on topics for their comprehensive supervision and management. In order to build the national IR4.0 framework, an HLTF was instructed with MOSTI, MOHE, and MITI, which is also participating in SME's efforts to embrace IoT and digitisation. In order to achieve corporate sustainability, SMEs must be able to cope with changes that use IoT as it is transformed into monetary value in the technology and the data generated. Furthermore, the economies of scale of SMEs might be strengthened by the adoption of IoT innovation in the conventional industry (SMECorp., 2021c). The HLTF provides information, awareness, and assistance for SMEs in Malaysia to boost digitalisation and overcome insecurities (SMECorp., 2016).

3.6 Discussion

When making decisions to accept IoT or not, the identification of the advantages of implementing IoT in SMEs is key. As long as inherited IT and information are reliable, SMEs will continue to use the same amount of time and money to deal with the effects of COVID-19 (Hanna, 2021). Business is constantly calculating risks that may be quantified and they seek chances to make a decision in connection with the organisation. Themes such as total quality management (TQM) generally highlight the difficulties of organisational transformations in many management issues. IoT strengthens an adaptable enterprise structure. TQM stated that according to Ono & Bodek (2019), the positives will emerge when firms chose to make the most of shift work. With the advantages of implementing IoT with the TQM issues in mind, waste and inefficiencies will always be eliminated, company productivity will be gradually enhanced. The definition of waste can be characterised as any improvements or decisions that don't enhance a company (Järvenpää & Lanz, 2020) by reducing SMEs' waste and inefficiencies

In connection to business ability, individuals, or employees need to be able to provide public support for the use of IoT systems to handle different applications. The IoT ecosystems that assist in reducing waste, and therefore, provide the efficiency required in SME enterprises are shown in Figure 3.1. The ecosystems included

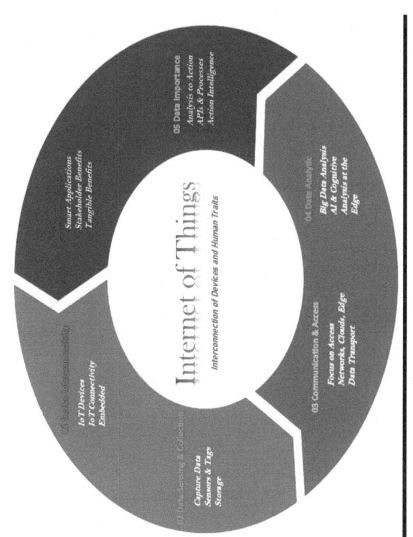

Figure 3.1 How IoT is inter-connected. The six cycle elements of an IoT interconnectivity created several benefits for the users

device connection, data sensing and raw data transmission, data processing, useful data collection, and the inclusion of stakeholder human value (Cook, 2018). SMEs can cross-reference with constant information and allow business and IT-associated undertakings to oversee measures with the most contextualised data.

Further, in buildings and structures, monitoring and detecting hazards may be monitored; via wasteful assets, materials, and implementations, operating expenses will decrease. SMEs may also directly link it with the association's detailed design by integrating information and knowledge into current natural, health, and security measures as well as in the HR department. IoT will assist SMEs to understand natural cycles and how ongoing information and research may help to reduce and manage their complexities.

3.6.1 Increasing SMEs' Productivity Effectiveness

As indicated by Končar et.al. (2020), the efficacy of an SME was enhanced by the utilisation of IoT in a specific business context. Indoor light, movement, and temperature differentials can, for example, be identified by IoT goods, such as smart metres or measurements. The planning of these components together with low-energy system management innovations, which are similar to Wi-Fi or Bluetooth advances, have begun to maintain IoT expansion in diverse indoor and outdoor environments. These arrangements can, therefore, be governed by microgrid or sun-based innovations, which makes drives alternatives that may be supportable free of charge. The IoT utilisation will bring better financial matters for energy and could effectively help in the following shortcomings that are present in lighting frameworks or resources.

In the larger context that suits SME's business acumen, SMEs will be able to strategise their organisation to expand the prominence and designation of these metrics into other functions through modifying existing framework integration to achieve a better quality of data. The better the data quality that SMEs have, the better the business strategy that is formulated. The relationship shown in Figure 3.2 shows the relationship between humans, the internet, and devices through IoT internetworking in virtual and existing real-world applications and scenarios.

3.6.2 Adoption Challenges

Operational structures and technical skills are difficulties that limit the progress of IoT and digitalisation (SMECorp., 2021c). Lorrette (2019) indicated that one of four main choices can be implemented by an SME: operating, divisional, matrix, or flat. However, SMEs need the know-how to determine the most typical facilities for the company. Businesses function differently by nature; therefore, for any SME as a whole, there will be no single way out. The best reaction under the circumstances for those SMEs is to initiate changes in the organisation and create a corporate

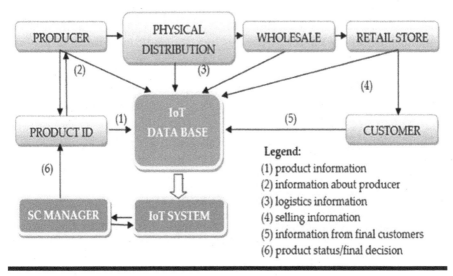

Figure 3.2   The IoT lifecycle in the SMEs business environment. The lifecycles and how IoT works towards fulfilling the customers' needs as well as the users

Source: Copyright by: Kon-ar et. al., (2020)

hierarchy that will improve company efficiency and operational efficacy. The charts and associated IT applications will lead to problems for SMEs. Technical skills are connected to entrepreneurs' and workers' knowledge. In the decision-making process, SMEs are conventional (Kyobe, Namirembe & Shongwe, 2015).

3.7 Limitations

In the following paragraphs, the discussion will be on the aspects of the impact of IoT adoption that would increase SME's business sustainability. In short, the well-being of SMEs under the current economic climate requires a technological component, which is necessary to legitimise the functioning of SMEs, as well as their commercial viability. The need to acquire IoT innovation means that the rest of the companies have competitive benefits. There is evidence that through these adoptions, that SMEs will start earning when being less concerned about what to waste. Productivity comes with the effectiveness of the adoption process.

In any new enterprise, SMEs will face various challenges. Whatever the size, it will make SMEs more sustainable to overcome these difficulties. Yet, SMEs do not stand alone, government agencies are quite supportive in their function. An SME's knowledge will ultimately have the most important role to play in ensuring that changing processes take place.

The main objective of this chapter was to highlight the implications when adopting IoT for SME business sustainability, therefore, enhancing the learning and understanding of the subject. References for the confirmatory factors in the field concerning SMEs and technology adoption are one of the main limitations of this chapter. It is advisable to spend more effort introducing SMEs to IoT and then the future study results could be better. There are a lot of deficiencies in the existing understanding of the subject. Research into IoT innovation issues for SMEs in the future might, as with government agencies, expand the knowledge across regulatory authorities as to how best to tackle SME challenges and processes.

3.8 Suggestions for Future Research

A more profound investigation into the relationship between innovation acknowledgement with and without government organisations' resistance would be an issue of interest. Future explorations into this issue should be possible by investigating past assessment results and examining the information gathered for connections. The relatively narrow but important question that might be identified after data collection was completed is: what is the impact in the long run of relative non-adopting SMEs following initial periods of more intense adoption carried out by most SMEs? The research outcomes might be utilised to give data to the MOF, MEDAC, and other related executive bodies on the requirements for advanced knowledge about SME development.

Discoveries from this specific chapter by reviewing the past research and articles have shown promising proof that utilising innovation-based applications, such as IoT and other activities do offer a worthwhile alternative to start charting SME's business sustainability approach. Additional time and endeavours when arranging and planning modern methodologies.

3.9 Conclusions

The facts and discussion tabled in this chapter reflected the reality of today's SMEs business environment. The findings showed that the SMEs have to achieve sustainability in order to not just help their business to survive the chaotic COVID-19 crisis, but also the national interest overall. Negligence in this aspect would cost SMEs severely. Rapid or continuous adoption of IoT by SMEs is about putting in more effort to learning and embracing organisational changes. It was reasoned that reality and time potentially affected the results of the achievements and is hoped that this chapter has contributed to and featured more knowledge and mindfulness on the understandings of each of the stakeholders, readers, academicians, as well as business owners, with regards to the significance of empowering SMEs with innovative technologies like the IoT innovation. This was the centre of attention during the COVID-19 crisis. Significantly, based on the suggestion from the theoretical adaptations and contributions of this chapter, SMEs, with the help of related government agencies, should start to enable the adoption process immediately in order to gain competitive advantages to sustain their business.

References

Alkhoraif, A., Rashid, H., & Mclaughlin, P. (2019). Lean implementation in small and medium enterprises: Literature review. *Operations Research Perspectives, 6*, 100089. doi:10.1016/j.orp.2018.100089

Annuar, A. (2020). Covid-19: After MCO, survey finds nearly 70pc SMEs lost half income. *Malay Mail.* Retrieved from www.malaymail.com/news/malaysia/2020/03/27/covid-19-after-mco-survey-finds-nearly-70pc-smes-lost-half-income/1850688

Avital, M., Dennis, A. R., Rossi, M., Sørensen, C., & French, A. (2019). The transformative effect of the internet of things on business and society. *Communications of the Association for Information Systems, 44*, 129–140. doi:10.17705/1cais.04405

Awan, U., Sroufe, R., & Shahbaz, M. (2021). Industry 4.0 and the circular economy: A literature review and recommendations for future research. *Business Strategy and the Environment, 30*(4), 2038–2060. doi:10.1002/bse.2731

Baumann, D. (2020). *Learning and Control Strategies for Cyber-Physical Systems from Wireless Control over Deep Reinforcement Learning to Causal Identification.* Stockholm: KTH Royal Institute of Technology.

Bharati, S. (2020). How artificial intelligence impacts businesses in the period of pandemics? *Journal of the International Academy for Case Studies, 26*(5).

Bhargava, S. (2007). *Developmental aspects of entrepreneurship.* Los Angeles: Response Books.

Bocken, N., Ingemarsdotter, E., & Gonzalez, D. (2018). Designing sustainable business models: Exploring IoT-enabled strategies to drive sustainable consumption. *Sustainable Business Models,* 61–88. doi:10.1007/978-3-319-93275-0_3

Broo, D. G., Boman, U., & Törngren, M. (2021). Cyber-physical systems research and education in 2030: Scenarios and strategies. *Journal of Industrial Information Integration, 21*, 100192. doi:10.1016/j.jii.2020.100192

Buntz, B. (2019). How IoT technology can help the environment. Retrieved from www.iotworldtoday.com/2019/12/19/how-iot-technology-can-help-the-environment/

Cook, K. (2018). 7 Ways to secure the IoT in your enterprise. Retrieved from www.houseofb ots.com/news-detail/3981-1-7-ways-to-secure-the-internet-of-things-iot-in-your-ent erprise

Dobrovič, J., & Timková, V. (2017). Examination of factors affecting the implementation of organizational changes. *Journal of Competitiveness, 9*(4), 5–17. doi:10.7441/joc.2017.04.01

Donnellan, M. B., & Lucas, R. E. (2013). Secondary data analysis. *Oxford Handbooks Online.* doi:10.1093/oxfordhb/9780199934898.013.0028

Donner, H., & Steep, M. (2021). Monetizing the IoT revolution. *Sustainability, 13*(4), 2195. doi:10.3390/su13042195

Feltham, T. S., Feltham, G., & Barnett, J. J. (2005). The dependence of family businesses on a single decision-maker. *Journal of Small Business Management, 43*(1), 1–15. doi:10.1111/j.1540-627x.2004.00122.x

Fukuda-Parr, S., & Muchhala, B. (2020). The southern origins of sustainable development goals: Ideas, actors, aspirations. *World Development, 126*, 104706. doi:10.1016/j.worlddev.2019.104706

Hanna, T. (2021). Veeam data protection report 2021 shows 58% of backups are failing. *Backup and Recovery Solutions News.* Retrieved from https://miniurl.li?s=FPXv

Haseeb, M., Hussain, H. I., Ślusarczyk, B., & Jermsittiparsert, K. (2019). Industry 4.0: A solution towards technology challenges of sustainable business performance. *Social Sciences, 8*(5), 154. doi:10.3390/socsci8050154

Hashim, H. (2021). Shape Up or Ship Out. Paper presented at IMM Webinar 2021 (Institute of Marketing Malaysia) in Putra Business School (UPM), Bangi, Malaysia.

Hassan, M. (2021). Critical Asset Protection. Paper presented at Simple and Smarter Cybersecurity for SMEs in National Cyber Security Agency (NACSA) & MDEC, Kuala Lumpur, Malaysia.

Hermawati, A., & Gunawan, E. (2020). The implementation of dynamic capabilities for small and medium-sized enterprises in creating innovation. *VINE Journal of Information and Knowledge Management Systems, 51*(1), 92–108. doi:10.1108/vjikms-08-2019-0121

Järvenpää, E., & Lanz, M. (2020). Lean manufacturing and sustainable development. *Encyclopedia of the UN Sustainable Development Goals Responsible Consumption and Production,* 423–432. doi:10.1007/978-3-319-95726-5_7

Johnston, M. (2014). Secondary data analysis: A method of which the time has come. *Qualitative and Quantitative Methods in Libraries (QQML), 3*(3), 619–626.

Karale, A. (2021). The challenges of IoT addressing security, ethics, privacy, and laws. *Internet of Things, 15*, 100420. doi:10.1016/j.iot.2021.100420

Končar, J., Grubor, A., Marić, R., Vučenović, S., & Vukmirović, G. (2020). Setbacks to IoT implementation in the function of FMCG supply chain sustainability during COVID-19 Pandemic. *Sustainability, 12*(18), 7391. doi:10.3390/su12187391

Krüger, N. A., & Meyer, N. (2021). The development of a small and medium-sized business risk management intervention tool. *Journal of Risk and Financial Management, 14*(7), 310. doi:10.3390/jrfm14070310

KSN. (n.d.). Retrieved from www.kaspersky.com/ksn

Kyobe, M., Namirembe, E., & Shongwe, M. (2015). The alignment of information technology applications with non-technological competencies of SMEs in Africa. *The Electronic Journal of Information Systems in Developing Countries, 67*(1), 1–22. doi:10.1002/j.1681-4835.2015.tb00483.x

Laarouchi, M. E. (2020). A safety approach for CPS-IoT (Master's thesis). Institut Polytechnique de Paris, Paris. Paris: Networking and Internet Architecture.

Lea, P. (2020). *IoT and edge computing for architects: Implementing edge and IoT systems from sensors to clouds with communication systems, analytics, and security.* Birmingham: Packt Publishing.

Lorette, K. (2019). Typical organizational structure of a small business. Retrieved from smallbusiness.chron.com/typical-organizational-structure-small-business-4895.html

Margherita, E. G., & Braccini, A. M. (2020). Industry 4.0 technologies in flexible manufacturing for sustainable organizational value: Reflections from a multiple case study of Italian manufacturers. *Information Systems Frontiers.* doi:10.1007/s10796-020-10047-y

Moore, M. (2019). What is Industry 4.0? Everything you need to know. Retrieved from www.techradar.com/news/what-is-industry-40-everything-you-need-to-know

Nasiri, M., Tura, N., & Ojanen, V. (2017). Developing disruptive innovations for sustainability: A review on impact of internet of things (IOT). *Portland International Conference on Management of Engineering and Technology (PICMET).* doi:10.23919/picmet.2017.8125369

Ōno, T., & Bodek, B. (2019). *Toyota production system: Beyond large-scale production.* New York: Productivity Press.

Paul, P. K., Bharati, S., Podder, P., & Mondal, M. R. (2021). 10 the role of IoMT during pandemics. *Computational Intelligence for Managing Pandemics,* 169–186. doi:10.1515/9783110712254-010

PEOPLE 4.0. (2021). *Data Protection Report 2021* (Rep.). Kuala Lumpur: VeeAM.

Podder, P., Khamparia, A., Mondal, M. R., Rahman, M. A., & Bharati, S. (2021). Forecasting the spread of COVID-19 and ICU requirements. *International Journal of Online and Biomedical Engineering, 17*(05), 81. doi:10.3991/ijoe.v17i05.20009

Romann, E. (2020). *Nonmarket strategy in Japan: How foreign firms lobby "inside the castle".* Singapore: Palgrave Macmillan.

Schranz, M., Caro, G. A., Schmickl, T., Elmenreich, W., Arvin, F., Şekercioğlu, A., & Sende, M. (2021). Swarm intelligence and cyber-physical systems: Concepts, challenges and future trends. *Swarm and Evolutionary Computation, 60,* 100762. doi:10.1016/j.swevo.2020.100762

SMECorp. (2016). High level task force meeting (HLTF). Retrieved from www.smecorp.gov.my/index.php/en/slides/182-events/1591-high-level-task-force-meeting-hltf

SMECorp. (2021a). SMEs must arm themselves with digital technology, says Wan Junaidi. Retrieved from www.smecorp.gov.my/index.php/en/resources/2015-12-21-10-55-22/news/4320-smes-must-arm-themselves-with-digital-technology-says-wan-junaidi

SMECorp. (2021b). Cybersecurity plays a crucial role in Malaysian SMEs' road to recovery SMEs. Retrieved from www.smecorp.gov.my/index.php/en/resources/2015-12-21-10-55-22/news/4317-cybersecurity-plays-a-crucial-role-in-malaysian-smes-road-to-recovery

SMECorp. (2021c). *SME Weekly News: Economics & Policy Division,* Retrieved from www.smecorp.gov.my/images/SME_Weekly_News/2021/SWN/SWN15_19feb.pdf

Sánchez-Báez, E. A., Fernández-Serrano, J., & Romero, I. (2020). Organizational culture and innovation in small businesses in Paraguay. *Regional Science Policy & Practice, 12*(2), 233–247. doi:10.1111/rsp3.12203

Tiong, Y. S. (2020). Cybersecurity plays a crucial role in Malaysian SMEs' road to recovery, note by General Manager for Southeast Asia at Kaspersky, Retrieved from www.smecorp.gov.my/index.php/en/resources/2015-12-21-10-55-22/news/4317-cybersecurity-plays-a-crucial-role-in-malaysian-smes-road-to-recovery

Tong, A., & Gong, R. (2020). The impact of COVID-19 on SME digitalisation in Malaysia. Retrieved from https://blogs.lse.ac.uk/seac/2020/10/20/the-impact-of-covid-19-on-sme-digitalisation-in-malaysia/

Tur-Porcar, A., Roig-Tierno, N., & Mestre, A. L. (2018). Factors affecting entrepreneurship and business sustainability. *Sustainability, 10*(2), 452. doi:10.3390/su10020452

Ungureanu, A. V. (2020). The transition from Industry 4.0 to Industry 5.0. The 4Cs of the global economic change. *16th Economic International Conference NCOE 4.0 2020.* doi:10.18662/lumproc/ncoe4.0.2020/07

Vanderstraeten, J., Loots, E., Hamelin, A., & Witteloostuijn, A. V. (2020). Micro-foundations of small business internationalization: Introduction to the special section. *Cross Cultural & Strategic Management, 27*(3), 265–283. doi:10.1108/ccsm-04-2020-0100

Ward, S. (2020). What Are SMEs? Retrieved from www.thebalancesmb.com/sme-small-to-medium-enterprise-definition-2947962

Welsh, J. A., White, J. F., & Dowell, P. (1982). A small business is not a little big business Harvard Business Review, 59(4). Retrieved from https://hbr.org/1981/07/a-small-business-is-not-a-little-big-business

Wiggen, J. (2020). The impact of COVID-19 on cyber-crime and state-sponsored cyber activities, *Konrad Adenauer Stiftung.* doi:10.2307/resrep25300

Winarsih, I. M., & Fuad, K. (2020). Impact of Covid-19 on digital transformation and sustainability in small and medium enterprises (SMEs): A conceptual framework. *Complex, Intelligent and Software Intensive Systems Advances in Intelligent Systems and Computing,* 471–476. doi:10.1007/978-3-030-50454-0_48

World Bank Group (2018). Malaysia's digital economy: A new driver of development, Retrieved from www.kkmm.gov.my/pdf/KPI/Laporan%207.pdf.

Xu, J., & Gao, X. (2021). E-Business enabling technologies and building capacities. *E-Business in the 21st Century Intelligent Information Systems,* 29–61. doi:10.1142/9789811231841_0002

Zhang, C., & Chen, Y. (2020). A review of research relevant to the emerging industry trends: Industry 4.0, IoT, blockchain, and business analytics. *Journal of Industrial Integration and Management, 05*(01), 165–180. doi:10.1142/s2424862219500192

Chapter 4

Impact of COVID-19: Insights from Key Sectors of the Indian Economy

Reena Malik

Chitkara Business School, Chitkara University, Punjab, India

Contents

DOI: 10.1201/9781003324447-4

4.1 Introduction

The corona outbreak has been a great menace worldwide affecting millions of people at large. It was not only detrimental to human life but also brought negative repercussions to business globally, harshly impacting economies and upending commercial activities. Since the identification of its first outbreak in Wuhan, China in 2020, it spread across the globe at a very fast rate. The World Health Organization declared a coronavirus pandemic on March 11, 2020. Most countries declared a complete lockdown to halt the spread of this deadly virus. The government of India also announced a lockdown on March 24, 2020, after the first case was identified in Kerala, India. COVID-19 has caused many disruptions to the economic system and halted the growth of the entire economic environment. The deadly virus has been regarded as worse than the Great Depression that was experienced in 1930. The chief of the International Monetary Fund said that "The entire world is uncertain about the duration and depth of this crisis; COVID-19 is such an economic fallout which is worst since Great Depression." Bigger economic trouble has been forecast by experts since the COVID-19 outbreak and with each passing day, the picture becomes gloomier than the previous. Coronavirus has placed the economy at standstill impacting almost every sector like tours and travel, hospitality, banks, retail, real estate, hotels, healthcare, media, education, and recreation.

Heavy loss in productivity has been witnessed that was caused by social distancing norms leading to a decrease in economic activities. Social distancing was the most effective tool to halt the ever-increasing spread of COVID-19. Developing economies were projected to face extreme economic disruptions owing to a fragile healthcare system and a weak macroeconomic framework with foreign spillovers. Former Reserve Bank of India (RBI) Governor Raghuram Rajan said, "This is the greatest emergency for the Indian economy since independence". India is already facing a downturn in the economy that was hit badly compared with disruptions faced by other countries. This chapter will focus on the damages attributed to the coronavirus in major sectors of the Indian economy and will recommend relevant policies to be adopted by the government in order to overcome the adverse circumstances. This chapter will also investigate the sectors that flourished during the pandemic and the impact of the pandemic on other economies across the world.

4.2 Sectoral Implications of the Pandemic

4.2.1 Primary Sector

This sector is composed of agriculture and industries involved in the production and extraction of raw materials. This sector contributes majorly to the gross domestic product (GDP) and provides bread and butter to millions of people. To halt the spread of the coronavirus India announced a lockdown like other economies worldwide. India announced a lockdown in March 2020, when harvesting of Rabi crops was at its peak, which was a major setback to farmers, especially in the northwest. It became even worse with restrictions on mobility, scarcity of labor (due to reverse migration), and transport despite some relaxations being allowed. A quick decline in demand owing to the closure of hotels and restaurants and businesses purchasing raw materials hit farmers badly and declining food prices became a major issue of concern for their livelihoods. There was already a decline in the income of workers before the pandemic but an increase in prices in 2020 showed some positive signs; however, this collapsed with the outbreak of the deadly virus in 2020 (Mukhopadhyay,2020). Farmers regarded the coronavirus as worse than demonetization in India (Saha & Bhattacharya, 2020). The pandemic-induced lockdown disrupted the food market causing the loss of food grains in production, marketing, distribution, and households. Perishable items were badly hit due to a lack of demand for milk, vegetables, and fruits.

4.2.2 Secondary Sector

The secondary sector is recognized as the creator of wealth and is the vibrant engine of a nation (Rele, 2020), contributing 20% to the GDP. Having both backward and forward links with other sectors, the secondary sector becomes even more significant because the impact on the secondary sector will be evident in other sectors. This pandemic has caused disruptions in demand and supply worldwide and manufacturing in India has come to standstill. The purchasing manufacturing index (PMI) slipped to 55.4 in March 2021. According to the Performance Results System Economic survey, the 2019–20220 manufacturing sector is expected to grow by 2.0%; however, due to the pandemic the share of the manufacturing sector in gross value added declined to 13.8% in the second quarter of 2019–2020 and the growth rate of this sector plunged to –39.3% in the quarter first of 2020–2021. According to the United Nations Industrial Development Organization survey, the most affected sectors in manufacturing were textiles, machinery and equipment, motor vehicles, chemical, and metal products. The auto sector contributes around 50% of the manufacturing sector's contribution to GDP; the manufacturing sector was estimated to decline between 22% and 35% across different industrial segments for the financial year 2021. Cuts in production due to less demand during the pandemic had a negative impact on the component industries in the form of suspending operations of medium and small enterprises (MSMEs) engaged in manufacturing small and spare parts. MSMEs form the major portion of manufacturing in India and provide employment and export opportunities. They contribute 30% of India's GDP. The interrupted supply chain reduced cash flow, and the reverse migration of workers hit businesses hard. MSMEs require financial assistance and the incapacity to deal with sudden disruptions makes them more vulnerable. It is very difficult to re-start medium and small-scale industries once they shut down (Chidambaram, 2021).

4.2.2.1 Mega Challenge

1. A high level of uncertainty has been created by COVID-19 in all aspects of the business. In order to halt the spread of COVID-19 further, the economy might return to a potential lockdown
2. In the future, when restrictions are relaxed, the market is going to experience cash constraints due to uncertainties and restrictions in deliveries created by the pandemic with respect to demand and their availability for MSMEs products. With lower business income and fixed charges to bear MSMEs will suffer
3. Human resources, especially unskilled labor, will be a major constraint, owing to the pandemic's reverse migration of labor that started. Even though labor is returning from their native homes, it is not building confidence for labor, which will be a major concern for MSMEs
4. The need for outstanding machinery maintenance will arise before resuming operations and MSMEs will have to bear significant costs with write-offs of stocks that were trapped on-site due to lockdown
5. Maintaining proper and timely supplies of essentials without price hikes is a matter of great concern. Most MSMEs have concerns about their vulnerability to supply shortages, especially those that are dependent on specialized parts from other states or different countries

4.2.3 Service Sector

The service sector employs millions of people in India and contributes a major portion of India's GDP. The sector is composed of industries like travel and tourism, hospitality, transportation, IT, retail, media, the banking and financial service industry, and others. Travel and transportation were the biggest hit sector due to the curtailment of transportation and restrictions on travel in order to halt the virus's spread. The closure of hotels and other services at tourist spots gave a crippling blow to the industry. Transportation was under a massive financial crisis and distress. The operations of all sorts of transportation were struck hard due to strict restrictions and border closures. A report by KPMG estimated job losses of approximately 38 million in India's travel, tourism, and hospitality industry. With a rise in nonperforming assets, the problem of twin balance sheets and an inadequately capitalized banking system, the financial sector was already decreasing with such massive problems and the pandemic made it even worse. Banks are considered a major help in times of crisis; however, some studies show that private sector firms are also financially weak and over-leveraged (Vardhan & Sengupta, 2019).

4.3 Becoming a Global Hub

The pandemic outbreak has sent shock waves across economies worldwide. At the same time, it brought a lucrative opportunity for India in the form of a reliability crisis in China. Accounting for one-third of the world's manufacturing, China has been considered an epicenter for manufacturing; however, with the outbreak of coronavirus, many economies are shifting their focus to other economies in order to avail cheap labor. India has a golden chance to take the initiative "Made in India" global. The COVID-19 virus originated in Wuhan, China and has created discomfort for the leading manufacturing hubs and the benefit of that discomfort and lack of reliability toward China could be turned into comfort for India. Economies shifting from China could put their focus on India, which is the second-largest populated country and has a huge domestic market, availability of a young and cheap workforce, strong transport networks, favorable government initiatives, and the availability of economic infrastructure.

4.4 Thriving amid COVID-19: Positive Implications

The pandemic outbreak has had a devastating impact on health, lives, and economies across the world. Respective governments put restrictions on movement and people had to remain in their homes due to lockdown. Businesses were shut; disruptions in demand and supply had negative repercussions on businesses and recovering from the torment inflicted by the pandemic is now a major concern. According to the Mckinsey, 2020 report (Sneader & Strenfels, 2020) to find a way forward, the next new normal business managers must possess five qualities of resolve, resilience, return, re-imagination, and reform.

Services that were flourishing during COVID-19.

1. Cleaning services
2. Delivery services
3. Grocery stores
4. Liquor stores

5. Telehealth companies
6. Tech companies
7. E-Learning
8. Healthcare workers

A positive impact of COVID-19 has also been seen on the environment (Sharma, 2020). Due to the restrictions on mobility and transportation, the positive impact was evident in better air and water quality, lower pollution, and improved wildlife. A sharp decline was registered within 7 days after the first lockdown phase, and a 30% reduction in electricity demand was noticed, port traffic was registered at 5% lower, and oil demand reduced by 70%. Indian rail activity compared with the previous year was <36% (Mahendra et. al., 2020). The major positive implication was decreased pollution in the Ganga River. The Chairman of the Mahamana Malaviya Research Centre for The Ganga, Prof. B. D. Tripathi, said the lockdown has been able to clean rivers in ways that large-scale projects could not.

4.5 Impact of the Second Wave

The pandemic has penetrated the deepest core of human civilization for almost 2 years now. During the first wave, we thought we have gained some control over this deadly virus, but the second wave has made us realize the importance of mother nature as people were buying oxygen to protect themselves. The second wave has completely shaken human lives and macroeconomics. The approach to dealing with the second wave was completely different from the first wave. It was more localized and was in the hands of the state governments, unlike the first one, which was centralized with a prolonged lockdown resulting in a smaller number of peak cases. Due to a smaller number of restrictions, the rural economy continued to move compared with the urban economy where manufacturing came to a grinding halt. The agricultural economy continued growing in the first wave and benefited from a good monsoon and the availability of labor (migrated laborers came back to work). The second wave hit rural areas compared with urban, unlike the first wave. The rural areas of Maharashtra, Kerala, and Andhra Pradesh, India were the worst hit. The inadequacy of the medical infrastructure was the biggest reason for the loss of lives (Kumar et. al, 2020).

4.5.1 Agriculture

Due to the lockdown, the second wave was gloomier for the farmers as the Agricultural Product Marketing Committee (Mandis) was closed and became nonoperational during the peak harvesting season, especially in Gujarat and Rajasthan, India, which had negative repercussions on farmers. A large number of crops were spoiled in fields as the Mandis have still not opened fully. As a result, processing industries and small vendors have been hit. A contrasting impact of the first and second waves registered growth in agricultural wages. It reduced to 2.9% in the second wave from November 2020 to March 2021 and from 8.5% in the first wave from April to August 2020.

4.5.2 Manufacturing

During both waves, manufacturing was at the receiving end working hard to halt the spread of the coronavirus at a lower capacity or was shut down. Undoubtedly, nonmanufacturing units were hit hard too with the long and stringent restrictions. Reverse migration started in the first wave, but fear of prolonged lockdowns is still there in the minds of workers. It will take time to build up their confidence again. Moreover, the supply chains at the local and global levels have not fully normalized after the first wave, which is increasing the burden on the increased cost of procuring raw materials for industries. As per the recent report by the Information Handling Services, the PMI slumped to 50.8 in May 2020, which is the lowest in the last 10 months.

4.5.3 Services

The service sector contributes more than half of the GDP and has become the bedrock of the Indian economy in the last two decades. With the advent of the internet, it became possible during lockdowns to work anywhere at any time. The pandemic has brought positive disruptions to the service sector as the workforce can be decentralized. A steep learning curve was required in the first wave in order to develop the infrastructure and processes for the organizations, especially for remote working. Lockdowns during the first wave were a new paradigm for employees and it took some time for them to adjust to working from a home environment and be productive at the same time. During the first wave, the prolonged lockdown and unlocking phases ensured that productivity reached prepandemic levels; however, the second wave destroyed almost everything although it was localized, and people started losing faith and confidence. The services sector was the least affected sector from the second wave from a standpoint of output (Table 4.1).

Table 4.1   Impact of First and Second Wave

Time Frame	GDP Growth (%)	GDP Growth (%)	Manufacturing GDP (%)	Agricultural GDP (%)
First wave (FY21)	–7.3	16 contracted	Contacted by 7.2	Grown by 3.4
Contribution to overall GDP	0	55	17.4	17.8
Expected from second wave	8.2 to 9.3 (due to base effect)	Lower than first wave	Lower than first wave	Higher than first wave

4.6 Overall Impact on GDP

It was evident from the data released by the Indian government on May 31, 2020, that GDP contracted by 7.3& during the financial year 2020–2021, which was considered the most severe contraction since India gained independence. The obvious reasons behind this trajectory were.

1. Closure of business units due to prolonged lockdown
2. Increase in unemployment rates
3. Significantly declining domestic consumption

A growth of 10.5% was anticipated by The Reserve Bank for the current financial year (2020), on the contrary, due to the impact of the second wave of COVID-19 global rating agencies have downgraded this estimation. Moody projected a 9.3% decline in growth for FY 2021–2022. The S&P Global Rating lowered the growth from 11% to 9.8% due to the moderate impact of the second wave. The forecasts for the third wave are showing a gloomier picture. Table 4.1 shows the COVID-19 global economic impact.

4.7 Revival Strategies for Businesses

In order to transform panic into proactive action, business houses must consider and follow some strategies.

1. Analyze the present (external) environment by conducting a Political, Economic, Sociological, Technological, Legal and Environmental (PESTLE) analysis. The analysis will throw light on political, economic, social, technological, ecological, and legal aspects to avail support extended by the government, and this will assist businesses to adjust their focus to compete and serve better
2. In the same way, to understand the current situation and position companies must undertake internal analysis in order to identify their core areas, and expertise and assess manpower requirements, especially during this turbulent time
3. After properly analyzing the internal and external environments, companies should assess their strengths, weaknesses, opportunities, and threats by conducting a SWOT analysis
4. Social distancing has made digitalization more prominent, and businesses are approaching their customers on digital platforms (social media platforms mainly) providing them with a seamless experience even in tough times
5. With the increased use of technology comes increased changes in crimes, and cyber security has to be taken care of as well

6. With the second wave of coronavirus and the third wave estimation, there may be potential lockdowns in the future, so marketing and e-commerce have to be promoted as the pandemic has changed the scenario in shopping behavior and has reduced purchasing power (gives an indication to focus on essentials)
7. Agility in business operations is required in order to reason swiftly and efficiently with the external environment
8. Businesses should emphasize carrying out essential tasks during COVID-19 and curtail nonessentials
9. In order to augment investment in local industries, businesses should localize some portion of their supply chain
10. Proper implementation and execution of business plans require skills and trained human resources, companies should focus on enhancing the skills of their workers by organizing some workshops and training programs
11. Companies should learn a lesson from this crisis and be ready for future uncertainties with a robust disaster management plan

4.8 Policies to Combat COVID-19

1. Policymakers should rethink the allocation of resources to various sectors and give impetus to those allocations that reduce inequalities. COVID-19 has made us realize the significance of and reliance on the agriculture sector
2. Available food stocks should be used properly, and a nutrition program should be formulated for the same
3. The government should include farmers and agricultural workers in assistance packages or formulate protection programs to address the crisis
4. As MSMEs cannot survive without financial assistance, repayment of loans should be delayed for them; even minimum support from the government should be extended to maintain daily expenses and retain employees
5. Trade should be smoother and in order to promote trade, the government should lift restrictions. Expenditure on public health should be raised in order to protect the public and maintain essential supply levels, and overdraft facilities should be increased by RBI
6. Low-income families should be supported by providing direct relief funds. Support facilities and infrastructure should be provided by the government for service and manufacturing continuation
7. A short-term skill program would be a great initiative from the government for unemployed and unskilled workers. Undoubtedly, the pandemic has widened the inequalities and the government should work to decrease them

The pandemic has had an economic impact; however, apart from this economic crisis, the social and health impacts cannot be ignored worldwide. Businesses collapsed, and mass unemployment, domestic violence, deaths, increasing poverty, income inequalities, and deteriorating health have become major challenges due to outbreaks of pandemics worldwide. The mental status of people has been hit hard from older to younger, rich to poor hard, everyone has been affected. Various health problems like anger, anxiety, depression, stress, fear, and many more have emerged as a result of the worldwide outbreak of COVID-19 (Torales et.al., 2020). An increase of 45% was recorded in the number of cases of domestic violence against women within 25 days following the lockdown, mainly in the states of Haryana, Bihar, Uttar Pradesh and Punjab, India according to the latest report by the National Commission for Women. As far as domestic violence is concerned, women in rural areas do not file cases and raise their voices, which makes the situation even worse (Kundu & Bhowmik, 2020). There was a significant decrease in the crime rate in India but in the aftermath of the crisis two monsters, poverty and inequality may lead to an increase in the crime rate (Uppal, 2020).

4.9 COVID-19 and Other Economies

The pandemic has created a need for urgent action for a lasting recovery, especially for developing economies. Many developing economies were already facing weaker growth before the pandemic crisis and COVID-19 makes the challenges these economies face even harder. Strengthening the public health system, and implementing reforms supporting sustainable growth is critical, especially for economies in developing countries facing daunting challenges. Exporters of industrial commodities, energy, oil, metals, and transport-related commodities have triggered an unprecedented collapse, and agriculture markets were well supplied globally.

4.10 Future Scope and Limitations

This bleak outlook is subject to great uncertainty due to the extent of persistence, restrictions, and prolonged disruptions due to the pandemic. However, restrictions have been lifted in various countries. It will be hard for businesses to service debt, and high borrowing costs might result in a financial crisis. Businesses might find it hard to service debt, and heightened risk aversion could lead to increased borrowing costs, and bankruptcies and defaults could result in financial crises in many countries. The economic forecast shows that policymakers will need to do more in the coming months to keep the economy going. Shifting to digital transactions propelled the growth in jobs relating to transportation, delivery, and warehouses. Owing to the pandemic, faster adoption of automation might be pushed into work arenas as many companies deployed artificial intelligence and automation in order to reduce workplace density.

COVID-19 has shaken the economies of every country in the world; this chapter only studied the impact of the pandemic on key sectors of the Indian economy. Further, for future research more economies should be analyzed for the impact of pandemics and comparisons could be made between developing and developed economies.

4.11 Conclusions

The world is in the grip of coronavirus. It has created a sense of uncertainty by shaking up the entire economic system worldwide. The pandemic has eroded wealth, disrupted workplaces, reduced confidence, and distorted markets. This chapter outlined the grip of coronavirus on the key sectors of the Indian economy and discussed the challenges and positive aspects of the pandemic. This chapter highlighted that the pandemic has shaken the entire economy; however, it has shown us a trend in increased automation, especially in workplaces. The Indian economy has been in a crisis phase since 2019 when its economy reduced by 4.9%, the lowest since 2013. Demonetization in November 2016 was the primary reason for this downfall, which made 86% of the money in the economy unusable (Mahendra, 2020). As a developing country, India had various plans in terms of providing employment opportunities, and promoting exports, programs like 'Make in India' aspired to achieve and reach USD 50 trillion economies by 2025. With the second wave, it has become more difficult for the government to choose between the health of the people and the health of the economy as prolonged lockdowns caused deteriorating conditions. High expenditure on building robust education and healthcare systems is crucial for dealing with uncertain problems in the future. MSMEs provide major employment and making investments in MSMEs could be milestones for an economy to achieve. However, every bad situation comes with something good; therefore, this pandemic has given us the unique opportunity to rethink the development of mankind and the environment. There is a great need to adopt sustainable developmental models, which should be based on an inclusive framework and self-reliance and be environmentally friendly, especially in developing economies like India.

References

Aggarwal A., Dhaliwal R. S., & Nobi K. (2018). Impact of structural empowerment on organizational commitment: Mediating role of women's psychological empowerment. *Vision.* 22(3), 284–294.

Aneja R., Ahuja V. (2021). An assessment of socioeconomic impact of COVID-19 pandemic in India. *Journal of Public Affairs*, e2266. doi.10.1002/pa.2266

Bharati, S. & Mondal, M. (2021). 12 Applicatons and challenges of AI- driven IOHT for combating pandemics: a review. In A. Khamparia, R. H. Mondal, P. Podder, B.

Bhushan, V. Albuquerque & S. Kumar (Eds.) *Computational Intelligence for Managing Pandemics*, pp. 213–230. Berlin, Boston: De Gruyter.

Bharati, S., Podder, P., Mondal, M. (2020). Hybrid deep learning for detecting lung diseases from X-ray images. *Informatics in Medicine Unlocked. 20*, 1–14.

Chidambaram, P. (2020). We will never know how many people died of starvation, because no state government will admit to starvation deaths. The Indian Express. Retrieved from https://indianexpress.com/article/opinion/columns/p-chidambaram-india-coro navirus-lockdownmigrants-hunger-6390882/

Jadhav, R. (2020). Lockdown impact: Maharastra farmers dump vegetables and fruits in trash containers. Hindu Business Line. Retrieved from www.thehindubusinessline.com/economy/agri-business/lockdown-impact-maharashtra-farmers-dump-vegetables-and-fruits-in-trash-in-garbage

Kumar, A. (2020). Impact on Indian economy after the COVID-19 second wave. Financial Express. Retrieved from www.financialexpress.com/economy/impact-on-indian-econ omy-after-the-COVID-19-second-wave/2275353/

Kumar, A., Nayar, K. R., & Koya, S. F. (2020). COVID-19: Challenges and its consequences for rural health care in India. *Public Health in Practice, 1*, 100009.

Kundu, B., & Bhowmik, D. (2020). Societal impact of novel coronavirus (COVID 19 pandemic) in India. *SocArXiv.* doi.org/10.31235/osf.io/vm5rz

Mahendra, Dev S., & Sengupta R. (2020). COVID-19: Impact on the Indian Economy. *Time.* Retrieved from https://time.com/5818819/imf-coronavirus-economic-collapse/.

Mondal, M. R. H., Bharati, S., & Podder, P. (2021). Diagnosis of COVID-19 using machine learning and deep learning: A review. *Current Medical Imaging, 17.* doi.10.2174/1573405617666210713113439

Mukhopadhyay, B. R. (2020). COVID-19 and the Indian farm sector: Ensuring everyone's seat at the table. *Agriculture and Human Values, 37*, 549–550. doi.10.1007/s10460-020

Podder, P., Khamparia, A., Mondel, M., Rahman, M., & Bharati, S. (2021). Forecasting the spread of COVID-19 and ICU requirements. *iJOE*, 17(5), 81–99.

Prabhu, S. (2020). Second wave of COVID-19 impacts economic recovery in India. Retrieved from https://economics.rabobank.com/publications/2021/may/second-wave-of-COVID-19-impacts-economic-recovery-in-india

Rele, S. (2020). Emerging outbreaks and epidemic threats: The practicality and limitations in the development and manufacturing of treatments for Coronavirus (COVID-19). *Polymorphism, 4*, 45–52.

Saha, T., & Bhattacharya, S. (2020). Consequences of lockdown amid COVID-19 pandemic on Indian agriculture. *Food and Scientific Reports. 1*(special issue), 47–50. Retrieved from https://foodandscientificreports.com/details/consequenceof-lockdown-amid-COVID-19-pandemic-on-indian-agriculture.html.

Sengupta, R., & Vardhan, H. (2019). Banking crisis is impeding India's economy. Retrieved from https://www.eastasiaforum.org/2019/10/03/banking-crisis-impedes-indias-economy/

Sharma, P., Kaur, M., & Narwal, G. (2020). Other side of the COVID-19 Pandemic: a review. *Pharma Innov, 9*, 366–369.

Sharma, V. (2020). The impact of COVID-19 on India's manufacturing sector. *The Wire.* Retrieved from https://thewire.in/economy/the-impact-of-COVID-19-on-indias-manufacturing-sector

Sneader, K. & Strenfels, B. (2020). From surviving to thriving: Reimagining the post-COVID-19 return. Retrieved from www.mckinsey.com/featured-insights/future-of-work/from-surviving-to-thriving-reimagining-the-post-COVID-19-return

Torales, J., O'Higgins, M., Castaldelli-Maia, J. M., & Ventriglio, A. (2020). The outbreak of COVID-19 coronavirus and its impact on global mental health. *International Journal of Social Psychiatry, 66*, 317–320.

Uppal, P. (2020). COVID-19 will lead to increased crime rates in India. *International Journal of Research, 8*(4), 72–78. Retrieved from https://economictimes.indiatimes.com/news/politics-and-nation/india-witnesses-steep-rise-in-crime-against-women-amid-lockdown-587-complaints-receivedncw/articleshow/75201412.cms

Chapter 5

Future Scope of Artificial Intelligence in Healthcare for COVID-19

Manas Kumar Yogi
Department of CSE, Pragati Engineering College, Surampalem, India

Jyotsna Garikipati
Department of IT, V R Siddhartha Engineering College, Vijayawada, India

Contents

DOI: 10.1201/9781003324447-5

5.1 Introduction

The COVID-19 pandemic has shaken the world with unanticipated outcomes. The world statistics as of October 6, 2021, showed that 220 countries and territories were affected due to COVID-19 with 237 million people infected and around 4.8 million deaths. The US, India, and Brazil were the worst affected countries (Statista, 2021) "Number of coronavirus (COVID-19) cases worldwide"). AI has attained significant importance in the past few months due to the COVID-19 pandemic. The use of this technology in day-to-day activities has skyrocketed in various sectors. In the healthcare sector, the technologies that have made an impact are artificial intelligence (AI), predictive analytics, the internet of medical things, telemedicine, robotics, cyber security, natural language generation, and speech recognition. In the context of COVID-19, AI can be used for the diagnosis and detection of COVID-19, thermal screening, CT scan analysis, drug design, and development. AI in healthcare can be used either virtually or physically. Virtual AI means using machine learning (ML), deep learning (DL), rule-based expert systems, and robot process automation, and physical AI means robots and brain–computer interfaces.

This chapter explains the role of AI in the pandemic and then moves to the use of AI in the post-pandemic era. This chapter starts with an overview of the important ML and DL algorithms in the context of COVID-19. Various algorithms like the convolutional neural networks (CNN), artificial neural networks (ANN), recurrent neural networks (RNN), and long short-term memory (LSTM) are explained briefly.

This chapter reviews how CT scans can be used for the diagnosis and detection of COVID-19 and a comparative analysis is done on the different algorithms that were presented by various researchers. In the following section, the future scope of AI will be discussed. As per the epidemiologists, the transmission of a virus will eventually stop if the community acquires herd immunity, which means that a certain threshold of people is immune to the virus. This can be achieved if the people are vaccinated. For drug design and development, it will take many years to complete the process. AI has helped on speeding up the process of drug design and development to get the vaccination. Various ML and DL algorithms that are used for drug design and development are discussed.

During this pandemic, everything went online. Storage and sharing of a huge amount of data in a secure way is a major concern in all the sectors like banking, healthcare, businesses, government, and e-commerce. In the healthcare sector, medical records, and patient details including insurance details are stored online. Any unauthorized access to such information is undesirable. DL when provided with lots of input can produce much better results. For that, the data needs to be shared across health organizations. This chapter explains how AI and blockchain can be integrated for secure data storage and sharing and analyzes different approaches for this.

To reduce the transmission of the virus to the maximum extent, people are opting for alternatives like contactless transactions. Therefore, how contactless healthcare services can be delivered using AI during and after the post-COVID-19 period is discussed. The authors propose a robust model for the contactless delivery of healthcare services and showed its applicability by using experimental case studies. Finally, the chapter concludes with a discussion on the ethical, legal, and societal aspects and issues of AI in healthcare.

5.2 Basic Terminology

In this subsection, an overview of different architectures in DL will be given.

1. ANN
   a. Similar to biological neural networks
   b. It has input, nodes, weights, and output
   c. Input is processed in one or more hidden layers
2. CNN
   a. It has multiple layers
   b. Common applications are image processing and object detection
   c. It has a convolutional layer, pooling layer, and fully connected layer
   d. Extraction of features is done from many hidden layers
   e. In the output layer, classification is performed
3. RNN
   a. It follows a set of directed cycles
   b. Can memorize previous inputs
   c. Has applications in image captioning, time series analysis, natural language processing, handwriting recognition, and machine translation
4. LSTM
   a. A type of RNN
   b. Holds the information for a long time
   c. Beneficial in the prediction of time series
   d. Has applications in Natural language processing, music composition, and drug manufacturing
5. Generative adversarial networks (GAN)
   a. Creates new instances similar to training data
   b. It has two components
      i. Generator, which generates fake data
      ii. Discriminator, which learns from the fake data

As we will be dealing with the chest X-ray images, a few architectures of CNN, like AlexNet, ResNet50, VGG16, and VGG19, are discussed.

1. AlexNet
   a. Eight layers (five convolutional and three fully connected)
   b. 60 million parameters

     c. First to use rectified linear units as activation functions

     d. Dropout.

  2. ResNet-50

     a. Skip connections, for example, shortcut connections and residuals

     b. 26 M parameters

     c. First to use batch normalization

  3. VGG-16

     a. 16 layers (13 convolutional + 3 fully connected)

     b. 138 M parameters

     c. Smaller size filters

     e. 500 MB storage space

     f. A deeper variant is VGG-19

The key contributions of the chapter are summarized below.

1. Analysis of how ML and DL algorithms are used for diagnosing COVID-19 using X-ray/CT images
2. Reviewed AI's role in gearing up the drug design and development process
3. Analysis of how AI and blockchain can be integrated for secure data storage and sharing
4. A novel robust model is developed to review AI's role in providing contactless healthcare services
5. Ethical, legal, and societal issues or aspects of AI are discussed

5.3 COVID-19 Diagnosis and Detection using Chest CT/X-Ray Scans

COVID-19 requires two types of testing: a diagnostic test and an antibody test. To identify whether or not someone is infected, diagnostic tests are employed. The real-time reverse transcription-polymerase chain reaction (RT-PCR) test is used to check whether a person is infected with the SARS-CoV2 virus. Antibody testing checks for antibodies that are produced by the immune system in response to the COVID-19 virus to determine a person's immunity. Antibody tests should never be used to identify whether someone has COVID-19. However, when testing a COVID-19 positive patient early in their sickness or after the virus has passed down the throat and into the lungs, the RT-PCR produces negative results, indicating that the material tested does not contain the virus. The lungs are the organs that are mostly affected by COVID-19. In such cases, chest X-ray, ultrasound, MRI, CT, and lung biopsy of the infected person using a needle are very helpful to determine the severity of the disease in the body. Compared with CT, chest X-rays are used to diagnose COVID-19, because CT takes a long time to image, is expensive, is limited in underdeveloped

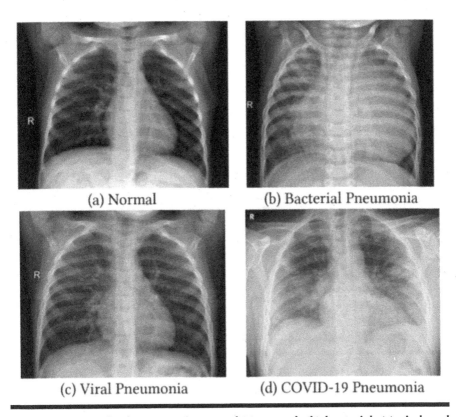

(a) Normal   (b) Bacterial Pneumonia

(c) Viral Pneumonia   (d) COVID-19 Pneumonia

Figure 5.1 **Sample chest X-ray images of (a) normal, (b) bacterial, (c) viral, and (d) COVID-19 pneumonia-affected patients, respectively**

Source: www.medrxiv.org/content/10.1101/2020.12.14.20248158v1.full.pdf

countries, and has severe health problems owing to high radiation. Figure 5.1 shows a sample of what the X-ray of : (a) normal; (b) bacterial pneumonia; (c) viral pneumonia; and (d) COVID-19 Pneumonia look like. X-ray images of four different persons are shown in a 2 × 2 square grid. Top left X-ray is of a normal person without any illness. In a normal X-ray, the lungs are blackish showing permanent markings of ribs, heart, and vascular shadows. The top right X-ray belongs to a person with bacterial pneumonia. Bacterial pneumonia X-ray shows diffused area of a whitish patch occupying considerable areas of lung fields, usually with well-defined margins. The bottom left X-ray belongs to a person with viral pneumonia. Viral pneumonia X-ray findings are small areas of white patchy segments all over the lung fields. The bottom right X-ray belongs to a person with COVID-19 pneumonia. COVID-19 pneumonia X-ray shows small areas of whitish patchy segments close to the ribcage, mostly in peripheral locations.

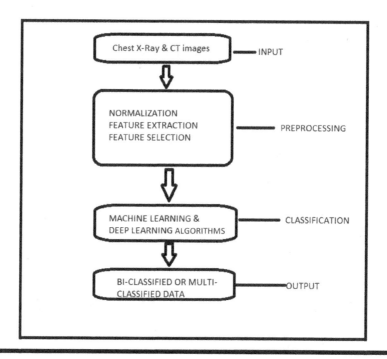

Figure 5.2   Flowchart for diagnosing COVID-19 using X-ray or CT images

Figure 5.2 shows the various stages that are involved when analyzing the CT or X-ray images. The output and the measuring metrics vary depending on the different techniques used in the intermediary stages. The flowchart shows the sequence of steps to be followed when diagnosing COVID-19 from X-ray or CT images. The chest X-ray or the CT image of the patient to be diagnosed will be given as input in the first step. With the given input X-ray/ CT image various preprocessing techniques like normalization, feature extraction, and feature selection will be applied based on the quality of the input. In the next stage, the preprocessed input will be fed to the ML or the DL algorithm based on the architecture chosen for classification. In the final step, the output will be obtained from the algorithm that can be either binary classified data or multiclassified data.

Various researchers have provided different frameworks or models to efficiently analyze the chest X-ray/CT for the detection of COVID-19. Mohammad-Rahimi et al. (2021) reviewed the work by various researchers for the diagnosis of COVID-19 from X-ray and CT image datasets using various ML and DL algorithms. The researchers concluded that among the ML algorithms support vector machine and random forest (RF) were widely used and among the DL algorithms, and CNN, LSTM, GAN, and RNNs were the popular ones.

Researchers (Nayak et al., 2021) evaluated eight CNN models for chest X-rays. Those include AlexNet, VGG-16, GoogleNet, MobileNet-V2, SqueezeNet,

ResNet-34, ResNet 50, and Inception V3. The researchers used the concept of transfer learning. A model that was trained for one activity was repurposed for a second task that is linked to t is called transfer learning. Transfer learning is used in cases where there are fewer data and the learning time is reduced as it is a pretrained model. Only the last layer or a few layers need to be trained. A binary classification has been carried out on the datasets from GitHub and a modified one from GitHub. In the preprocessing stage, the data is normalized in the range of zero and one and then augmented to get larger and variable data. The last layer is replaced with a fully connected layer with output for two classes. Among the others, ResNet-34 outscored the others, and the Adam optimizer outperformed the others in training.

Researchers (Karakanis et al., 2021) used lightweight architecture for binary and multiclassification in chest X-ray images. GAN was used to get synthetic data as the original dataset was limited. Jain et al. (2021) compared DL CNN models, InceptionV3, Xception net, and ResNxt. Augmentation is used to enhance accuracy and prevent overfitting. Instead of the normal Relu activation function, the Leaky Relu activation function was used to accelerate the training and eliminate the issue of dead neurons. Softmax classification is used here to assign decimal probabilities to each class in a multiclass problem. Manjunath Aradhya et al. (2020) used an ensemble of generalized regression neural s (GRNNs) and probabilistic neural networks (PNNs) to perform multiclassification. The GRNN and PNN provided a better generalization. A new concept of a one-shot cluster-based approach was proposed. One-shot learning means learning or classifying from a single or a few examples for each class. Nur-A-Alam et al. (2021) used the concept of feature fusion using DL to detect COVID from chest X-rays. Feature fusion is done by integrating features from different sources to get better feature-rich information. Their proposed model gave better results than the individual feature extraction methods like a histogram-oriented gradient (HOG) and the VGG19 CNN model. The Watershed segmentation technique is useful in spotting the fractured areas, which are very helpful for detecting COVID-19. The limitation of their work was a small data set and imbalanced data was considered.

Saygili. (2021) proposed an approach to detect COVID-19 from X-ray and CT scans claiming that COVID detection can be achieved within a minute using image processing and classical learning methods. The HOG and the local binary patterns methods gave the best results for feature extraction. For selecting features, principal component analysis is employed as it removes correlation between features and reduces overfitting. The data set is trained using classical learning methods, such as K-nearest neighbor (K-NN), support vector machine (SVM), bag of tree (improved decision tree), and kernel-extreme learning machine (K-ELM) where a single hidden layer feeds forward NN with kernels).

Bharati et al. (2021) developed a new DL algorithm on top of conventional ResNet101. The authors applied different augmentation techniques and fine-tuned the hyperparameters, and their model was optimized for COVID-19 detection.

5.4 Contactless Healthcare Services with AI

The outbreak of the COVID-19 pandemic has caused a move to remote working across multiple companies to prevent further transmission of the virus. Distancing oneself from others and washing one's hands regularly have become commonplace. The constant increase in cases has additionally reduced consultations with doctors, particularly for patients who are going through ordinary treatment. These patients should be observed by a specialist for their standard registration. Therefore, this has influenced the entire interaction by preventing the virus. Subsequently, medical services associations have generally received trend-setting innovations to empower contactless monitoring (Wang et al., 2016). Contactless observing frameworks have arisen as a significant advance in medical care conveyance. Joined with most recent advances like AI, ML, and the Internet of Things (IoT), contactless patient observing is assuming a major role in fighting COVID-19. By transitioning to contactless patient health checks as soon as possible and observation frameworks, emergency clinics and medical care associations are moving toward adopting flexible platforms to reshape the global medical care landscape. Due to the need to limit social contact, there has been a major change in the plans of the medical care foundations. Lounge areas in the clinics are being expanded to prevent the spread of the infection. Touchpoints are gradually being phased out in favor of contactless devices. Sensor-based sanitizers and contactless thermometers for standard temperature checks, for example, have been installed in emergency clinics and other strategic locations.

The previous prototype has three major concepts that need to be implemented as part of the proposed contactless healthcare service system (Figure 5.3).

1. Defining the scope of contactless healthcare service. The scope of contactless healthcare services must be measured and defined by the stakeholders of the system. The stakeholders are the representative users and healthcare service providers who may be potential elements in the proposed ecosystem. The limit to which contact must be established should be analyzed with great care. The challenge here is the factors that need to be considered to measure the degree of contactless service might be outside the control of the stakeholder. Technological constraints might hinder the scope of the contactless service. Once the scope is defined, the next stage is to formulate the concerned healthcare problem

2. Healthcare problem formulation. When formulating the healthcare problem, data must be collected. This data might be the risk rates of a patient, the average healing time, and the treatment period for a specific health problem. This data is important because the nature of the data collected decides how fast the contactless service may be delivered as an outcome

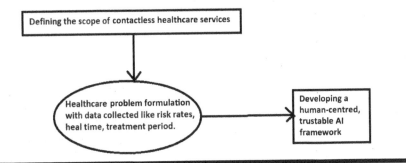

Figure 5.3   Proposed contactless healthcare service system prototype

3. Developing a human-centered, trustable AI framework. A utilitarian trust structure would assist with explaining specialist organizations' and framework designers' obligations and give guidance on what segments can explore IoT-based frameworks in detail. To assure the success of IoT integration, IoT has to be considered as a form of change management. Organization security and information protection and wellbeing will assume a critical part in the overall reception of IoT and related advances. IoT is quite powerless against insurance and protection against threats, because of its uncertainty and variety. IoT-based frameworks need a scalable trust structure to ensure security and control allocation (Strielkina et al., 2018). One other part of the IoT system is that it will help with managing huge volumes of information, and the use of the IoT model guides programming program appropriations. Application engineers should keep their plans basic and guarantee that threats are overseen inside a trust system that has manual configuration options. This trust structure could likewise incorporate inventive segments into the framework, which could be added safely when required, instead of using unrestricted parts of the whole framework (Linn et.al., 2019). Moreover, frameworks could be told to initiate a generally simple reference control when interfacing with different frameworks in the organization's channels for availability purposes. Securing client protection, important frameworks, and sites from the huge scope of threats implies that they should be interconnected IoT PCs. Potential threats, such as IoT botnets can submerge designated sites or organizations with huge traffic, which can expand their transmission capacity ability (Aghili et al., 2019). Designers and suppliers of the IoT-based framework should be creative in guaranteeing that potential security insurance hazards have been appropriately verified. The IoT model will probably require upscaling to such an extent that the demonstration cycle is associated enough with singular segments. This could comprise the normalized names and references, and the standards enabled to part with varying capacities to connect to the proposed framework.

5.5 Future Scope

5.5.1 ML and DL in Drug Design

The main purpose of drug discovery is to cure and treat diseases. The drug discovery process requires the identification of candidates, synthesis, characterization, validation of the chosen candidates, optimizing the validated candidates, screening, and assays for therapeutic efficacy. The major hurdles in drug design and development are time and cost. Nearly 12–15 years are needed to get a drug for a disease to the market requiring an investment of USD 1 billion. By employing various ML and DL algorithms we can reduce the time and cost of discovery and development of drugs for various diseases (e.g., Insilico Medicine designed, synthesized, and validated new drug candidates in 46 days)). The synthesis of peptides, virtual screening based on ligands and structures, single nucleotide polymorphism discoveries, drug repurposing, lead identification, toxicity, prediction of toxicity, drug monitoring and release, pharmacophore modeling, quantitative structure-activity relationship, repositioning of drug, poly pharmacology, and physiochemical activity, can all be implemented using ML and DL algorithms
(Gupta et al., 2021).

Vaccines for COVID 19 are being developed in a handful of countries. As per the statistics of the World Health Organisation up to October 8, 2021, 126 vaccines were in clinical development, and around 194 vaccines were in the preclinical development stage. Some vaccines (i.e., Pfizer) need low-temperature storage, which is not possible when transporting and storing in underdeveloped countries. Furthermore, mass vaccination on a global scale remains a significant barrier. Large-scale vaccine production is the need of the hour to produce the vaccine for the world's population. Also, no one is sure about the efficacy of the vaccines against the new emerging variants. RF, SVM, and recursive feature selection (RFE) are examples of ML algorithms that have been used to identify antigens from protein sequences for COVID-19 vaccines (Arshadi et al., 2020). To find possible SARS-CoV-2 virus T cell epitopes, researchers used supervised neural network-based methods. To find potential vaccination targets, researchers used DL RNN. Natural language processing models are helpful in protein interactions and model–molecular reactions in COVID-19 vaccine discovery. AI can help by identifying the potential elements for the vaccine, which is an important step in vaccine design. However, AI cannot replace or speed up animal and human trials, which are very crucial and time-consuming parts of vaccine development.

Precision medicine is a new concept that is being discussed these days. In precision medicine, in addition to medical reports, the patient's genetic factors, environment, and lifestyle will be considered when recommending a treatment. For that purpose, data from different domains need to be collected, which results in a huge amount of heterogeneous data. Various ML algorithms (MacEachern et al., 2021) have been used with genomics data: (1) the SVM model to identify Type 1 diabetes based on the genome-wide association studies; (2) anticancer drug sensitivity prediction using an SVM classifier based on genetic information; (3) DL algorithms in pharmacogenomics, a relatively new research field, where drug response will be predicted to get personalized drug design; (4) identifying biomarkers for specific diseases; and (5) RF is used for pathway analysis, genetic association, and epistasis detection.

5.5.2 Addressing Security and Privacy Issues with Blockchain

The combination of AI with blockchain creates what is arguably the world's most dependable innovation-enabled dynamic framework, which is fundamentally well-designed and provides solid pieces of knowledge and options. AI gathers information about the world and events that occur because of it through information. The information takes care of AI, and AI wants to improve itself because of it. On the other hand, blockchain is essentially an invention that considers the scrambled storage of information on a disseminated record. It considers the creation of entirely accurate databases that can be examined by parties that have been endorsed to do so. Clinical information is far too sensitive to entrust to a single organization and its computations. Putting this data on a blockchain, which can be accessed by AI with consent, could (after it has gone through the proper procedures) provide us with numerous benefits, such as personalized recommendations when securely storing delicate data.

Thanks to blockchain technology, there are consistent records of the abundance of information, elements, and cycles employed by AIs for their activity cycles. This makes reviewing the entire interactions much easier. All approaches to passing information can be observed with suitable blockchain programming. It creates faith in the aims of AI programs. This is a significant step forward because consumers and businesses will be hesitant to use AI systems if they don't understand how they work or the data they use to make decisions. Information is recorded in a decentralized fashion in blockchain, with each node contributing to the overall ledger. Users (who conduct transactions) and miners (who validate blocks in a distributed ledger) make up the network nodes that make up the peer-to-peer infrastructure (that facilitate the transactions in a distributed ledger).

Medical services partners have distinguished various appealing uses for this profoundly trustworthy information obtained through blockchain, including overseeing claims transactions, checking pharmaceutical inventory chains, and following proficient accreditations or affirmations. Blockchain ties together different associations and establishes a protected climate for significant data trading on collective wellbeing to create AI.

Blockchain could be used as an instrument to deliver metadata on the datasets that are accessible at numerous associations. The metadata for a common blockchain works with the disclosure of data and the ensuing security, and the distributed trade of that data. A lightweight blockchain that records metadata has a gigantic incentive for AI scientists, particularly with regards to handling probably the greatest fault: the accidental bias in the information that can slant the aftereffects of a clinical decision support model or other calculation. Metadata put on blockchain permits us to follow the provenance of information that is used to prepare an AI model. On the off chance that bias creeps into the model eventually, you could look back through the blockchain to perceive what information is causing the bias and change the model as needed. As well as forestalling bias during advancement and preparation, blockchain can help medical services associations approve the aftereffects of AI models as they develop. To date, approval is an arduous cycle. Clinical calculations, for instance, should commonly be approved against information explained by specialists, which can be questionable or difficult to gather at scale. Devices that imply that they offer decision support should be completely confirmed for precision and security before they can be incorporated into the clinical climate, giving motivation to specialists and designers to accelerate the approval process.

5.5 Future Challenges

Fundamentally, blockchain applications in medical care should be secure. Research must concentrate on identification verification. Numerous tests focused on the patient's ability to permit access to patient records in advance; but, in the event of an emergency, what backup plans or emergency protocols can be implemented to provide physicians access to the records without authorization?

Moral issues might likewise be a worry when joining AI and blockchain. Although the characteristics of the partners are private, the public availability of clinical information in a blockchain ledger may not generally be appealing. By and large, clinical information should not be openly accessible; however, maybe the rundown of encoded transactions or squares containing access authorizations to the information could be; then, clinical information would stay with approved workers. Blockchain may likewise be helpless against a purported 51% of threats, a situation wherein a malignant client acquires a larger part of the control. This has been found in the Bitcoin organization, in which four mining pools contributed the most computational force. Although medical care associations would not be viewed as malignant, they may unavoidably contribute to >51% of hacks. Finally, ICT policy experts should think about the exceptionally wide scope of issues on information security, adaptability, information integrity, morals, and computational assets.

The combination of blockchain and AI is a natural fit that has the potential to accelerate advances in personalized cardiovascular medicine by vastly increasing the availability of data for AI development and preparation, sharing exclusive AI calculations for estimation, decentralizing data sets from various sellers or healthcare systems, and enhancing agreements that improve results over time. In any event, such applications are still in their early stages, and there are concerns about their implementation. More research is needed in areas related to trust at the specialized level, regardless of whether competing associations would express a desire for this development of knowledge, repayment, and moral considerations.

Some questions that arise when AI demonstrates its impact in various fields are (Gandhi, 2018).

1. Will AI eventually be a substitute for humans?
2. Will people become increasingly reliant on machines?
3. What should we do if AI becomes uncontrollable and does irrevocable harm to humanity?
4. How can we accept AI if we don't know how it makes its decisions?

Numerous jobs are lost during automation. Losing a job does not only imply losing work and income but also reputation and status. As with every other technology, the impact of AI is tremendous.

Technology's very nature is to be disruptive. Technology creates new ways and opportunities; however, it also replaces established methods and processes, like a two-edged sword. Technology, disruption, and change are strongly intertwined. The same happened with AI. Furthermore, technology cannot be slowed down. It can be monitored, and restricted to a degree based on ethical values, but it will never be banished from the world. When developing AI models, special care should be taken to ensure that, in addition to reaping the benefits of AI, ethical and legal concerns are addressed.

5.6 Conclusions

Regardless of the various advantages given by AI applications in different fields, AI raises a few ethical, lawful, and cultural worries. Even though a large number of the issues are being addressed by AI, a considerable number of concerned moral inquiries are not dealt with. Engineers should plan AI applications so that they are moral, fair, and safe for individuals who are utilizing them. AI-driven algorithms are logically being used to determine the choices that influence our daily lives. Subsequently, if a calculation is wrong, the outcomes could be catastrophic. Huge innovative partnerships have even given rapid alerts to financial backers about the ethical ambiguities around AI. Certain ethical aspects like transparency, justice and fairness, accountability and responsibility, and security and privacy should be taken into consideration when developing AI applications and certain ethical aspects like transparency, justice and fairness, accountability and responsibility, security and privacy need to be focused on when AI is applied in design. The transparent AI concept must be included in a trustable AI framework; therefore, medical personnel and patients can involve themselves in this type of system. Unbiased AI models must be embedded in the core of all operations that take place in the healthcare environment. The design of chatbots for healthcare should not jeopardize the security and privacy of patients and care should be taken by the chatbot designers so that the conversational agents do not transmit any negative messages. The AI models that are used in healthcare should be accountable and responsible for any unintended incident that endangers the patient's life. In our opinion, by 2030, AI applications will be able to access multiple data sources to predict patterns in disease and help in the treatment of patients. Healthcare systems could easily gauge an individual's risk from certain diseases and suggest preventive measures. The waiting times for patients will reduce significantly; therefore, improving the efficiency of healthcare institutions.

References

Aghili, S. F., Mala, H., Shojafar, M., & Peris-Lopez, P. (2019). Laco: Lightweight three-factor authentication, access control, and ownership transfer scheme for e-health systems in iot. *Future Generation Computer Systems, 96,* 410–424.

Arshadi, A. K., Webb, J., Salem, M., Cruz, E., Calad-Thomson, S., Ghadirian, N., & Collins J. (2020) Artificial intelligence for COVID-19 drug discovery and vaccine development. *Frontiers in Artificial Intelligence, 18.* doi:10.3389/frai.2020.00065

Bharati, S., Podder, P., Mondal, M. R. H., & Prasath, V. B. S. (2021). CO-ResNet: Optimized ResNet model for COVID-19 diagnosis from X-ray images. *International Journal of Hybrid Intelligent Systems, 17,* 71–85. doi:10.3233/his-210008

Gupta, R., Srivastava, D., Sahu, M., Tiwari, S., Ambasta R. K., & Kumar, P. (2021). Artificial intelligence to deep learning: machine intelligence approach for drug discovery. *Molecular Diversity.* doi:10.1007/s11030-021-10217-3

Jain, R., Gupta, M., Taneja, S., & Hemanth, D. J. (2021). Deep learning based detection and analysis of C0vid-19 on chest X-ray images. *Applied Intelligence,* 51:1690-1700. doi:10.1007/s10489-020-01902-1.

Karakanis, S., & Leontidis, G. (2021). Lightweight deep learning models for detecting COVID-19 from chest X-ray images. *Computers in Biology and Medicine, 130,* 104181. doi:10.1016/j.compbiomed.2020.104181

Leslie, D. (2019). Understanding artificial intelligence ethics and safety: A guide for the responsible design and implementation of AI systems in the public sector. *The Alan Turing Institute.* doi:10.5281/zenodo.3240529.

MacEachern, S. J., & Forkert, N. D. (2021). Machine learning for precision medicine. *Genome, 64*(4), doi: 10.1139/gen-2020-0131

Manjunath Aradhya, V. N., Mufti Mahmud, D. S. Guru, B. A., & Shamim Kaiser, M. (2020) . One-shot cluster-based approach for the detection of COVID-19 from chest X-ray images. *Cognitive Computation.* doi:10.007/s12559-020-09774-w

Mohammad-Rahimi, H., Nadimi, M., Ghalyanchi-Langeroudi, A., Taheri, M., & Ghafouri-Fard, S. (2021). Application of machine learning in diagnosis of COVID-19 through X-ray and CT images: A scoping review. *Frontiers in Cardiovascular Medicine.* doi:10.3389/fcvm.2021.638011

Nayak, S. R., Nayak, D. R., Sinha, U., Arora, V., & Pachori, R. B. (2021). Applications of deep learning techniques for the detection of COVID-19 cases using chest x-rays: A comprehensive study. *BioMedical Signal Processing and Control,* 64. doi:10.1016/j.bspc.2020.102365

Nur-A-Alam, M. Ahsan, M. D., Based, A., Haider, J., & Kowalski, M. (2021). COVID-19 detection from chest X-ray images using feature fusion and deep learning. *Sensors,* 21(4) 1480. doi:10.3390/s21041480

Saygili, A. (2021). A new approach for computer-aided detection of coronavirus (COVID-19) from CT and X-ray images using machine learning methods. *Applied Soft Computing,* 105. doi: 10.1016/j.asoc.2021.107323

Statista. (2021) Number of coronavirus (COVID-19) cases worldwide as of July 30, 2021, by country. www.statista.com/statistics/1043366/novel-coronavirus-2019ncov-cases-worldwide-by-country/

Strielkina, A., Kharchenko, V., & Uzun, D. (2018). Availability models for healthcare iot systems: Classification and research considering attacks on vulnerabilities, in: 9th International Conference on Dependable Systems, Services and Technologies (DESSERT), IEEE, Kyiv, Ukraine. pp. 58–62.

Wang, H., Li, K., Ota, K., & Shen J. (2016). Remote data integrity checking and sharing in cloud-based health internet of things. *IEICE Transactions on information and systems* 99(8) (2016), 1966–1973.

Chapter 6

Patient Recovery and Tracing Repercussions for COVID-19 in Discharged Patients

B. Patel, K. Patel, M. Bohara, and A. Ganatra
Computer Science and Engineering, Devang Patel Institute of
Advance Technology and Research, CHARUSAT, India

D. Patel
Computer Engineering, Chandubhai S. Patel Institute of Technology,
CHARUSAT, India

Contents

DOI: 10.1201/9781003324447-6

6.1 Introduction: Patient Recovery and Tracing Repercussions of Coronavirus in Discharged Patients

Many countries have been forced to implement austere lockdown policies due to the coronavirus COVID-2019 (COVID-19), a pandemic which has slowed down the infection rate in many European countries, which includes many countries such as Japan, China, Singapore, Italy, Hong Kong, and Spain. Given the lack of immunisation, most of these restrictions will certainly be extended in the coming months, particularly for youngsters and the elderly; however, it is too early to say for how long.

In this environment, many countries are witnessing extraordinary changes in social habits and medical (Garrigues et al. 2020) attention for individuals of all ages, and youngsters. School, athletics, and other social activities are being disrupted, pushing youngsters to spend the majority of their time at home, in direct contact with their (often inactive) family. Furthermore, the lockdown has had a direct impact on lowering the activity in non-COVID intensive care units (ICUs) and hospital department wards, as a result of personnel changes in COVID units and widespread germaphobia (dread of germs and illnesses, as an outcome of hospitalisation). Many COVID units (including COVID-paediatric units) have been quickly formed in most hospitals, and operations in other units have focused on patients (Garrigues, et al 2020) with severe and acute issues, care, and assistance for patients (Garrigues, et al. 2020) with chronic or (Garrigues et al. 2020) unusual diseases has been limited. Apart from that, this motionless revolution is having several drawbacks for healthcare staff and patients, with unquantifiable effects, as well as certain opportunities that will be unique and impossible to replicate once the emergency has passed.

Even though the vast majority of COVID-19 (Carretta, et al. 2021) patients get better weeks after getting ill, some people experience post-COVID (Carretta, et al. 2021) indications. Citizens might acquire a large number of new, returning, or persistent medical issues, which are known as post-COVID diseases, ≥4 weeks after being affected by the disease-causing virus COVID-19 (Truffaut, 2021). It can take days or weeks for a person who does not present with any COVID-19 symptoms, following their infection to develop post-COVID complications. At various times, these disorders can cause various types and combinations of health problems.

Long COVID, long-haul COVID, post-acute COVID-19 (Truffaut, 2021), long-term COVID effects, and chronic COVID are all terms used to describe these post-COVID problems. The Center for Disease Control and Prevention (CDC) and (Hall, 2021) specialists from around the world (Hall, 2021) are seeking to understand more about COVID-19's short- and long-term health impacts, as well as who gets them and why.

The following are the issues considered in this chapter.

1. COVID-related symptoms and post-COVID requirements
2. Impact of the coronavirus on multiple organs
3. The coronavirus has the greatest impact on several organs
4. The risk of post-COVID problems and long-term coronavirus impacts
5. The steps to take after recovering from COVID, and the need for self-observation after COVID-19 recovery

6.2 Post-COVID Conditions: What Are They?

A virus is one of the factors that caused COVID-19, which infects people (Munnangi, et al.2021) and is transmitted from person to person, some people deal with a wide variety of new or severe symptoms that can remain for some weeks or months. The patient has mild or no symptoms (Mondal, Bharati, & Podder, 2020) at all, and everyone who has had COVID-19 potentially develops these symptoms, unlike certain other post-COVID difficulties that primarily affect people who have had a severe illness. Figure 6.1 shows the patients' health conditions after coronavirus. Different combinations of the following symptoms are regularly reported by people (Table 6.1).

Coronavirus 2 (SARS-CoV-2) can induce significant inflammation, which can stimulate an immune system's response to injury by increasing the activity of the blood clotting system. The lungs, kidneys, liver, heart, and legs are among the organs affected by blood clots (Spruit, 2020). COVID-19 can also weaken (Spruit, 2020) and cause leaky blood vessels, potentially leading to long-term liver and kidney problems (Spruit, 2020). Many COVID-19 survivors are at risk of getting chronic fatigue syndrome (Xing, 2020), extreme tiredness that worsens with physical or mental exertion but does not improve with rest and is a chronic condition (Xing, 2020).

Although it is impossible to foresee the long-term effects of coronavirus (Bharati & Podder, 2021a), experts are still trying to figure out why patients' symptoms persist for so long after they have recovered.

6.2.1 COVID-19's Multiorgan Impact

Multiorgan effects or autoimmune illnesses can emerge in people who have had a severe COVID-19 infection over time, with symptoms lasting weeks or months. Most, if not all, body systems (Carretta, et al .2021), involving the heart, brain, kidneys, skin, and lungs, can (Carretta, et al. 2021) be affected by multiorgan effects. When the immune system targets the body's healthy cells, it causes inflammation (painful swelling) and tissue damage in the affected areas, resulting in autoimmune illnesses.

It is extremely uncommon, for some people, especially children, to develop multisystem inflammatory syndrome (MIS) during or shortly after contracting COVID-19. Different body parts can become inflamed as a result of MIS. If a person continues to have multiorgan effects or other symptoms, MIS can progress to post-COVID problems.

6.2.1.1 COVID-19 Organ Damage over Time (Multiorgan Dysfunction)

Severe acute respiratory distress syndrome is a severe form of acute respiratory distress in which infection by SARS-CoV-2 produces long-term immune system changes,

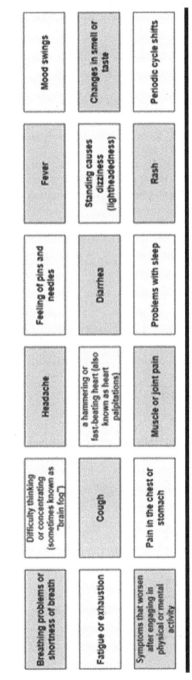

Figure 6.1 Post-COVID related symptoms: The patients' health condition after coronavirus

Table 6.1   Significant Criteria of Post-COVID

Criteria
Body and joint pain or headache
High blood sugar (hyperglycemia)
Fever
Fatigue, feeling of tiredness, or lack of energy
Loss of taste or smell
Breathing problems or shortness of breath
Coughing or chest pain
New-onset diabetes
Myalgia (muscle pain) for a long period
Inability to focus or difficulty thinking or a lack of mental clarity (brain fog)
Rapid or fast heartbeat (heart palpitations)
Red bumps or rash on a flat, red patch of skin (maculopapular rash)
Symptoms that worsen after exercising
Insomnia, anxiety disorder, or depression
Dizziness or light-headedness when you stand up from sitting or lying down (orthostatic hypotension)

Table 6.2   Post-Acute COVID-19 Syndrome is Characterised as When Patients Who Have Been Infected with COVID-19 and Have Recovered May Face the Following Severe Problems in Addition to Other Post-COVID Symptoms

Problems and post-COVID 19 Symptoms
MI: chest discomfort with or without dyspnoea, nausea, and diaphoresis
Chronic fatigue syndrome
Deep vein thrombosis is a blood clot in a deep vein
Neurological symptoms: seizures, stroke, muscle weakness, tingling, or numbness in the hands and feet
GI symptoms include a lack of weight, nausea, puking, diarrhoea, and intestinal pain or discomfort are all symptoms to look out for.
Pancreatitis
Haemothorax: a blood clot that forms between the chest wall and the lung.
Pneumothorax: when air seeps into the gap between the lungs and the chest wall
Pulmonary fibrosis: progressive lung fibrosis due to respiratory infections
Arthritis: swelling and tenderness in one or more of your joints
Fungal infections like mucormycosis, aspergillosis, yellow fungus, and many more

Table 6.3   COVID-19 Mostly Affects the Following Organs and Body Components

Number	Human Organ	How They Are Affected
1	Lungs	The tiny branches of air passages in the lungs (alveoli), which exchange oxygen and carbon dioxide between the lungs and the blood when breathing in and out, might be disrupted for a long time by COVID-19-induced pneumonia (Balbiab, 2021). Long-term respiratory difficulties can be caused by scar tissue in the lungs
2	Heart	Even though they only experienced minor symptoms, COVID-19 patients who recovered had irreversible tissue loss of the heart muscle. In the future, this could increase the risk of MI, heart failure, and other life-threatening heart disorders
3	Brain	COVID-19 has been related to neurological symptoms in many young people, including muscle weakness, tingling, or numbness in their hands and feet, which can develop into paralysis (Guillain-Barré syndrome), dizziness, abrupt blackout, confusion, delirium, seizures, and stroke. COVID-19 has also been connected to Alzheimer's and Parkinson's disease (Bharati, 2020)
4	Kidneys	Acute kidney injury can occur in COVID-19 patients who have a sudden decrease in renal function. Dialysis may be required in extreme cases; however, this type of kidney impairment can sometimes be reversed. After recovering from COVID-19, people with chronic kidney disease(CKD)are more prone to experience severe symptoms. As a result, taking all necessary precautions to avoid infection is crucial

primarily in the lungs. Multiple organs, including the lungs, brain (Bozkurt, 2021), blood vessels, skin, nerves, kidneys, and heart, may be injured as a result of long-term COVID-19 infection. Metabolic, musculoskeletal, cardiovascular, and neurological problems are all possible side effects of the condition. Long-term health difficulties may be exacerbated by organ damage. Post-acute COVID-19 Syndrome is shown in Table 6.2. Patients who have been infected with COVID-19 and have since recovered may experience the following severe problems in addition to other post-COVID symptoms. Table 6.3 shows the organs and parts of the body that are most often affected.

6.2.1.2 Clots in the Blood and Difficulties with the Blood Vessels

COVID-19 has the potential to cause blood cells to clump together and coagulate blood cells. Heart attacks and strokes can be caused by big clots (Weerahandi, 2021), COVID-19 is considered to cause the majority of heart damage by forming minute clots that constrict microscopic blood arteries (capillaries) in the heart muscle (Mondal, 2021). Blood clots can harm the lungs, legs, liver, and kidneys (Xing, 2020), as well as other organs. COVID-19 weakens and causes leaky blood vessels, which can lead to long-term liver and renal problems.

6.2.2.3 Problems with Mood Changes and Exhaustion

COVID-19 patients with severe symptoms are frequently treated in the critical care unit of a hospital, requiring artificial breathing assistance, such as ventilators. Surviving this catastrophe can put a person at risk of acquiring post-traumatic stress disorder (PTSD), depression, or anxiousness in the future. Because the long-term consequences of (Paul, 2021) COVID-19 are (Xing, 2020) tough to anticipate, researchers are examining the long-term effects of related viruses, and viruses that cause severe acute respiratory syndrome (SARS) are included (Xing, 2020).

Many people who have been cured of SARS have developed chronic fatigue syndrome, which is characterised by excessive exhaustion that worsens with physical or mental exertion but does not (Xing, 2020) improve with rest. COVID-19 sufferers are probably the same.

6.2.1.4 COVID-19 has Several Long-Term Consequences That Are Still Unclear

Much remains unknown regarding COVID-19's long-term consequences (Anaya, 2021), but research is ongoing. Doctors should see patients frequently and monitor individuals who have undergone COVID-19 to evaluate how their organs work once they have recovered, according to researchers.

Many prestigious medical institutes are establishing specific clinics to treat people who have persistent symptoms or illnesses after recovering from COVID-19. A variety of additional support groups are available.

It's important to remember that most COVID-19 (Balbiab, 2021) patients recover quickly (Balbiab, 2021). However, due to COVID-19's long-term implications, it is vital to take precautions to prevent COVID-19 from spreading (Weerahandi, 2021). Masks should be worn, social distancing should be maintained, crowds should be avoided, vaccines should be obtained when possible, and hands should be kept clean.

6.2.1.5 Inability to Tolerate Physical Activity

This is primarily a result of the coronavirus infection and decreased physical mobility. This could be due to the virus's impact or harm to the lungs, heart, blood vessels, or muscle alterations.

6.2.1.6 Complications in the Lungs or Respiratory System

Lung diseases are the most common long-term consequence of COVID-19 (Garg, 2021). Aside from minor issues like shortness of breath, colds, and coughs (Kothadiya, 2021) the vast majority of COVID-19 patients fully recover. However, a small percentage of patients suffer from severe lung injuries, and some acquire pulmonary fibrosis. Patients may also experience symptoms similar to asthma as a result of post-viral bronchial hyperresponsiveness. Bacterial, fungal (mucormycosis, aspergillosis), and tuberculosis (TB) secondary infections are common.

6.2.1.7 Cardiac Complications

Recent research has connected patients with coronavirus COVID-19 to an increased risk of heart failure. This has been linked to dysrhythmias (Mondal, 2021a), acute coronary syndrome, prolonged hypotension, acute myocardial infarction (MI) (stroke), and infective myocarditis.

6.2.1.8 Injury to Cardiac Muscle

After several days or weeks of recuperation, heart damage or cardiac muscle injury can occur. COVID-19 infections can induce inflammation in numerous areas of the body, which can weaken the heart muscle and produce irregular cardiac rhythms, in addition to the risk of blood clots forming in blood vessels. Myocarditis (Bharati, 2021b), or cardiac inflammation, occurs when the heart fails to efficiently pump blood, narrowing the arteries, causing high blood pressure, and putting the patient at risk of a heart attack.

6.2.1.9 Complications of Renal Injury or Failure

Even in patients who didn't have kidney problems before COVID-19. High levels of protein in the urine could be considered the primary sign of kidney problems (Podder, 2021). COVID-19 patients who are hypertensive or diabetic have an increased risk of kidney complications after infection. Some difficulties may necessitate the use of dialysis. By removing excess water, poisons, and waste products from the body, the kidneys act as filters for the body. As a result, their proper operation is critical. Blood clots can block the kidneys' tiny blood veins, causing damage.

6.2.1.10 Diabetes

Even though it is a common condition, diabetes is considered a complication of COVID. It's a long-term condition in which blood glucose or sugar levels become dangerously high. Insulin, a pancreatic hormone, aids glucose entry into cells. However, when the body does not produce enough insulin, glucose remains in the bloodstream, creating a variety of health problems.

6.2.1.11 Brain Disease: Acute Necrotising Encephalopathy

Acute necrotising encephalopathy (ANE) is an immune-mediated disease that is caused by mycoplasma, influenza A, or the herpes simplex virus infection (Abdullah, 2020). However, it has recently been described in post-COVID patients, and it is rarely encountered in youngsters. Neurological symptoms and post-COVID difficulties are typical because ACE receptors are located in arterial smooth and glial cells in the brain (Podder, 2021), and the coronavirus interacts with them. A cribriform plate of ethmoid bone or hematogenous (Bohara, 2021) dispersion would be the method of entry into the central nervous system (CNS).

COVID 19 in combination with a cytokine storm causes immune-mediated harm with a preference for the CNS, and the specific pathogenesis is unknown. ANE in children manifests as focal seizures, hemiparesis, agitation, and shifting awareness. Multisystem inflammatory system in children (MIS-C) causes seizures, restlessness, and food intolerance, as well as hypotension and shortness of breath. Because they are immune-mediated as well as originate from post-COVID issues, they are frequently misunderstood.

Hyperintensities FLAIR and T2 can be seen in the cerebellum, internal capsule, basal ganglia, thalamus, and, on rare occasions, the occipital and parietal lobes in ANE. Fever, rash, breathing trouble, hypotension, vomiting, and coagulation problems are among the symptoms of MIS-C. It arises as a result of a sustained increase in immunoglobulin G (IgG), which activates monocytes and causes T lymphocytes to become more activated. Children have a high prevalence of ANE. In the paediatric population, multiple cases of MIS-C have been reported. These consequences tend to be equated with a direct attack on the CNS because COVID-19 is a pro-inflammatory condition. Another possibility is viral infiltration directly. ANE is a condition that can be fatal. It requires rapid ICU admission, magnetic resonance imaging to check for brain abnormalities, to check for subclinical seizures an electroencephalogram is used, and to rule out a CNS infection a cerebrospinal fluid investigation can be used.

6.2.1.12 Complications in the Vascular System

COVID-19 is a virus that induces pro-inflammatory and prothrombotic states that led to macrovascular and micro thrombosis, as well as venous thrombotic and arterial events. Macrovascular thrombotic events, such as venous thromboembolism, cardiac injury or infarction, and stroke, affected one-third of patients (Liu, 2021) who were hospitalised due to extreme COVID-19 (Liu, 2021). Common consequences include acute limb ischaemia or gangrene, acute pulmonary thromboembolism, mesenteric ischaemia, and deep vein thrombosis.

6.2.1.13 Complications with Psychiatric Illness

Anxiety, despair, insomnia, inability to concentrate, anhedonia, and suicidal ideation have all been documented.

6.2.1.14 Depression and Anxiety

As a result of the pandemic's stress and combatting the disease, these might be noticed in patients. COVID-19 isn't only a respiratory infection; it has a significant impact on a person's mental health.

6.2.1.15 Insomnia

This is a sleep condition that affects the CNS and disturbs a person's sleeping cycle, causing them to recover more slowly. Anxiety, stress, and loneliness are some of the elements that might cause this. This is especially true for patients who are isolated or hospitalised for weeks, making insomnia a post-COVID consequence.

The pandemic's unpredictability has become a part of our daily lives, and the list of challenges increases by the day. It is best to avoid infection by taking the appropriate procedures to reduce complications.

6.2.1.16 Complications in Other Organs

Acute liver failure can lead to gangrene and acute bowel ischaemia, as well as gastrointestinal (GI) complications like gangrene. Petechial rash, dissecting hematomas, haemorrhagic bullae with intra-bullae blood clots, and isolated herpetiform lesions are all skin issues.

6.2.1.17 Adult MIS and MIS-C

MIS is an uncommon but deadly illness caused by COVID-19 in which numerous bodily components are affected, and inflammation occurs in different organs, such as the brain, heart, lungs, eyes, kidneys, skin, and GI organs (Truffaut, 2021). MIS can (Truffaut, 2021) affect youngsters (MIS-C) and adults (MIS-A) (Hall, 2021). MIS-C case definition includes people <21 years old, whereas the MIS-A case definition (Hall, 2021) includes those >21 years old. Figure 6.2 shows the available signs of MIS-C and MIS-A that are present in kids and adults.

Currently, the best method to avoid contracting MIS-C or MIS-A is to protect yourself from COVID-19, which includes the COVID-19 vaccine for those aged ≥12 years old.

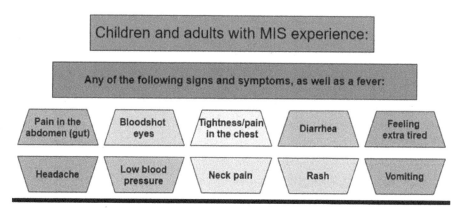

Figure 6.2 Signs that are available in children and adults

6.2.2 COVID-19 Illness or Hospitalisation Effects

During the recovery phase, for lung-related diseases, such as COVID-19, hospitalisations and severe illnesses are common, and can cause extreme weakness and weariness.

Another result of hospitalisation is post-intensive care syndrome (PICS), which describes the health effects that begin when a patient is in the ICU and may persist after they return home. The side effects include severe weakness, difficulty with thinking and judgement, and PTSD. Long-term reactions to a traumatic event cause PTSD.

Some of the symptoms that people with mild or no symptoms may experience many weeks after receiving COVID-19 are very similar to the symptoms that people with mild or no symptoms may experience. It's difficult to say whether they're caused by hospitalisation, the virus's long-term consequences, or a mix of both. Other impacts of the COVID-19 pandemic (Holmes, et al. 2020) such as mental health (Holmes, et al. 2020) the effects of isolation, unfavourable economic situations, and a lack of access to treatment for managing underlying problems, may exacerbate these conditions. People that have had COVID-19 and those who have not might have been affected by these circumstances.

PICS, which refers to health (Xing, 2020) consequences that persist after a critical illness, can be a side effect of COVID-19 treatment and hospitalisation. Severe weakness and PTSD (Garrigues et al. 2020) are examples of these side effects. Immunosuppressive medications can cause fulminant secondary infections and opportunistic infections in people with PTSD. Long-term use of steroids (Werthman-Ehrenreich, 2021) might cause hyperglycaemia and subsequent infections.

6.2.3 Long-Term Effects of Coronavirus after Recovery, Post-COVID Complications

People infected with COVID-19 may have moderate symptoms or be completely asymptomatic, according to current research. The duration of the coronavirus infection in the body varies from person to person, as does the virus's exposure and intensity of infection. According to the World Health Organisation, patients will recover totally after an initial infection of 10–4 days, and sometimes more. COVID-19 cases that are mild to moderate will heal in about 14 days. COVID-19 symptoms might last anywhere from 20–45 days in some cases. Patients may develop post-COVID problems as a result of the coronavirus's long-term effects.

SARS caused by COVID-19 (SARS-CoV-2) (Abdullah, 2020) can harm the lungs, brain, blood vessels, skin, nerves, kidneys, and heart, and increases the risk of long-term health problems. The virus; however, can stay in the body for ≤ 3 months following diagnosis. This could result in some people receiving a second positive test result after they have recovered, although this does not necessarily mean the virus is still contagious (Mondal, 2021b).

6.2.3.1 What is Long COVID Syndrome or Post-COVID Syndrome?

The majority of patients infected with COVID-19 get better within 10 days of becoming ill. People who continue to experience mild symptoms after recovery, which is referred to as post-COVID Syndrome (Anaya, 2021) or long COVID, may develop post-COVID problems as well as long-term organ concerns. Post-COVID effects are a wide range of new, ongoing, or returning health disorders that individuals might get after being infected with the coronavirus for >28 days (4 weeks).

Even those who were asymptomatic when infected could have the complication of post-COVID-19. Due to this, different types of health problems occur.

6.2.3.2 Who are at Risk of Post-COVID Problems, as well as Long-term Coronavirus Effects?

People in their eighties and nineties, as well as those with major medical illnesses, such as diabetes, immunodeficiency disorders, malignancies, or chronic diseases, are at risk of experiencing post-COVID. According to new evidence, even if a young individual recovers from COVID-19 feeling healthy, the virus can have long-term impacts, with symptoms lasting weeks to months after infection. Figure 6.3 shows the causes of post-COVID post-syndrome or long-term COVID.

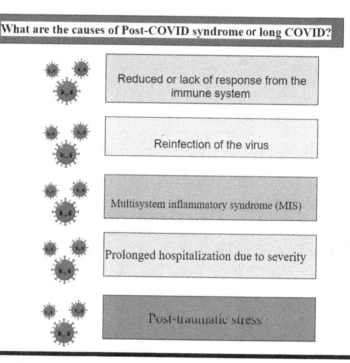

Figure 6.3 Causes of post-COVID: According to new evidence, even if a young individual recovers from COVID-19 feeling healthy, the virus can have long-term impacts, with symptoms lasting weeks to months after infection

6.3 Diagnosis of Post-COVID Syndrome or Long COVID

If someone develops symptoms after COVID-19, it is not necessary to double-check the positive results. The physician may need the patient's complete medical history and previous COVID-19 treatment to make a diagnosis. A physician may order these tests in addition to evaluating temperature, blood pressure, pulse rate, oxygen saturation (SpO_2) level, and respiratory function to determine the severity of symptoms as shown in Figure 6.4.

6.4 What Measures Should You Take After You've Recovered from COVID?

Because the immune system has been impaired by the virus, it is recommended that people stay hydrated by drinking enough fluids, practice meditation and breathing

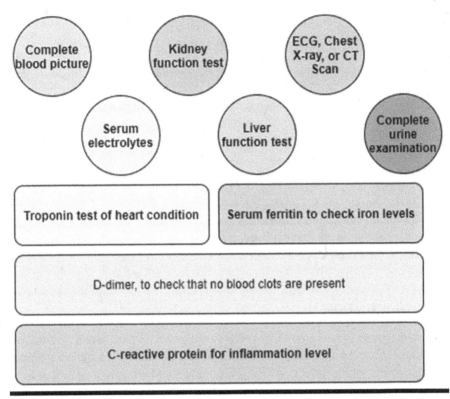

Figure 6.4 Post-COVID syndrome diagnosis: The physician may need the patient's complete medical history and previous COVID-19 treatment to make a diagnosis

exercises, eating healthy foods, getting enough sleep, and avoiding alcohol and smoking.

Those who have recovered from COVID-19 and have comorbidities, such as diabetes, hypertension, cardiovascular, kidney, or liver diseases, or other chronic medical illnesses (Garg, 2021) should return to their pre-COVID medication as soon as possible. After 45 days of recovery, they should be immunised.

Many people who have survived COVID-19 infectious disease are at risk of other long-term health issues. These people must follow-up with their primary care doctors to monitor their organ function once they've recovered.

Specialised medical centres are developing post-COVID care support to assist these folks in overcoming persistent problems. If somebody is experiencing any of the previous symptoms, they should contact their primary care physician or schedule an appointment with their team for treatment and management through mental and physical rehabilitation.

6.5 Importance of Self-Observation after Recovering from COVID-19

For at ≤3–4 months, patients should monitor critical factors, such as blood oxygen level and blood pressure. If they experience a prolonged headache, chest pains, or difficulty breathing, they should see a doctor. It's crucial to keep an eye on symptoms because they could indicate major problems. The appropriate consultation and management could help to avoid unnecessary healthcare costs and lower the chances of death.

People who attempt to push themselves hard and put a strain on their bodies soon after they have recovered from COVID-19, might deplete their bodies and make them worse. Mild, slow-paced workouts should be recommended, with enough time for the body to rebuild its strength. Although long-term COVID-19 can be debilitating, early diagnosis and good care can help people heal faster and relieve the symptoms.

6.6 Conclusions

This chapter provided a study of COVID-19 patients who have tested positive for the coronavirus and produced theoretical analyses on the various small and big health issues. It clearly outlined the post-COVID problems and symptoms, as well as how to take the necessary actions for a quick recovery. Researchers have compiled data on the effects of COVID-19 on people's lungs, hearts, brains, and kidneys. This virus has been shown to attack blood cells and harm the heart. This chapter also portrayed the long-term consequences of COVID-19 and offered a solution to stay healthy through physical activity, yoga, social distancing, and taking some supplements every day to enhance immunity. Initially, older individuals were affected, and then this virus began to attack young people's immunity, and it is now affecting small children. As a result, an age-based study was thoroughly explained in this chapter.

References

Anaya, J. M., Rojas, M., Salinas, M. L., Rodriguez, Y., Roa, G., Lozano, M., ... Zapata. E. (2021). Post-COVID study group. Post-COVID syndrome: A case series and comprehensive review. *Autoimmunity Reviews*, *20*(11). doi.10.1016/j.autrev.2021.102947

Abdullah, M. S., Chong, P. L., Asli, R., Momin, R. N., Mani, B. I., Metussin, D., & Chong, V. H. (2020). Post discharge positive re-tests in COVID-19: common but clinically non-significant. *Infectious Diseases, 52*(10), 743–745.

Balbi, M., Conti, C., Imeri, G., Caroli, A., Surace, A., Corsi, A., ... Sironi, S. (2021). Post-discharge chest CT findings and pulmonary function tests in severe COVID-19 patients. *European Journal of Radiology, 138*, 109676.

Bharati, S., & Mondal, M. R. H. (2021). 12 Applications and challenges of AI-driven IoHT for combating pandemics: a review. *Intelligence for Managing Pandemics, 213*.

· Bharati, S., Podder, P., & Mondal, M. R. H. (2020). Hybrid deep learning for detecting lung diseases from X-ray images. *Informatics in Medicine Unlocked, 20*, 100391.

Bharati, S., Podder, P., Mondal, M., & Prasath, V. B. (2021a). *Medical Imaging with Deep Learning for COVID-19 Diagnosis: A Comprehensive Review.* preprint *arXiv:2107.09602*.

Bharati, S., Podder, P., Mondal, M., & Prasath, V. B. (2021b). CO-ResNet: Optimized ResNet model for COVID-19 diagnosis from X-ray images. *International Journal of Hybrid Intelligent Systems*, 1–15. Manuscript submitted for publication.

Bohara, M., Patel, K., Patel, B., & Desai, J. (2021). An AI based web portal for cotton price analysis and prediction. Paper presented at the proceeding of the 3rd International Conference on Integrated Intelligent Computing Communication & Security (ICIIC 2021) (pp. 33–39). Atlantis Press.

Bozkurt, B., Kamat, I., & Hotez, P. J. (2021). Myocarditis with COVID-19 mRNA vaccines. *Circulation, 144*(6), 471–484.

Carretta, D. M., Silva, A. M., D'Agostino, D., Topi, S., Lovero, R., Charitos, I. A., ... Santacroce, L. (2021). Cardiac involvement in COVID-19 patients: A contemporary review. *Infectious Disease Reports, 13*(2), 494–517.

Erdem, H., & Lucey, D. R. (2021). Healthcare worker infections and deaths due to COVID-19: A survey from 37 nations and a call for WHO to post national data on their website. *International Journal of Infectious Diseases, 102*, 239.

Garg, D., Muthu, V., Sehgal, I. S., Ramachandran, R., Kaur, H., Bhalla, A., ... Agarwal, R. (2021). Coronavirus disease (Covid-19) associated mucormycosis (CAM): Case report and systematic review of literature. *Mycopathologia, 186* (2), 289–298.

Garg, M., Maralakunte, M., Garg, S., Dhooria, S., Sehgal, I., Bhalla, A. S., ... Sandhu, M. S. (2021). The conundrum of 'Long-COVID-19': A narrative rreview. *International Journal of General Medicine, 14*, 2491.

Garrigues, E., Janvier, P., Kherabi, Y., Le Bot, A., Hamon, A., Gouze, H., ...Nguyen, Y. (2020). Post-discharge persistent symptoms and health-related quality of life after hospitalization for COVID-19. *Journal of Infection, 81*(6), e4–e6.

Hall, J., Myall, K., Lam, J. L., Mason, T., Mukherjee, B., West, A., & Dewar, A. (2021). Identifying patients at risk of post-discharge complications related to COVID-19 infection. *Thorax, 76*(4), 408–411.

Heneka, M. T., Golenbock, D., Latz, E., Morgan, D., & Brown, R. (2020). Immediate and long-term consequences of COVID-19 infections for the development of neurological disease. *Alzheimer's Research & Therapy, 12*(1), 1–3.

Holmes, E. A., O'Connor, R. C., Perry, V. H., Tracey, I., Wessely, S., Arseneault, L., ... Bullmore, E. (2020). Multidisciplinary research priorities for the COVID-19 pandemic: a call for action for mental health science. *The Lancet Psychiatry*, 7(6), 547–560.

Iqbal, F. M., Lam, K., Sounderajah, V., Clarke, J. M., Ashrafian, H., & Darzi, A. (2021). Characteristics and predictors of acute and chronic post-COVID syndrome: A systematic review and meta-analysis. *EClinicalMedicine, 36*, 100899.

Kothadiya D., Chaudhari A., Macwan R., Patel K., Bhatt C. (2021). The convergence of deep learning and computer vision: Smart city applications and research Challenges. Paper presented at the Proceedings of the 3rd International Conference on Integrated Intelligent Computing Communication & Security (ICIIC 2021). Atlantis Press (pp. 14–22)

Liu, F., Cai, Z. B., Huang, J. S., Niu, H. Y., Yu, W. Y., Zhang, Y., … Xu, A. F. (2021). Repeated COVID-19 relapse during post-discharge surveillance with viral shedding lasting for 67 days in a recovered patient infected with SARS-CoV-2. *Journal of Microbiology, Immunology and Infection, 54*(1), 101–104.

Mondal, M. R. H., Bharati, S., & Podder, P. (2020). Data analytics for novel coronavirus disease. *Informatics in Medicine Unlocked, 20*, 100374.

Mondal, M. R. H., Bharati, S., & Podder, P. (2021a). Diagnosis of COVID-19 using machine learning and deep learning: A review. *Current Medical Imaging, 17*(12), 1403–1418

Mondal, M. R. H., Bharati, S., & Podder, P. (2021b). CO-IRv2: Optimized InceptionResNetV2 for COVID-19 detection from chest CT images. *PLoS One, 16*(10), e0259179.

Munnangi, A. K., Sekaran, R., Rajeyyagari, S., Ramachandran, M., Kannan, S., & Bharati, S. (2022). Nonlinear Cosine Neighborhood Time Series-Based Deep Learning for the Prediction and Analysis of COVID-19 in India. *Wireless Communications and Mobile Computing.*

Paul, P., Bharati S. Podder, P., & Mondal, M. R. H. (2021). 10 The role of IoMT during pandemics. In A. Khamparia, R. Hossain Mondal, P., Podder, B. Bushan, V. Albuquerque, & S. Kumar (Eds.) *Computational Intelligence for Managing Pandemics.* Berlin, Boston: De Gruyter.

Podder, P., Bharati, S., Mondal, M. R. H., & Kose, U. (2021). Application of machine learning for the diagnosis of COVID-19. *Data Science for COVID-19,* 175-194). doi. org/10.1016/B978-0-12-824536-1.00008-3

Podder, P., Khamparia, A., Mondal, M. R. H., Rahman, M. A., & Bharati, S. (2021). Forecasting the Spread of COVID-19 and ICU Requirements. *International Journal of Online and Biomedical Engineering, 17*(5), 81–99.

Praticò, A. D. (2021). COVID-19 pandemic for Pediatric Health Care: Disadvantages and opportunities. *Pediatric Research, 89*(4), 709–710.

Singh, S., Kaur, R., & Singh, R. K. (2020). Revisiting the role of vitamin D levels in the prevention of COVID-19 infection and mortality in European countries post infections peak. *Aging Clinical and Experimental Research, 32*(8), 1609–1612.

Shi, Y., Wang, Y., Shao, C., Huang, J., Gan, J., Huang, X., … Melino, G. (2020). COVID-19 infection: the perspectives on immune responses. *Cell Death & Differentiation, 27*(5), 1451–1454.

Spruit, M. A., Holland, A. E., Singh, S. J., Tonia, T., Wilson, K. C., & Troosters, T. (2020). COVID-19: interim guidance on rehabilitation in the hospital and post-hospital phase from a European Respiratory Society-and American Thoracic Society-coordinated international task force. *European Respiratory Journal, 56*(6).

Truffaut, L., Demey, L., Bruyneel, A. V., Roman, A., Alard, S., De Vos, N., & Bruyneel, M. (2021). Post-discharge critical COVID-19 lung function related to severity of radiologic lung involvement at admission. *Respiratory Research, 22*(1), 1–6.

von Meijenfeldt, F. A., Havervall, S., Adelmeijer, J., Lundström, A., Magnusson, M., Mackman, N., … Lisman, T. (2021). Sustained prothrombotic changes in COVID-19 patients 4 months after hospital discharge. *Blood Advances, 5*(3), 756–759.

Weerahandi, H., Hochman, K. A., Simon, E., Blaum, C., Chodosh, J., Duan, E., … Horwitz, L. I. (2021). Post-discharge health status and symptoms in patients with severe COVID-19. *Journal of General Internal Medicine, 36*(3), 738–745.

Werthman-Ehrenreich, A. (2021). Mucormycosis with orbital compartment syndrome in a patient with COVID-19. *The American Journal of Emergency Medicine, 42*, 264-e5.

Wu, Y., Xu, X., Chen, Z., Duan, J., Hashimoto, K., Yang, L., ... Yang, C. (2020). Nervous system involvement after infection with COVID-19 and other coronaviruses. *Brain, Behavior, and Immunity, 87,* 18–22.

Xing, Y., Mo, P., Xiao, Y., Zhao, O., Zhang, Y., & Wang, F. (2020). Post-discharge surveillance and positive virus detection in two medical staff recovered from coronavirus disease 2019 (COVID-19), China, January to February 2020. *Eurosurveillance, 25*(10), 2000191.

Chapter 7

The Impact of COVID-19 on the Maritime Economy: A Study on Bangladesh

Bornali Rahman, Mohammad Tameem Hossain Azmi, and Jakir Hosain

Department of Shipping and Maritime Science, Canadian University of Bangladesh, Dhaka, Bangladesh

Contents

DOI: 10.1201/9781003324447-7

7.1 Introduction

Shipping is considered one of the oldest industries, with >5, 000 years of history. It was stated that by using water as a carrier, a more extensive market opened up to every sort of industry than what land carriage solely afforded (Smith, 2008). Maritime transportation played a more vital role in global trading than the previous land transportation earlier. Most business hubs and industries were established around port cities, where shipping added value to the economy. Maritime transportation connects the global supply chain. With shipping and ports handling >80% of worldwide product trade by volume and >70% by value, maritime transportation enables global supply chain connections and economic interconnectivity (Millefiori et al., 2021; Schnurr & Walker, 2019; UNCTAD, 2021)

Since the outbreak of COVID-19 at the start of 2020, the whole world has been going through the most challenging and crucial period of the century. The virus has spread globally very quickly; as of March 11, 2020, World Health Organization (WHO) declared the novel coronavirus a pandemic (Bharati et al., 2021). The virus is an unknown and complicated variant; effective medication and vaccination are currently being researched. According to WHO, in 2020, 82,661,954 cases were confirmed, and 732,373 deaths were confirmed. Until January 1, 2021, the virus spread worldwide with >35,695,922 confirmed and probable cases and 956,150 deaths caused by COVID-19 (Bansal & Upadhyay, 2017; Bharati et al., 2020) This huge number of cases and death ratio supports the nature and unpredictability of this disease. Coronavirus is indeed a life-threatening virus (Fan et al., 2019; Lan et al., 2020; Mondal et al., 2020; Podder et al., 2021). Expertise suggests that initial and precise analysis and efficient treatment procedures could be beneficial to cure the patients. (Mondal, 2021).The concerned nations used various measures to contain the pandemic, including movement restriction orders, and partial and entire lockdowns. Some cities took interventions like social restrictions, quarantines, and curfews orders to stop mass gatherings of people, which eventually reduced the spreading of COVID-19. Nation-wise, nonpharmaceutical interventions were first imposed in Italy in March 2020; later followed by many countries around the world (Ebrahim et al., 2020; Hellewell, 2020; Sarkis, 2020; Perra, 2021; Sanche et al., 2020). Records have been confirming this pandemic situation as being similar to a war, where humans are fighting against the novel coronavirus. Human life is now greatly threatened due to this infectious virus, which can easily be transmitted by proximity to COVID-19 infected people. Lung damage and breathing problems are the common symptoms of coronavirus (Bharati et al., 2020). Research is being continued by WHO; when infected individuals cough or sneeze, COVID-19 is transmitted largely through droplets of saliva or discharges from the nose (Liu et al., 2020; Stadnytskyi et al., 2020; Xu et al., 2020). Therefore, lockdowns and shutdowns are being used to prevent the spreading of coronavirus; the sudden shock of COVID-19 resulted in discontinuation in the world's economic supply and demand chain. According to the World Bank report, the world's growth rate has decreased from 2.336% (2019) to -3.593% (2020), which is the highest decline in GDP declination in the last 50 years. This reduction shows that in 2020 the world economy went through a global recession due to the sudden shock of COVID-19 (World Bank, 2020). The United Nations Conference on Trade and Development (UNCTAD) reported that, in a scenario of this kind, where the major developed economies will lose an average of 0.5% of their GDP, the world economy would experience a further decrease of about 0.6% of GDP (UNCTAD, 2021). The trend in developed countries is alarming as trading with foreign consumers is being reduced; therefore, having an impact on the world economy. World GDP growth can heavily influence the number of goods transported via sea routes (Michail, 2020). A Baltic and International Maritime Council report shows that the declination in world GDP proportionally reduced the seaborne trade growth by -2.8%. The COVID-19 pandemic resulted in a significant drop in foreign direct investment (FDI). Global FDI fell by 20% in 2020, which was USD 1.5 trillion in 2019 (UNCTAD, 2021). At the end of the first quarter of 2020, the novel coronavirus appeared in Bangladesh and spread with time. Bangladesh's population is equivalent to 2.11% of the total world population, and the density is 1,265/km² (3,277 people/mile²). As of January 1, 2021, the confirmed and probable cases of COVID-19 in Bangladesh were 82,164. In March 2020, the first COVID-19 case was suspected in Bangladesh. The high population density resulted in the rapid transmission of coronavirus; therefore, the government announced lockdowns and shutdowns several times in 2020 to resist the infectious disease, thus, affecting the national economy; the GDP growth rate was reduced to 2.36% (2020) from 8.153% (2020). Although the growth rate is positive, GDP is increasing but at a slow growth rate. As the sea carries >90% of trade in Bangladesh, the seaborne trade has a significant influence over the national economy. The government has been trying to continue trading during this pandemic; however, the global recession has affected trade volume. In this chapter, an empirical model is presented using linear regression analysis to show a relationship between COVID-19 and trade volume. The impacts of COVID-19 on the all-export and import commodities, and total seaborne trade, where confirmed COVID-19 cases are used to measure COVID-19 intensity was assessed. In order to estimate the pandemic consequences, COVID-19 is considered as the independent variable where the export–import commodities are the dependent variables in this chapter. Descriptive statistical analysis was made through exploratory data analysis (EDA); then, a simple linear regression model is constructed between the independent and dependent variables to describe the impact of COVID-19 on the major commodities of the seaborne trade. This chapter tries to explain how the intensity of COVID-19 cases influences the seaborne trade volume.

The chapter contributions are summarized as follows.

1. The theoretical concept of the maritime economy is described and reviewed from the related literature. Additionally, the seaborne trade of Bangladesh is briefly described
2. The empirical model associated with EDA and linear regression analyses were applied to determine the impact of COVID-19 on the maritime economy
3. The data analysis explained the impact of COVID-19 impact on all trade commodities
4. This work elaborately described the future research prospects for the maritime economy of Bangladesh.

7.2 Maritime Economy of Bangladesh

7.2.1 Economy and Maritime Economy

The economy is considered the basis of worldwide development. Adam Smith explained economics as "an inquiry into the nature and causes of the wealth of nations"(Smith, 2008). The concept of resource scarcity, allocation, and resource utilization is not abstracted in the definition, which emphasizes natural resources for wealth. In 1932 Lionel Robbin said, "Economics is the science which studies human behavior as a relationship between ends and scarce means which have alternative uses" (Cowell & Witztum, 2007; Lipsey, 2009). Macroeconomic concepts of national income and aggregate supply and demand are not provided in the definition; furthermore, normative social science transformed it into positive science using the stylized mathematical model. Paul Samuelson gives the most appropriate definition for economics; he aggregated the previous concept and added the modern commodity production and distribution concept. As per Samuelson, "Economics is the study of how people and society choose, with or without the use of money, to employ scarce productive resources which could have alternative uses, to produce various commodities over time and distribute them for consumption now and in the future among various persons and groups of society." (Samuelson & Nordhaus, 2009). In contrast, overseas resource distribution results in the demand for the transportation mode. As per Martin Stopford, energy, mining, and agriculture are the building blocks of the economy; the shipping industry was the primary market for moving large parcels from one place to another, which helped to decrease transport costs (List et al., 2010). Maritime transportation is essential and the most accepted among all transportation modes, because it is efficient and effective due to its high-volume carrying capacity. The maritime economy encompasses all the activities connected to the sea or whose development is influenced by water (Kalaydjian, 2014). The total range of the maritime economy is broad, and it raises the question of the possibility of giving a proper definition of this range.

The rise in globalization has expanded trade exchange across the world and created the importance of maritime transportation. The maritime economy is the process of economic activities and results connected with an environment of a sea and its basins, involving production and processing, allocation and spending of goods and services (Kalaydjian, 2014; Kronfeld-Goharani, 2018; List et al., 2010). The world economy is the most crucial determinant of seaborne trade, which is related to the global demand-supply chain. A large economy has more significant needs for raw materials and manufactured goods that are shipped by sea (List et al., 2010). As per Martin Stopford, the main differences between international economists and maritime economists are that trade economists concentrate on the value of trade, and maritime economists focus on the trade volume; maritime economists pay special attention to the way of trade exchange; however, international economists cover the whole trade spectrum; the geographical region is more important than political nation-states in maritime trade assessment (List et al., 2010). Stopford also provides three fundamental reasons for trade. These are: (1) differences in manufacturing costs; (2) differences in natural resources; and (3) temporary local imbalances. The factors are related to the quantity and commodity of any country's seaborne trade.

Figure 7.1 shows the role of maritime transportation in international trade exchanges. Individual demand creates the market demand for any goods: the goods or resources results in overseas trade flow. Maritime transportation acts as a link between two different markets; geographical position plays a vital role in transportation. The distance and freight rate have a comparative effect on the commodity price that controls commodity supply and demand; on the other hand, the vessel demand proportionally depends on the commodity's demand. Nevertheless, seaborne trade is the basis of the maritime economy and affects the world economy. Therefore, this chapter focused on seaborne trade to assess the maritime economy of Bangladesh.

7.2.2 Seaborne Trade in Bangladesh

Bangladesh has the oldest maritime history for their geographical position; using the example of Chattogram Port, Chattogram, Bangladesh, the maritime history started as long ago as the ninth century. A variety of economic sectors are explored around the current maritime boundary of Bangladesh (Hussain et al., 2018). Maritime trade and shipping are focus areas in Bangladesh's blue economy vision. Regarding the importance of globalization, Bangladesh's external freight trade is seaborne Approximately >92% of total national trade is made by sea, where Chattogram Port contributed to 90% of the seaborne trade. Another seaport of Bangladesh is Mongla Port, located in Khulna. Due to draft restrictions and poor hinterland connectivity, this port contributed only 10% to the trade exchange. During the COVID-19 pandemic, flights and foreign immigration were restricted in several COVID-19 affected countries. Nevertheless, port activities and cargo handling continued; therefore, global maritime trade connectivity was not interrupted. Consumers for goods determine sea transport (Lun, 2010). The COVID-19 impact on the demands for goods resulted in slow growth in vessel number at Chattogram Port.

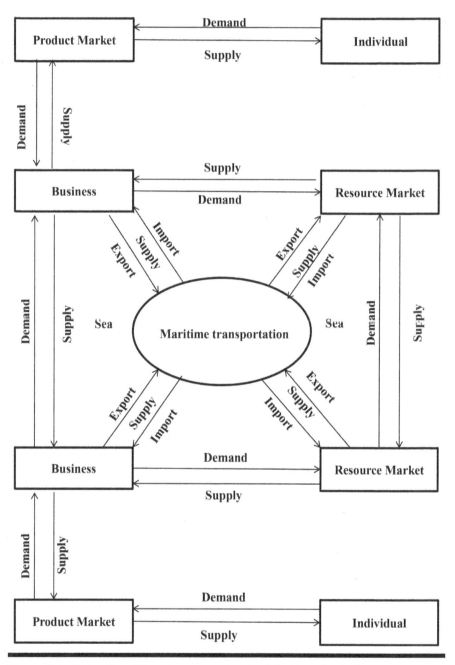

Figure 7.1 Role of maritime transportation in global supply chain

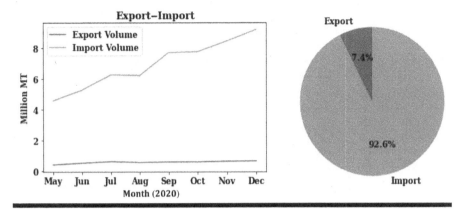

Figure 7.2   Export–import at Chattogram Port in 2020

Figure 7.2 shows the growth in export–import volumes during 2020. The total export–import volume had several fluctuation phases; the average import volume is accountable for 93% of the seaborne trade volume. In Bangladesh, major seaborne commodities are bulk cargoes, such as rice, urea, naphtha, ammonia, food grain, fertilizer, coal, salt, sugar, edible oil, petroleum oil, and other raw materials. Industrial cargoes such as container cargoes included jute, jute goods, leather, tea, ready-made garments, frozen goods, knitted or crocheted fabrics, dairy products, machinery, and many others. Heckscher-Ohlin's theory said that countries with plentiful capital would export capital-intensive products and import labor-intensive products, and vice-versa for a country with plenty of labor. Bangladesh has a dense population of 1,265/km²; due to the dense population, natural resources are not plentiful; however, labor is plentiful. That results in the import of high volumes of grain, sugar, salt, and other capital-intensive commodities and raw materials; on the other hand, export goods are labor-intensive, like jute goods and ready-made garments (RMG). As Bangladesh has achieved the second position in Global Market Share (6.5%) in RMG, seaborne trade is highly influenced by this sector. Among the import commodities, textile raw materials are high volume, and in return, the sector accounts for 45% of total exports. As several development projects are ongoing, C/Clinker is the highest import commodity. After the outbreak of COVID-19 in March 2020, the effect of panic on the demand chain was apparent from April 2020. A decline in supply resulted in decreased export–import volumes. The export volume depends on the demand from overseas countries. A large economy has more significant requirements for raw materials and manufactured goods that are shipped by sea (List et al., 2010). Because GDP growth is the indicator of any country's economic health., the export volume of one country is highly influenced by the GDP of importer countries. The USA, Germany, UK, Spain, France, Italy, Poland, India, Netherlands,

Canada, Japan, Denmark, Australia, Belgium, and Sweden are the major buying countries for goods from Bangladesh; as per the report in *Trading Economics*, these countries experienced negative GDP growth in 2020. The Bangladesh Bank data presents the countrywide income of Bangladesh, where export income declined in line with other significant countries except for Poland. Among all European countries, only Poland recovered its economy and achieved positive economic growth in 2020. As Bangladesh exports manufactured goods, with the decline in export volume, a decline occurs in the import of raw materials. Therefore, the impact of COVID-19 on the economy of overseas countries had a proportional impact on the seaborne trade volume of Bangladesh.

7.3 The Empirical Model

The novel coronavirus has expanded since the end of March 2020. In order to understand the impact of COVID-19 on the maritime economy and examine the pandemic impacts on major export–import commodities separately, this section applied a data analysis model. Python3 was used to construct the empirical model for data analysis and visualization. This data analysis aims to determine the effect of the COVID-19 pandemic on the seaborne trade in Bangladesh. Equation 7.1 calculates the growth rate of COVID-19.

$$\text{growth rate of COVID-19} = \{(b-a)/a\} \times 100 \tag{7.1}$$

where:
a = COVID-19 confirmed cases in the previous month
b = COVID-19 confirmed cases in the following month

The data on COVID-19 confirmed cases were obtained from the WHO. In addition, the volume of export–imports were collected from the Chittagong Port Authority (CPA) website. The full dataset is presented in Appendix 7.A (Table 7.7). Then, EDA was performed to investigate the data set's initial investigation to check assumptions using descriptive statistics and graphical representation. Finally, simple linear regression was used to estimate the model to calculate the impact of COVID-19 on the seaborne trade.

7.3.1 EDA

The dataset of this study contained the total export–import volume of Chattogram Port in 2020 from May to December. The volume of the major export–import commodities were recorded for this study. The description of the variables is presented in Table 7.1.

Table 7.1   Variables Applied in EDA

Variable Name	Variable Description
Export_Jute	The volume of exported jute cargoes in the container
Export_Jute goods	The volume of exported jute goods in the container
Export_Leather	The volume of exported leather cargoes in the container
Export-RMG	The volume of exported ready-made garments in the container
Export-Frozen goods	The volume of exported frozen goods in the container
Export_Container_Others	The volume of exported other container cargoes
Export_Ammonia	The volume of exported ammonia cargoes in bulk
Export_Bulk_Others	The volume of exported other bulk cargoes
Total_Export	The volume of total exported cargoes
Import_Grain	The volume of imported grain in bulk
Import_Clinker	The volume of imported Clinker in bulk
Import_Fertilizer	The volume of imported fertilizers in bulk
Import_Coal	The volume of imported coal in bulk
Import_Salt	The volume of imported salt in bulk
Import_Sugar	The volume of imported sugar in bulk
Import_Eidible_Oil	The volume of imported edible oil in bulk
Import_Petrolium_Oil	The volume of imported petroleum oil bulk
Import_Bulk_ Others	The volume of imported other bulk cargoes
Import_Container	The volume of imported container cargoes
Covid-19_Rate	% of COVID-19 increasing rate
Total	Tola Volume of export and import

In this chapter, an analysis was conducted on 22 variables. The variables were grouped into four sections: (1) COVID-19 rate: COVID-19_Rate; (2) export commodities: Export_Jute, Export_Jute_Goods, Export_Leather, Export RMG, Export, FrozenGoods, Export_Container_Others, Export_Ammonia, Export_Bulk_Others; (3) import commodities: Import_Fertilizer, Import_Coal, Import_Salt, Import_Sugar, Import_Eidible_Oil, Import_Petrolium_Oil, Import_Bulk_Others, Import_Container; and (4) total: Total_Export, Total_Import, Total. Figure 7.3 shows the heatmap correlation matrix of total export volume, total import volume, and total volume. The heatmap shows that total volume was related more to total import

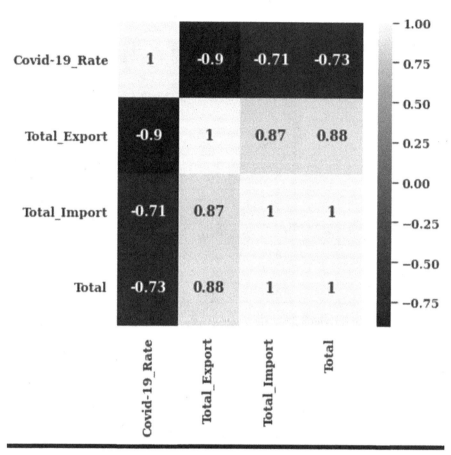

Figure 7.3 Correlation heat map of COVID-19 rate, total export, total import, and total export–import

volume than export, indicating a higher import volume. The correlation between import and export volume was also evident, because exporting manufacturing products is related to imported raw materials. COVID-19 has a negative correlation with these three, which shows the increasing COVID-19 rate resulted in decreasing export–imports in Bangladesh. From the correlation matrix, COVID-19 impact on the seaborne trade of Bangladesh was evident.

7.3.2 Linear Regression Analysis

In this chapter, simple linear regression was applied for quantitative analysis of the COVID-19 impact. The analysis was conducted using seaborne and matplotlib library in PYTHON3. The simple linear regression equation is expressed in Equation 7.2:

$$y = \beta_0 + \beta_1 X_1 + \epsilon \tag{7.2}$$

where:

y = dependent variable

X_1 = independent variable

b_0 = intercept, where the line crosses the y-axis

b_1 = slope that describes the line's direction and inclines

$b_1 X_1$ = linear effect of X_1

ϵ = error

7.3.2.1 Import Volume and COVID-19

The regression analysis report given in Table 7.2 illustrates that the value of the correlation coefficient (R^2) was higher in clinker, petroleum oil, and most commodities had a low R^2 value. Thus, for container cargo R^2 = 0.248, and container import was significantly less affected by the COVID-19 pandemic.

Table 7.3 gives the summary of the regression result; from the analysis, the estimated equation for import volume was: $y = 7.400 - 0.074x$. $R^2=0.516$ indicates that 51.6% of the import volume can be explained by COVID-19. The downward slope in Figure 7.4 shows a negative relationship between both variables. With the increasing Covid cases, import volume was declining.

7.3.2.2 Export Volume and COVID-19

Table 7.4 shows the linear relationship between export cargoes and COVID-19. Among all the export commodities, RMG and jute goods had a high R^2 value, and

Table 7.2 Results of Simple Linear Regression with Different Import Commodities

Major Commodities	R	R^2	p-value
Bulk Cargo-Grain	0.409	0.167	0.34
Bulk Cargo-Clinker	0.762	0.581	0.028
Bulk Cargo-Fertilizer	0.594	0.353	0.12
Bulk Cargo-Coal	0.278	0.077	0.506
Bulk Cargo-Salt	0.002	0.000	0.997
Bulk Cargo-Sugar	0.486	0.237	0.22
Bulk Cargo-Edible Oil	0.240	0.058	0.567
Petroleum Oil	0.811	0.658	0.014
Bulk Others	0.463	0.214	0.248
Container	0.498	0.248	0.209

Table 7.3   Summary of Regression Result for Total Import

	Coefficient	p-value	R^2
Intercept	7.4001	0.000	0.516
X = COVID-19 Rate	-0.0074	0.044	

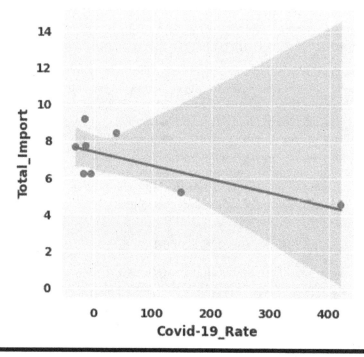

Figure 7.4   Scatter plot of COVID-19 and total import volume

Table 7.4   Result of Simple Linear Regression with Different Export Commodities

Major Commodities	R	R^2	p-value
Container Cargo-Jute	0.529	0.280	0.170
Container Cargo-Jute goods	0.873	0.762	0.005
Container Cargo-Leather	0.562	0.316	0.147
Container Cargo-RMG	0.794	0.631	0.019
Container Cargo-Frozen goods	0.256	0.066	0.540
Container Cargo-Others	0.006	0.00	0.986
Bulk Cargo-Ammonia	0.067	0.004	0.876
Bulk Cargo-Others	0.377	0.142	0.357

Table 7.5 Summary of Regression Result for Total Export

	Coefficient	p-value	R^2
Intercept	0.5856	0.000	0.808
X = COVID-19 Rate	-0.0005	0.002	

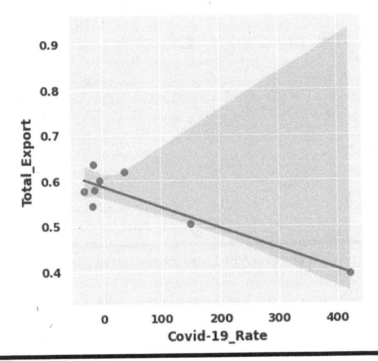

Figure 7.5 Scatter plot of COVID-19 and total export volume

$p<0.05$. On the other hand, other export commodities, especially bulk cargo, had a low Covid impact. From Table 7.5, the estimated regression equation for total export values was: $y = 0.5856 - 0.0005x$, and the p-value was 0.002 ($p<0.05$); therefore, the null hypothesis was rejected at 5% significance. The obtained value of R^2 for total export volume was 0.808; therefore, the equation could predict the export volume by 80.8%, where the independent variable was COVID-19. Figure 7.5 shows a downward slope that indicates that the growth of COVID-19 decreased export volume.

7.3.2.3 Total Seaborne Trade Volume and COVID-19

From the linear regression model, the $p = 0.042$ ($p<0.05$); therefore, the null hypothesis was rejected at the 5% level of significance, so the H_0 = null hypothesis was

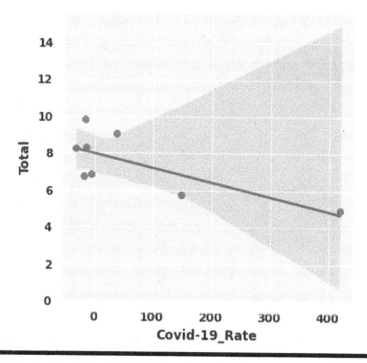

Figure 7.6 Scatter plot of COVID-19 and total seaborne trade

Table 7.6 Summary of Regression Result for Total Seaborne

	Coefficient	p-value	R²
Intercept	7.9857	0.000	0.526
X = COVID-19 Rate	-0.0078	0.042	

rejected. Figure 7.6 shows a downward slope that indicated a negative relationship between both variables. Table 7.6 shows the regression result summary of total seaborne cargoes with COVID-19; the following fitted model from the python output was obtained $y = 7.9857 - 0.0078 \times 0.0070$. $R^2 = 0.526$, hence the equation was 52.5% fitted to predict the total seaborne trade volume using the COVID-19 rate. The fitted model indicated that COVID-19 had a moderate impact on the total seaborne trade.

7.4 Discussion

The maritime sector in Bangladesh has added significant value to the revenue earnings, as most of the commodities in Bangladesh are exchanged by sea. However, the COVID-19 pandemic has created a random shock worldwide; therefore, affecting the world's economic supply and demand chain. In this chapter, an empirical model was made by EDA and simple linear regression to conduct a quantitative analysis of the effect of Covid on the maritime economy of Bangladesh. Major export and import commodities volume, total export volume, total import volume, and total seaborne trade volume were used as dependent variables where the growth in COVID-19 cases was independent.

In Bangladesh, import commodities are around 93% higher than export commodities; consequently, import volumes greatly impact the maritime and national economies. From the EDA, the correlation matrix showed a -71% correlation between COVID-19 and import volume. The high and negative values indicated that increasing the COVID-19 rate decreased the import volume. The regression analysis demonstrated that, for petroleum oil, $R^2 = 0.658$, and $R = 0.811$, and a significant relationship between COVID-19 and petroleum oil was evident. The R^2 with C/Clinker was 0.581 and $R = 0.762$, and a moderate Covid effect appeared in the C/Clinker import. The lockdown interrupted several construction projects; therefore, impacting demand and proportionally the imported C/Clinker volume. Consumable and necessary goods, such as grain ($R^2 = 0.167$, $R = 0.409$), salt ($R^2 = 0.237$, $R = 0.486$), sugar ($R^2 = 0.058$, $R = 0.240$) were not affected Covid. Because around 30% of total import volume was necessary goods, Covid moderately influenced the total import volume ($R^2 = 0.516$). From the simple linear regression model, the import volume of 52% could be explained by COVID-19.

Bangladesh exports several commodities, and among them, the container cargo share is higher than the bulk cargoes. According to EDA, the correlation value of COVID-19 and export volume was -90%. The linear regression gave a significant relation between jute goods ($R^2 = 0.762$, $R = 0.873$), and RMG ($R^2 = 0.794$, $R = 0.631$). As Bangladesh is a labor-intensive country goods, such as RMG, textiles, jute goods, leather products, and footwear are the major export commodities. The RMG sector contributes around 45% of the total export goods. As per the simple linear regression calculation, $R^2 = 0.808$ proved a strong COVID-19 effect on the seaborne export volume. The economic recession in the major buying countries due to COVID-19 adversely affected the supply of the goods and demanded chain in 2020. That resulted in a decreased export volume in Bangladesh.

The EDA report presents the negative correlation between (-73%) COVID-19 and total seaborne trade. A simple linear regression model showed that the total volume could be 52.5% predicted by COVID-19. Thus, there was a moderate negative relationship between the total seaborne trade and COVID-19. In future studies, the descriptive statistics and linear regression will determine the COVID-19 impact on the seaborne trade in Bangladesh.

7.5 Limitations and Future Research

This chapter tried to conduct a quantitative analysis to estimate the COVID-19 impact on the seaborne trade in Bangladesh. Although the chapter explained the impact with descriptive statistics and a simple linear regression model, some limitations are associated with the research. The limitations are described as follows.

1. Restriction in data collection: the data was collected from the CPA website only due to the visit restriction for the COVID-19 pandemic
2. Data availability: The prediction was made on the CPA data from 2020, because the new data for 2021 was unavailable on the website
3. Uneven COVID-19 rate: As COVID-19 is not spreading uniformly and the observations were made over 8 months, the prediction could be varied in some cases

This chapter focused on using the data science approach in economic analysis. Descriptive statistics analysis and a simple linear regression model were applied in the research to co-relate COVID-19 and seaborne trade in Bangladesh, the estimated equation from the regression model, could be used to predict the trade volume in a COVID-19 recession. The limitation of our study could be a benefit for further research. In the future, the following analysis should be applied to enhance the research.

1. To predict more accurately, a questionnaire survey of experts' opinions could be assessed
2. This chapter focused on the data from the COVID-19 first wave. The model from this chapter could assess the second-wave scenario
3. Data science approach could be made to compare the COVID-19 impact on the maritime economy in 2020 and 2021
4. Decision tree could be applied to the research to define the COVID-19 recession

Furthermore, research is required on the commodities separately to assess the international demand and supply chain and the decreased world GDP growth. The COVID-19 recession has had a revolutionary change in the world economy and the maritime sector. There are significant prospects for research on the COVID-19 affected shipping and logistic sectors.

7.6 Conclusions

After the outbreak of COVID-19, the world has been going through a challenging time. The health, social affairs, and economy were affected by the COVID-19 pandemic. This chapter described the pandemic impact on the maritime economy in Bangladesh, and data science was used to accomplish the research. This chapter has provided an estimated relationship between COVID-19 and the total seaborne trade volume to assess the pandemic's impact on Bangladesh's maritime economy. Furthermore, a theoretical description of the maritime economy was described, and the maritime area of Bangladesh was briefly drawn in this chapter. The descriptive statistics and regression analysis were applied to examine the COVID-19 pandemic impact. Overall, the results showed that the COVID-19 shock moderately influenced the total seaborne trade volume, except for some commodities. In addition, this chapter discovered that consumable and necessary goods volume remained the same as in previous years. Lockdowns and shutdowns interrupted transportation movement worldwide, and in Bangladesh, the continuous reduction in oil demand resulted in a decrease in oil imports. The GDP growth rate in major buyer countries accounted for the lower export volume; then, the imported raw materials volume also declined. Although some limitations were perceived in the research in this chapter, these are a source of further research. Moreover, this chapter successfully demonstrated the research purpose and achieved all contributions of the chapter.

The findings are essential for business decision-making, and the commodity analysis could help shippers, ship charterers, and brokers. Furthermore, the key findings from this chapter highlighted that consumer demand has a substantial influence on the maritime economy; therefore, the export market of Bangladesh was highly affected during this pandemic. Therefore, this chapter suggests that Bangladesh might adjust its trade pattern by considering the prevalence of COVID-19 in different countries. Additionally, as long as the COVID-19 recession exists, the manufacturers must focus more on consumables and necessary products than durable and luxury products. Nevertheless, the maritime economy in Bangladesh maintained its position during this most challenging time. Therefore, we should see great prosperity in the maritime economy of Bangladesh in the future.

Appendix 7.A

Table 7.7 Data used for Empirical Model

Month (2020)	May	June	July	August	September	October	November	December	Total (t)	Total (million t)
Export Commodities										
Jute	11,325	9,042	21,162	18,836	17,540	15,427	13,434	32,969	139,735	0.139735
Jute goods	16,130	28,750	40,795	40,427	47,038	54,271	53,712	47,834	328,957	0.328957
Leather	1,065	1,959	2,953	1,844	1,456	1,811	1,904	2,793	15,785	0.015785
RMG	145,354	247,531	359,833	253,082	256,789	260,403	271,012	300,715	2,094,719	2.094719
Frozen goods	8,913	6,865	8,756	8,383	6,819	6,920	6,848	9,067	62,571	0.062571
Cont. others	209390	186885	166163	176045	246465	212716	221440	203.590	1,622,694	1.622694
Ammonia	0	13,650	0	13,000	0	0	0	6.300	32,950	0.03295
Bulk others	248	9997	105	31500	0	27436	51629	32.326	153,241	0.153241
Import Commodities										
Food grain	277,226	487,983	287,319	322,421	989,580	797,195	276,325	547.182	3,985,231	3.985231
C/Clinker	1,181,976	976,242	2,414,564	1,948,138	2,450,219	2,399,872	2,687,171	2,654,402	16,712,584	16.712584
Fertilizer	24,770	33,430	105,430	75,368	138,401	122,306	143,638	282,659	926,002	0.926002
Coal	80,855	25,750	63,950	31,775	124,100	252,243	676,844	895,321	2,150,838	2.150838
Salt	0	39300	14000	0	85400	600	44199	28,800	212,299	0.212299
Sugar	84,101	136,806	166,027	189,175	201,339	142,397	332,395	151,231	1,403,471	1.403471
Edible oil	156,626	305,135	200,315	93,696	149,137	134,498	181,066	158,920	1,379,393	1.379393
Petroleum oil	259,690	461,398	448,010	513,598	753,414	680,481	543,449	588,411	4,248,451	4.248451

Bulk others	1,137,471	1,403,378	1,139,754	1,600,175	1,365,225	1,783,568	2,059,576	2,216,170	12,705,317	12.705317
Container others	1,361,890	1,393,482	1,419,088	1,439,991	1,443,104	1,443,104	1,504,409	1,670,866	11,675,934	11.675934
Total (t)	4,957,030	5,767,583	6,858,224	6,757,454	8,276,026	8,335,248	9,069,051	9,829,556	5,985,0172	
Total (million t)	4.95703	5.767583	6.858224	6.757454	8.276026	8.335248	9.069051	9.829556	59.850172	
Growth during Covid	421%	149%	-6%	-18%	-33%	-15%	37%	-17%		

Month	Bulk Import	Bulk Export	Cont Import	Cont-Export	ICD-Import	ICD-Export	ICT-Import	ICT-EXPORT	TOTAL IMPRT	TOTAL EXPRT	TOTAL (t)	TOTAL (MILLION t)
January	7,567,844	8,651	1,830,793	62,6222	35,445	15,597	10,011	1,351	9,444,093	651,821	10,095,914	10.095914
February	6,775,532	180	1,536,896	542,017	34,550	13,785	10,402	777	8,357,380	556,759	8,914,139	8.914139
March	7,426,460	58,473	1,643,279	590,277	32,335	13,474	6,402	787	9,108,476	663,011	9,771,487	9.771487
April	5,209,926	10,840	925,869	288,807	6,041	3,047	23,310	302	6,165,146	302,996	6,468,142	6.468142
May	3,202,715	248	1,361,890	392,177	18,419	8,594	10,637	0	4,593,661	401,019	4,994,680	4.99468
June	3,869,422	23,647	1,393,482	481,032	26,014	11,259	6,693	468	5,295,611	516,406	5,812,017	5.812017
July	4,839,369	105	1,419,088	599,662	22,599	13,697	12,520	433	6,293,576	613,897	6,907,473	6.907473
August	4,774,346	44,500	1,439,991	498,617	16,672	8,127	15,120	338	6,246,129	551,582	6,797,711	6.797711
September	6,256,815	0	1,430,044	576,107	24,698	9,944	15,132	107	7,726,689	586,158	8,312,847	8.312847
October	6,313,160	27,436	1,443,104	551,548	32,380	10,191	18,840	77	7,807,484	589,252	8,396,736	8.396736
November	6,944,663	51,629	1,504,409	568,350	35,860	10,674	13,371	479	8,498,303	631,132	9,129,435	9.129435
December	7,523,096	38,626	1,670,866	596,968	32,850	9,821	25,040	610	9,251,852	646,025	9,897,877	9.897877

Source: www.cpa.gov.bd/; www.who.int/

References

Bansal, A., & Upadhyay, A. K. (2017). Microsoft Power BI. *International Journal of Soft Computing and Engineering*. Retrieved from https://app.powerbi.com/view?r=eyJrIjo iYWRiZWVkNWUtNmM0Ni00MDAwLTljYWMtN2EwNTM3YjQzYmRmIiwi dCI6ImY2MTBjMGI3LWJkMjQtNGIzOS04MTBiLTNkYzI4MGFmYjU5MCIsI mMiOjh9

Bharati, S., Podder, P., & Mondal, M. R. H. (2020). Hybrid deep learning for detecting lung diseases from X-ray images. *Informatics in Medicine Unlocked, 20*, 100391. doi.10.1016/j.imu.2020.100391

Bharati, S., Podder, P., Mondal, M. R. H., & Prasath, V. B. S. (2021). Medical imaging with deep Learning for COVID- 19 diagnosis: A comprehensive review. *International Journal of Computer Information Systems and Industrial Management Applications, 13*, 91–112.

Cowell, F., & Witztum, A. (Eds). (2007). Lionel Robbins essay on the nature and significance of economic science. *75th Anniversary Conference*, 1–500.

Ebrahim, S. H., Ahmed, Q. A., Gozzer, E., Schlagenhauf, P., & Memish, Z. A. (2020). Covid-19 and community mitigation strategies in a pandemic. *The BMJ, 368*. doi.10.1136/ BMJ.M1066

Fan, Y., Zhao, K., Shi, Z.-L., & Zhou, P. (2019). Bat Coronaviruses in China. *Viruses, 11*(3), e210. doi.10.3390/V11030210

Hellewell, J. (2020). Feasibility of controlling COVID-19 outbreaks by isolation of cases and contacts. *Lancet Global Health, 8*(4), e488–e496. doi.10.1016/s2214-109x(20)30074-7

Hussain, M. G., Failler, P., Karim, A. Al, & Alam, M. K. (2018). Major opportunities of blue economy development in Bangladesh. *Journal of the Indian Ocean Region, 14*(1), 88–99. doi.10.1080/19480881.2017.1368250

Kalaydjian, R. (2014). Maritime economy: Definition and main aspects. *Value and Economy of Marine Resources*, 233–290. doi.1002/9781119007791.ch4

Kronfeld-Goharani, U. (2018). Maritime economy: Insights on corporate visions and strategies towards sustainability. *Ocean and Coastal Management, 165*, 126–140. doi.10.1016/j.ocecoaman.2018.08.010

Lan, F.-Y., Wei, C.-F., Hsu, Y.-T., Christiani, D. C., & Kales, S. N. (2020). Work-related COVID-19 transmission in six Asian countries/areas: A follow-up study. *PlosOne, 15*(5), e0233588. doi.10.1371/JOURNAL.PONE.0233588

Lipsey, R. G. (2009). Some legacies of robbins' an essay on the nature and significance of economic science. *Economica, 76*(S1), 845–856. doi.10.1111/j.1468-0335.2009.00792.x

List, L., Economics, M., & Economics, M. (2010). Maritime economics. *Choice Reviews Online, 47*(7). doi.10.5860/choice.47-3934

Liu, J., Liao, X., Qian, S., Yuan, J., Wang, F., Liu, Y., ...Zhang, Z. (2020). Community transmission of severe acute respiratory syndrome Coronavirus 2, Shenzhen, China, 2020. *Emerging Infectious Diseases, 26*(6), 1320–1323. doi.10.3201/EID2606.200239

Lun, K.-H. L. (2010). Bulk shipping market. In K.-H. L. Lun (Ed.) *Shipping and Logistics Management* (p. 33). London: Springer.

Michail, N. A. (2020). World economic growth and seaborne trade volume: Quantifying the relationship. *Transportation Research Interdisciplinary Perspectives, 4*, 100108. doi.10.1016/j.trip.2020.100108

Millefiori, L. M., Braca, P., Zissis, D., Spiliopoulos, G., Marano, S., Willett, P. K., & Carniel, S. (2021). COVID-19 impact on global maritime mobility. *Scientific Reports, 11*(1), 1–16. doi.10.1038/s41598-021-97461-7

Mondal, M. R. H., Bharati, S., Podder, P., & Podder, P. (2020). Data analytics for novel coronavirus disease. *Informatics in Medicine Unlocked, 20*, 100374.

Mondal, M. R. H., Bharati, S., & Podder, P. (2021). CO-IRv2: Optimized InceptionResNetV2 for COVID-19 detection from chest CT images. *PlosOne, 16*(10), e0259179. doi.10.1371/journal.pone.0259179

Perra, N. (2021). Non-pharmaceutical interventions during the COVID-19 pandemic: A review. *Physics Reports, 913*, 1–52. doi.10.1016/j.physrep.2021.02.001

Podder, P., Khamparia, A., Rubaiyat Hossain Mondal, M., Rahman, M. A., & Bharati, S. (2021). Forecasting the spread of COVID-19 and ICU requirements. *International Journal of Online and Biomedical Engineering, 17*(5), 81–99. doi.10.3991/ijoe.v17i05.20009

Samuelson, P. A., & Nordhaus, W. D. (2009). *Economics* (19th ed.). McGraw Hill: New York. Retrieved from www.mhhe.com

Sanche, S., Lin, Y. T., Xu, C., Romero-Severson, E., Hengartner, N., & Ke, R. (2020). The novel Coronavirus, 2019-nCoV, is highly contagious and more infectious than initially estimated. *MedRxiv.* doi.10.1101/2020.02.07.20021154

Sarkis, J., Cohen, M. J., Dewick, P., & Schroder, P. (2020). A brave new world: Lessons from the COVID-19 pandemic for transitioning to sustainable supply and production. *Resources, Conservation, Recycling, 159*, 104894. doi.10.1016/j.resconrec.2020.104894

Schnurr, R. E. J., & Walker, T. R. (2019). Marine transportation and energy use. *Reference Module in Earth Systems and Environmental Sciences.* doi.10.1016/B978-0-12-409548-9.09270-8

Smith, A. (2008). An inquiry into the nature and causes of the wealth of nations. *Readings in Economic Sociology, 1776*, 6–17. doi.10.1002/9780470755679.ch1

Stadnytskyi, V., Bax, C. E., Bax, A., & Anfinrud, P. (2020). The airborne lifetime of small speech droplets and their potential importance in SARS-CoV-2 transmission. *Proceedings of the National Academy of Sciences of the United States of America, 117*(22). doi.10.1073/PNAS.2006874117

UNCTAD. (2021). World investment report UNCTAD. *United Nations Conference on Trade and Development.* Retrieved from https://unctad.org/topic/investment/world-investment-report

World Bank. (2020). Supporting countries in unprecedented times. *Annual Report 2020*, 1–106. Retrieved from www.worldbank.org/en/about/annual-report/world-bank-group-downloads

Xu, R., Cui, B., Duan, X., Zhang, P., Zhou, X., & Yuan, Q. (2020). Saliva: potential diagnostic value and transmission of 2019-nCoV. *International Journal of Oral Science, 12*(1), 1–6. doi.10.1038/s4368-020-0080-z

Chapter 8

Intelligent Optimization and Computational Learning Techniques for Mitigating Pandemics

Kayode Abiodun Oladapo
Babcock University, Ilisan-Remo, Ogun, Nigeria

Jide Ebenezer Taiwo Akinsola, Moruf Adeagbo, and Fathia Onipede
First Technical University, Ibadan, Nigeria

Samuel Ayomikun Akinseinde
The Amateur Polymath, Lagos, Nigeria

Adebola Abdulwaheed Yusuf
Federal University of Petroleum Resources, Effurun, Nigeria

Contents

DOI: 10.1201/9781003324447-8

143

8.1 Introduction

For the past few decades, the use of emerging technologies has rapidly increased its application in various disciplines. In particular, the recent COVID-19 pandemics, it was shown to be effective in the process of mitigating it. The advances in new technologies on the Internet of Things (IoT) frameworks, and sensor technologies together with artificial intelligence (AI), such as the Internet of Medical Things, can be about innovative solutions to assist when mitigating pandemics. SARS-CoV-2 is the infectious virus that triggered the disease called coronavirus, which belongs to the family of coronaviridae. This means that flue and indications like fatigue, cough, shortness of breath, and fever are associated with coronavirus, which is popularly known as COVID-19. The cause of this virus is not known, and it is still under discussion (Tayarani, 2021).

The widespread of the disease in almost every country has caused the death of >2,271,000 people and nearly 104,371,000 confirmed cases according to World

Health Organization (WHO) statistics. Significant implementations have been provided by technology and science toward the anticipated restrictive strategies by the governments of many countries to ease the COVID-19 pandemic effects. For instance, the development of drones to sterilize public places and robots could be applied to the distribution of medicine and food to hospitals (Nguyen et al., 2020). Machine learning (ML) techniques can be defined as the gathering of tools that are used to recognize patterns in data that are opposed to the traditional methods of recognizing patterns, the tools used in ML depend on AI to know when new data becomes accessible, how to draw patterns from a large amount of data, and when new data is achieving these tasks rapidly and is available (Bansal et al., 2020). The ML analytics approaches are now being utilized in many fields (Akinsola et al., 2019). Evolving and recurring transferable diseases have destroyed societies, which is taking place with extraordinary speed. Nonetheless, formal approaches for performance assessment compared with conventional methodologies have been demonstrated to be profound (Akinsola et al., 2020). Therefore, this chapter focuses on the employment of intelligent optimization and computational learning techniques (IOCLT) for mitigating pandemics.

The contributions of this chapter are summarized below.

1. A categorization of a deep learning algorithm for computational intelligence
2. A new approach termed a nonlinear optimized empirical model is proposed in this chapter. It was centered on the convolutional neural networks (CNNs) framework and optimization algorithm (Adam optimizer) when optimizing the weights of the model
3. A dataset of 25,266 instances and nine columns from COVID-19 circumstances and mortality rates
4. A description is provided of how an epoch can be used to give a holistic view of how a model has performed

The rest of the chapter is organized as follows. Section 8.2 provides a review that established the important aspects of the use of IOCLT for mitigating pandemics. Section 8.3 discusses the application of deep learning to computational learning techniques. Section 8.4 discusses the data description, analysis, and results. Section 8.5 highlights some limitations and the future scope. Finally, Section 8.6 provides the concluding remarks

8.2 Review on IOCLT for Mitigating Pandemics

Over the past decade, the world has seen epidemics and outbreaks of numerous diseases according to WHO, which were caused by >20 infectious agents. Different communicable agents caused the majority of these epidemics, for example, MERS.3 and H1N12 (Balkhair, 2020). A pandemic is an epidemic of a disease that is transferable, which spreads universally, or through multiple landmasses, or human populations across a large area, for instance, diseases that can spread and contaminate humans easily (WHO, 2020). A pandemic causes significant political, economic, and social disruption and an increase in deaths and illness over a wide geographical area (Madhav et al., 2017). When there is a large number of illnesses, economic effects, deaths, and severe social effects it means that the pandemic is becoming a tragedy. The pandemic diseases known in the past include smallpox, polio, leprosy, yellow fever, cholera, and measles.

A pandemic spread can be reduced by following some strategies that include (Madhav et al., 2017).

1. The vulnerability of uninfected individuals should be reduced, which can be achieved through the provision of vaccines
2. Interactions should be restrained between uninfected and infected populations through the practice of social distancing, patient isolation, school closures, and quarantine
3. Infection of the symptomatic patient should be reduced through the use of infection control practices, antibiotics, and antiviral treatments

Plans for executing these actions should be verified and established through imitation exercises. Emerging technology and innovations and technologies are providing substantial activities to eradicate the spread of a pandemic, for example, vaccine development, designing targeted response, population screening, effective quarantine, infection tracking, and prioritizing the use and allocation of resources. ML was developed to help computers understand the past or present and anticipate or predict what will occur in future in unidentified situations (Akinsola et al., 2019) and this has been of great influence when treating pandemics, especially COVID-19. An intelligent user interface (IUI) anchored on ML paradigms is essential for intelligent optimized solutions (Akinsola et al., 2021).

Innovations and technologies are also supporting the extension of social and economic activities during a pandemic by ensuring that education and delivery services are carried out remotely, business activities are restored, and employees are safe. Some of the emerging innovations and advanced technologies are big data, 5G- based smart applications, advanced robotics, AI, wearable technologies, and the IoT, (Guangzhou University, 2020). Robots, AI, and drones are being installed to help implement preventive measures and track the disease and nanotechnologies, synthetic biology, and gene editing are being applied by scientists in order to test and prepare diagnostics, vaccines, and treatments. Insurance payments can be managed, medical supply chains are upheld, and contagion can be tracked through the application of blockchain. The increasing need for medical hardware is met by sustaining the effort by hospitals and governments around the world through the use of open source and three-dimensional (3D) printing technologies, for example, breathing filters, facemasks, ventilators, and necessary medical equipment are optimized and supplied. The spread of the virus is reduced through the use of telehealth technologies and this ensures that those with symptoms remain at home and worse cases are sent to the hospital. It also helps to maintain hospital capacity by operating as a possible filter (Kritikos, 2020). The approaches in the following sections can be used in the mitigation of pandemics.

8.2.1 AI

This is a useful technology because COVID-19 is identified using chest computed tomography (CT) images. It provides machines to detect COVID-19 patients through the detection of some symptoms. It predicts, tracks, and screens the present and future of COVID-19 patients. ML (Akinsola et al., 2019) has been largely used as a component of AI (Osisanwo et al., 2017; Oladapo et al, 2021). Information is provided about the identified individuals for testing, pathology and prevalence, isolation, and contact tracing (Whitelaw et al., 2020). AI is a disruptive technology that is creating a new path for information technology (IT) explorers with the use of ML (Akinsola et al., 2020). The significance of pattern-driven datasets on supervised ML makes AI achieve its objective (Akinsola et al., 2020).

8.2.2 Blockchain

A key technology that emerged in the critical domain of epidemic management is known as blockchain technology. An economical, transparent, and faster means of enabling operative decision-making can be made available through the use of this technology, and as a result, faster replies can be possible during emergencies of this kind. Blockchain can become a vital part of the worldwide reply to coronavirus by handling insurance payments, tracking the spread of the disease, and maintaining the availability of various donations and medical supply chains (Kritikos, 2020).

8.2.3 Open Source Technologies

For a better understanding of the origins and to prevent the spread of the infection, rapid data sharing is critical, and it can serve as a basis for effective care, prevention, and treatment. A multitude of IT platforms for data sharing has been recognized due to the capability of IT to allow for low costs and the distribution of data (Kritikos, 2020).

8.2.4 3D Printing

Governments around the world are taking progressively extreme actions to improve the supply of essential medical equipment and to increase production. 3D printing can play a significant part as a disruptive digital manufacturing technology when supporting the struggles of hospital workers in the middle of this emergency. In addition, it can keep patients alive as coronavirus continues to place stress on hospitals around the world (Kritikos, 2020). A crucial role could be performed by 3D printing through the production of equipment, which is very important when it is hard to source; thus, deficiencies in the supply of medical equipment in times of emergency are eased (Kritikos, 2020).

8.2.5 Telehealth Technologies

The patient is seen and diagnosed by doctors via a two-way interactive, real time, and audiovisual communication system. This includes video visits through tablets, smartphones, automated algorithms, webcam-enabled computers, and chatbots (Kritikos, 2020).

8.2.6 Comparative Analysis of IOCT

Epoch development, problem target, multipoint, run time, solution guarantee, and variable state are six characteristics that must be considered when considering IOCLT, as shown in Table 8.1. The problem targets are optimization problems and are focused on as multi-objective, nonlinear, continuous, combinatorial, and global. The variations in optimization problems as shown in Table 8.1 indicate that in combinatorial optimization an optimal solution is selected from a finite number of solutions, which gives an advantage to IOCLT. The runtime for IOCLT is short because it works on subset selection from the actual data with the use of an optimizer. The guarantee from the solution deals with the algorithm efficiency, its evaluation is based on the optimality and computational cost. The number of search points is used in all computational learning techniques, because it gives a framework to construct an optimal solution to every problem among the existing

Table 8.1   Comparative Analysis of IOCLT

Number	Assessment	Computational Learning Techniques	IOCLT
1	Epoch development	1983	2000
2	Problem target	Optimal solution	Combinatorial optimization
3	Search point	Multipoint search	Multipoint search
4	Run time	Medium	Short
5	Solution guarantee	Appropriate	Precise
6	Variable state	Mixed variable	Discrete, continuous, and mixed variables

solutions when finding an optimal result (Bezdek, 2013; Montes-Castañeda et al., 2015; Chawla & Goswami, 2015; Olyaie et al., 2017; Abdulrahman et al., 2020; Chawla & Goswami, 2015).

8.3 Materials and Methods

8.3.1 Deep Learning for Computational Learning Techniques

The application of deep learning techniques is continuously growing and attracting a lot of attention in various fields, such as speech, image, and voice recognition (Wang & Lin, 2019) as well as in the health sector when mitigating the spread of diseases. Several approaches for learning techniques, which have proved to be efficient and were used in computational intelligence, are active learning, online learning, multitasking learning, ensemble learning, and transfer learning. These learning approaches belong to ML, which are referred to as learning techniques. These approaches are implanted in the deep learning algorithm and subsequently are deployed into computational intelligence and used in a number of systems to mitigate the underlying challenges and reduce the spread of diseases such as MERS, influenzas, and SARS.

Furthermore, the sudden appearance and exponential outbreak of COVID-19 has increased the attention of researchers in making an intensive effort toward developing different methods of computational intelligence, especially by an epidemiologist in the health sector to mitigate the pandemics (Tseng et al., 2020). Computational intelligence deals with the basic level of data, such as image pixels without giving recourse the prior knowledge as in the case of AI. Both have the same goal of realizing general intelligence. However, the former is developed utilizing the concept of soft computing technologies the latter utilizes the hard computing technologies concept (Marks, 1993). The techniques of computational intelligence are varied because the problem it intends to tackle also varies, which requires a different form of approach.

Therefore, the integration of computational intelligence depends on the problem, devices, systems, and their underlying conditions. These techniques include computational modeling, data analytics, AI, high performance computing, and some fields of ML in relation to AI, which have received a lot of attention, specifically when combating pandemics (Tseng et al., 2020). There are many benefits embedded in computational intelligence because of its capabilities to adapt to various forms or conditions and the ability to handle uncertainties. These capabilities in the long run allow the aggregation of data to form partial facts, which can be transformed into something that mimics and acts like the human brain (Marks, 1993).

8.3.2 Categorization of Deep Learning Algorithm for Computational Intelligence

Various forms of computational intelligence have, over the years, been applied to deal with different kinds of underlying effects of diseases. During this period, the nature of the problem, the device to use, and the systems in which computational intelligence was deployed and their underlying conditions have necessitated the emergence of different types of deep learning algorithms, which are currently reinforcing the domain. The evidence from the achievement of deep learning when controlling past pandemics has given a new direction and inspired experts on the use of different algorithms. Deep learning technologies are used to treat infected patients through the use of radiological images to diagnose patients, discover medicines, and create new drugs that can be used to produce vaccines (Asraf et al., 2020).

Deep learning is composed of several layers of data analysis that have been filtered, such that the preceding layer outcomes serve as the successive layer input. Disease tracking, drug discovery, medical imaging, and analysis of protein structures are some of the focuses of deep learning when combating the severity of pandemics. Figure 8.1 shows different ways deep learning applications have been used recently

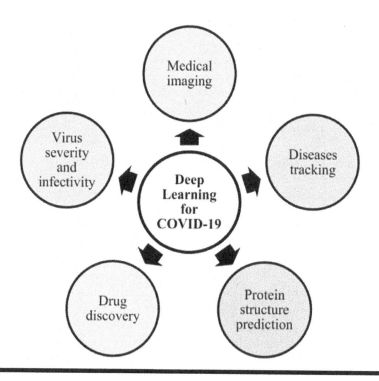

Figure 8.1 Deep learning application for COVID-19

to mitigate pandemics. Wu et al., (2020) used deep learning to diagnose medical imaging by analyzing X-rays and computing tomography which helped doctors when predicting COVID-19 infections. Disease tracking has been frequently achieved by experts through the use of deep learning techniques, which employed depth footage of the camera instead of medical imaging to analyze the patterns of respiration when predicting tachypnea (Wang et al., 2020). In the same vein, epidemiologists model the dynamics of diseases intending to identify parameters that are essentially responsible for infections spreading among the populace and the mediation impacts that govern the pandemic (Ferguson et al., 2020).

Deep learning approaches for predicting protein structures have advanced, implying that they can be used to analyze RNA structures. RNA, as a crucial component in the core dogma, is required for gene expression. By base pairing, RNAs fold into RNA secondary structures, which can then fold further to generate RNA tertiary structures. This RNA folding is critical for the numerous and intricate biological functions of RNA (Joynt & Wu, 2020). Zhavoronkov et al. (2020) employed deep learning architecture that used a pipeline for the detection of inhibitors to effectively discover drugs that could be used to handle the COVID-19 pandemic. During the discovery of virus infectivity and severity, Bartoszewicz et al. (2020) employed deep learning techniques to propose a novel approach that predicted the possibility of a virus directly infecting the human body. This approach used a sequence of the next generation with the outcome showing that CNN and long term-short memory (LSTM) networks outperformed the contemporary ML algorithms. Based on the previous discussion, various categories of deep learning algorithms for computational intelligence are stated discussed in the following sections.

8.3.2.1 CNNs

A CNN is a neural network that is considered a subcategory of ML and is the core of deep learning algorithms. What mainly distinguishes CNNs from other neural networks is the superiority of their performance in the inputs of speech, image, and audio signals. The main categories of the layers in CNNs are convolutional, pooling, and fully connected layers (IBM Cloud Education, 2020). CNNs have produced an array of research breakthroughs in computer vision, speech recognition, and other domains that have subsequently been incorporated into marketing, healthcare, retail, and automotive industries.

The performance of deep CNNs have been remarkable, especially in computer vision-related tasks and when deployed in real time through the use of models and fixed dataset that have been trained (Roy et al., 2019). Zhou (2020) proposed a theoretical framework to provide answers to questions regarding learning theory. The answers provided clarity on the ability of deep learning methods to provide generalization and approximations produced by the architecture of the network in deep CNNs. The approach showed that CNNs were universal and could be deployed for the approximation of a continuous function to generate arbitrary accuracy in a deep neural network. The automatic discovery of a COVID-19 infection model using the images of chest X-rays with an accuracy, recall rate, and precision of 89.6%, 98.2%, and 93% respectively was also proposed by Khan et al., (2020). The model used a COVID-19 trained dataset and other pneumonia chest X-ray images as well as pretrained datasets on ImageNet. A system that provided a detailed analysis of lung conditions using X-ray images was introduced by Wang et al. (2020) to differentiate the cases of COVID-19 from others through the use of CNNs, which was called COVID-Net. This evaluates the performance of the classification of the medical images using state-of-the-art architecture in the CNNs. This study used the dataset that was composed of 1,427 cases of infected X-ray images with COVID-19, pneumonia, and some other diseases for the automatic detection of coronavirus cases with specificity, accuracy, and sensitivity results of 96.46%, 96.78%, and 98.66%, respectively.

8.3.2.2 LSTMs

LSTMs are advanced recurrent neural networks (RNN) that allow information to be stored (Saxena, 2021). It has the capabilities to manage the disappearing gradient problem facing the RNN and was explicitly created for the circumvention of continuing dependency problems. LSTM has the required behavior to handle complex problems in a domain, such as speech recognition, ML, and many more (Brownlee, 2017). Several researchers have capitalized on these capabilities to bring about novel research in different domains of study. Some of the areas where LSTMs have been successfully deployed are energy consumption forecasting (Somu et al., 2020), enhancement of streamflow forecast and insight extraction (Feng et al., 2020), forecasting demand in multichannel retail (Punia et al., 2020), and fault diagnosis (Hao et al., 2020).

Also, the application of LSTM in the health sector cannot be underestimated. LSTMs have been proved to be useful in sequential observation modeling, especially in medical imaging and natural language processing, which have been applied in the screening of lung protocols for the interpretation of CTs. In the novel approach when predicting if the human body can be infected directly with a virus or not, Bartoszewicz et al. (2020) proved CNNs and LSTMs to be of optimum performance when compared with other ML algorithms. Similarly, Gao et al. (2020) proposed a time-distanced gate using LSTM that emphasized temporal models to diagnose lung cancer by evaluating pulmonary nodules based on malignancy. The study also corrected the irregularity in the sampling and acquisition of clinical imaging, which may be combined with clinical uses. Sharma et al. (2020) forecasted the risks in public health that may originate from airborne pollutants by amalgamating CNNs with LSTM models for the prediction of hourly total suspended particulate values using the encapsulation of a new feature mapping scheme. Because pollution of the air is regarded as a public health threat. However, this study could capture air quality at a high temporal resolution.

8.3.2.3 RNNs

RNNs use persistent memory that remembers the information from the previous process or output and uses it in the processing of the present input. However, RNNs are deficient because of their vanishing gradient problems and inability to remember long-term dependencies (Saxena, 2021). RNNs were deployed in health management and prognosis for the construction of smart health systems. This approach brought about intelligence and the construction of a health indicator by combining the structural benefits of CNN and RNN-based methods. It chronologically maintains the order in the arrangement of a convolution feature map by converting the data input into an array of local features.

The sequential local features are then neatly linked by an RNN, resulting in extracted features in the recurrent layer including global semantic information with time series (Chen et al., 2020). Ye et al. (2020) used the hybridization of LSTM, RNN, and bidirectional LSTM to design a risk-adapted model that could be deployed in the prediction of the possibility of getting blood pressure (BP) control targets associated with regimens of BP treatments. It employed 245,499 instances of datasets of a patient diagnosed with hypertension and that were receiving treatment, with results showing the pathway potential of the predictive model giving the optimum hypertension treatment.

Also, in an attempt to fight against the pandemic, a system that detected COVID-19 was developed by Hassan et al. (2020) using RNNs. In this study, the system took advantage of the important and recognized architecture that was embedded in the RNN as well as analyzing the features of breathing, voice, and coughing of the patients using LSTMs. Liu et al. (2020) proposed framework models that used the billing codes to predict medications utilizing RNNs. The work creates a model of pollution by utilizing a decay mechanism, and the introduction of noise into recurrent veiled states.

8.3.2.4 Generative Adversarial Networks

The essential foundations of generative adversarial networks (GANs) are made up of a generator, input vector, and discriminator with the discriminator and generator adjudged to be implicit function expressions that are mostly implemented using deep neural networks (Creswell et al., 2018). All distribution of data can be learned by the generative model with outstanding performance using adversarial methods. GANs can be used for digital image processing, cycle-GAN, and analysis of medical imaging as well as bioinformatics and medical informatics (Lan et al., 2020). Bao et al. (2020) proposed a conflict resolution between the economic resilience and public health caused by the COVID-19 pandemic. It used spatiotemporal conditional GANs to establish the mobility, such as variations in points of interest visits considering various conditions in the real world, for example, the severity of COVID-19, interventions of existing policies with a combination of data from multiple sources.

COVID-19 was detected using GANs and transfer learning models that utilized 5,863 datasets of chest X-ray images infected with pneumonia. The modeled GAN proved to be efficient as it used 10% of the trained data of the dataset and 90% of the images were generated (Khalifa et al., 2020). Waheed et al. (2020) developed an auxiliary classifier GAN-based model that produced synthetic image chest X-rays used to enhance the detection of COVID-19. Adding Covid-GAN increased the performance from the 85% classification accuracy generated by CNNs to 95% accuracy. In the same vein, the GAN technologies that diagnosed glaucoma and other eye disorders in the middle of the COVID-19 pandemic showed a high performance in the detection of retinal disease (Saeed et al., 2021).

8.3.3 Optimization Techniques

Optimization can be regarded as the process of discovering an optimal solution that is acceptable for a particular problem among various possible ones (Fouad et al., 2020). Optimization problems in the real world are complex. The tasks in optimization are mostly transformed into a multidimensional space of search problems. The search in this context is practically regarded as the maximization or minimization of the objective function. This resulting objective function evaluates the solution candidate quality, which is mostly signified by the search space vectors. The general standard optimization problem is composed of a nonlinear, single objective and the constraint of the optimization problem (Venter, 2010), as represented in Equation 8.1.

$$
\begin{aligned}
\text{Minimize: } & f(x) \\
\text{Subject to: } & g_j(x) \leq \quad j = l, m \\
& h_k(x) \quad k = l, p \\
& X_{iL} < X_i, X, X_{iu} \, I = l, n
\end{aligned}
\tag{8.1}
$$

*w*here:
$f(x)$ = goal or objective function
$g_j(x)$ = constraint in the inequality
$h_k(x)$ = constraint in the equality function; and
x = vector representing the n modified designed variables to achieve the optimum.

The design variables X_{iU} and X_{iL} represent the side constraints of the lower and upper bounds in the design space that can be searched. The objective function and constraint function can be in general terms either nonlinear or linear and an implicit function or explicit function. The implicit functions mostly occur when utilizing a numerical simulation when evaluating the response function, such as the value of stress. The optimization problem that involves the use of discrete or integer values as a design variable is regarded as a discrete or integer optimization problem. The optimization problem can be generally solved using either local or global algorithms. The difficulties encountered when solving an optimization problem that involves the use of discrete or integer variables using local algorithms can be successfully solved using global algorithms.

The side constraints are mostly considered separately by the optimization algorithms from the inequality and equality constraints. The implementation of the algorithm directly has the possibility of efficiently handling the side constraints, because side constraints can never be violated by an excellent algorithm. Thus, an optimization problem with an unconstrained function may have a side constraint but has no inequality or equality constraints when the optimization problem with a constraint has one or more inequality, or equality constraint, or both and with or without the possibility of having side constraints. Either violation or satisfaction can be achieved in a constrained optimization problem with an equality constraint and the same can occur in an inequality constraint and can be active. The active inequality constraint is the one in which $gj(x) = 0$. The general form of optimization problems specifically stated in Equation 8.1 is what optimization algorithms find solutions to. The approach is composed of looking for combinational values of design variables, which give the desired objective function that satisfies the side constraints, inequality, and equality. The various optimization algorithm can be deployed to attain the best rate for the objective function that satisfies all the conditions. The four major optimization algorithms considered are discussed in the following section.

8.3.3.1 Genetic Algorithm

A genetic algorithm is an evolutionary algorithms class that looks for approximate solutions to a search and optimization problems using the technique of a local search. This evolutionary class of algorithms (GAs) uses techniques stimulated by biology, and evolutionary biology processes, such as crossover, inheritance, mutation, and selection. The implementation of GAs is based on computer simulation in which a population of abstract representations of candidate solutions to an optimization problem evolved toward better solutions. The inspired techniques of GAs in the evolutionary algorithms in evolutionary biology start with a population of fully random individuals and happens in a generation. There is, in an individual generation, an evaluation of the whole population's fitness and the stochastic selection of multiple individuals based on fitness from the present population as well as modified either recombined or mutated. The diagram in Figure 8.2 shows the GA flow.

A GA is efficient, powerful, and can be utilized in various applications, such as ML and automatic programming as well as modeling in the immune system of humans,

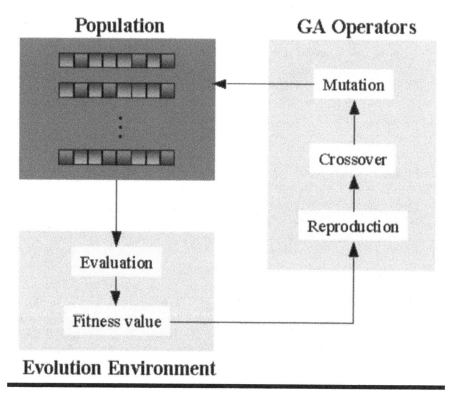

Figure 8.2 The flow of GAs

economics, population genetics, ecology, and social systems (Carr, 2014). It has a feature to solve problems that cannot be solved with other optimization methods because of their inability to handle problems with derivatives, continuity, linearity, and many more. GAs have been utilized as adaptive algorithms in engineering and science to practically solve problems as well as the computational modeling of evolutionary systems (Mitchell, 1999). GAs are utilized by genetic programming where programs represent each individual. An example of where genetic programming has been applied is in the prediction model for mortality cases and confirmed cases of COVID-19 in India (Salgotra et al., 2020).

8.3.3.2 Adam Algorithm

The Adam optimization algorithm is an alternative procedure as a replacement for stochastic gradient descent (SGD) to update the network weights iterative based on the training data (Brownlee, 2021). Adam is a prevalent algorithm and an extension of stochastic GD with great adoption in deep learning applications, because of its ability to attain excellent output within a short time. An example of the area of deep learning where the Adam optimization algorithm can be deployed is natural language processing, computer vision, and many more. The Adam algorithm is embedded with numerous attractive benefits in terms of low memory requirements, computational efficiency, ease of implementation, and intuitiveness in interpretation to mention but a few.

In the study (Khan et al., 2020) the main features were utilized in the Adam algorithm rule for the adjustment of step size against the use of the same step size for each dimension to enhance the algorithm of the Beetle Antennae search to increase the rate of convergence (Khan et al., 2020). Also, the inability of stochastic GD to handle vectors with high dimensions to achieve full gradient computation was resolved by introducing the Adam in an optimization algorithm for online learning (Zhou et al., 2020). Shams et al. (2020) utilized the Adam optimizer and stochastic GD to generate large datasets, which were required for effective results in deep neural networks in ML. The results were adjudged to be of the lowest loss function for COVID-19 detection using the generated X-ray chest images.

8.3.3.3 GD Algorithm

GD is another prevalent algorithm that performs optimization, especially in neural networks and various other algorithms in ML. However, this optimization algorithm is usually used in a block box optimizer, because its weaknesses and strengths are practically hard to explain (Ruder, 2020). The GD has three variants, which are batch GD, stochastic GD, and mini-batch GD. Each varies in terms of the size of the data required for the computation of the objective function gradient. The possibility of a trade-off between the performance time of the update and parameter update based on accuracy depends on the size of the data. Batch GD (otherwise called Vanilla GD) is used for the cost function gradient computation and is relative to the parameters of the whole data in the training dataset.

The limitation of batch GD is the memory unsuitability of difficult datasets and the possibility of being very slow, because the whole dataset calculation requires the gradient for the performance of just one update. In stochastic GD, data are fitted to an objective function using the iterative method (Plagianakos et al., 2013). Stochastic GD executes a parameter update for every individual training example; however, batch GD makes needless computations for substantial datasets because of the gradient recomputation before every individual parameter update for similar examples. The single rate of learning is maintained for all the weight updates in stochastic GD and there is no change in the learning rate during the training (Brownlee, 2021).

The mini-batch GD uses matrix optimization that is highly optimized and similar to the advanced deep learning libraries, which makes it very efficient for mini-batch of gradient computation. The mini-batch GD makes updates to the training example for each mini-batch, which subsequently gives convergence that is more stable because of the variance reduction in the parameter update. Newhagen & Bucy

(2020) utilized the information g from professionals, such as scientists and doctors during the COVID-19 pandemic on a training map for GD. GD was utilized in a neural network visualization tool as an iterative optimization algorithm to overcome the resistance to the adoption of the COVID-19 vaccine.

An attempt was made to deploy an epidemiological model to visualize the trends and evolution of COVID-19 infections based on region. GD optimization was utilized to help gain a better approximation of the parameters of the model for a particular region or country by optimizing the root mean square error on the available data for the minimization of the loss function (Barai et al., 2020).

8.3.3.4 Adaptive Gradient Algorithm

Adagrad is a gradient-based algorithm for optimization with the adaptation of the learning rate to the parameters (Duchi et al., 2011). Fewer updates are performed for each parameter associated with features that occur frequently and more updates are performed for parameters associated with features that are not frequent. Based on the previous discussion, Adagrad can be utilized to handle sparse data. In the research conducted by Dean et al. (2012), Adagrad was advantageous in the sense that it enhanced the robustness of the SGD, which was subsequently used in the large-scale training of the neural net by Google. Also, Adagrad was used by Pennington et al. (2014) for the training of words embedded in Glove since higher updates of infrequent words are required more than those that are frequent.

Zokaeinikoo et al. (2020) used Adagrad to optimize the categorization of the cross-entropy, which is a loss function in the classification of radiography chest images into categories of normal, COVID-19, and other functions. This was combined in an attempt to model interpretable AI that detected COVID-19 using radiography chest images. The benefits embedded in root mean square propagation (RMSprop) and Adagrad were also capitalized on in the artificial neural network model proposed by Ahmad & Asad (2020) for the prediction of individual COVID-19 cases in Pakistan. In the analysis model proposed by Alruwaili et al. (2021) to diagnose COVID-19 utilizing improved Inception-ResNetV2, the result adjudged the Adam and Adagrad optimizer to be of the highest performance comparison with other optimizers.

8.3.4 Evaluation Metrics

When evaluating the performance of the proposed CNN model, the epoch was used to give a holistic view of how well the model performed. Epoch is a method of hyperparameters, which shows an integral part in the training process. With the application of the epoch, the accuracy was computed as shown in Equation 8.2.

$$\text{Accuracy} = \frac{TP + TN}{TP + TN + FP + FN} \tag{8.2}$$

where:

TN and *TP* = true negative and positive, respectively

FN and *FP* = false negative and positive, respectively

The epoch processing time and loss function were also used in performance evaluation.

8.3.5 IOCLT

This chapter proposed an IOCLT framework when mitigating the pandemic. Many approaches are classified as learning techniques. Online, active, ensemble, multitask, and transfer learning are ML groups referred to as learning techniques. Therefore, IOCLT was centered on the CNNs, and optimization algorithms as characterized using the learning techniques when considering the accuracy performance metric. The CNNs framework was made up of convolutional pooling and fully connected layers. This was used to carry out feature extraction, and the fully connected layers map the extracted features into the output, which, in this chapter, was classification. The input vectors were resized to 28 × 28 pixels. A four-layered CNN with an Adam optimizer was employed when optimizing the weights of the model. The learning rate was set to 0.0001, the epoch value was 10 and the Re_{LU} and soft-max activation functions were used. The labels were transformed using one-hot encoder. Then, the data was split into a training set to train the network and a validation set for cross-validation of the model during the training phase. The validation set kept an eye on the model performance using the fine-tuned parameters and a final framework was picked. The IOCLT framework was implemented using Python, Keras with Tensorflow. The general framework of the nonlinear optimized empirical model of the proposed prediction model is shown in Figure 8.3.

8.4 Results and Discussion

8.4.1 Data Description

The considered dataset was gathered from European Centre for Disease Prevention and Control. It is the historical date (to 14 December 2020) on the daily total of COVID-19 cases and mortality rates by country worldwide. It is composed of 25,266 instances and nine columns.

8.4.2 Data Analysis and Modeling

When obtaining a correct result, and for the substantial evaluation of the nonlinear optimized empirical model, the CNN was fed with testing data. The data was trained, validated, and evaluated based on the performance of the model. This

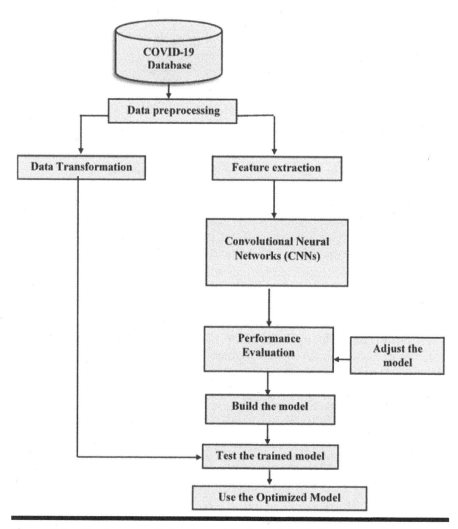

Figure 8.3 Nonlinear optimized empirical model of the proposed prediction algorithm

chapter proposed an intelligent and computation learning model for mitigating pandemics. A deep learning algorithm for computational learning techniques along-side an optimization algorithm was applied to the datasets. This was carried out in two main phases: training and testing. In the first phase, the data was preprocessed and standardized and then used to construct a nonlinear optimized empirical model. The optimization techniques were selected, such that the loss function was minimized during the training. In the testing phase, the model with the selected parameters was used for mitigation. The performance metrics were used to verify the model. The key underlying idea of this chapter was to employ an IOCLT for mitigating pandemics

8.4.3 Results Analysis

A straightforward approach without data augmentation was used and the experiments were carried out on the daily number of COVID-19 cases and deaths by country worldwide using various hyperparameters and with various epoch values for training the model. The computational speed along the accuracy of the model based on the different epochs was calculated and compared. This was carried out to determine what the accuracy effects were and if there was any overfitting.

Figure 8.4 shows the increase in the loss function as a result of the increase in the epochs. At epoch = 1, it was noticed that the loss function was 0.3652 for training and 0.0741 for validation. Also, at epoch = 2, the loss function was 0.059 for training and 0.0593 for validation with slight changes. At epoch = 3, there was a slight increment in the loss function to 0.0332 for training at the same time as 0.0506 for validation. When epoch = 4, the loss function for training was 0.0204 with a reduced value of 0.0512 for validation. At epoch = 5, the loss function was 0.0142 for training and 0.0573 for validation. The loss function for the 10 epoch shows that there were variations from the first epoch and there was consistency in the trained and validation data toward epochs 8–10.

From Figure 8.5, at epoch = 1, it was noticed that the accuracy was 89.36%. Also, at epoch = 2, the accuracy was 98.36%. At epoch = 3, there was a slight increase in the accuracy to 99.04%. When epoch = 4, the accuracy was 99.4%. At epoch = 5, the accuracy was 99.61%. In addition, as epoch = 6, the accuracy was 99.71%. At epoch = 7, the accuracy was 99.88%. At epoch = 8, the accuracy was 99.74%. Furthermore, at epochs = 9 and 10, the accuracy was 99.84% and 99.91%, respectively. The epoch was finally allocated as 10 to train the model and there was a very good accuracy of 99.91%.

From Figure 8.6, at epoch = 1, it was noticed that the accuracy was 89.36% at 59. 91 s. Also, at epoch = 2, the accuracy was 98.36% at 43.91 s. At epoch = 3, there was a slight increase in the accuracy to 99.04% at the same time of 43.91 s. When epoch = 4, the accuracy was 99.4% at a reduced time of 43.92 s. At epoch = 5, the accuracy was 99.61% at 43.91 s. In addition, at epoch = 6, the accuracy was 99.71% at the same time. At epoch = 7, the accuracy was 99.88% with the same time limit of 43.92 s. At epoch = 8, the accuracy was 99.74% at the same average time. Furthermore, at epochs = 9 and 10, the accuracy was 99.84% and 99.91%, respectively at the same time of 43.92 s. The epoch was finally allocated as 10 to train the model at an average time of 43.92 s because there was consistency in the trained and validation data toward epochs 8–10.

From Figure 8.7, at epoch = 1, it was noticed that the accuracy was 89.36% at 59.91 s. Also, at epoch = 2, the accuracy was 98.36% at 43.91 s. At epoch = 3, there was a slight increase in the accuracy to 99.04% at the same time of 43.91 s. When epoch = 4, the accuracy was 99.4% at a reduced time of 43.92 s. At epoch = 5, the accuracy was 99.61% at 43.91 s. In addition, as epoch = 6, the accuracy was 99.71% at the same time. At epoch = 7, the accuracy was 99.88% with the same

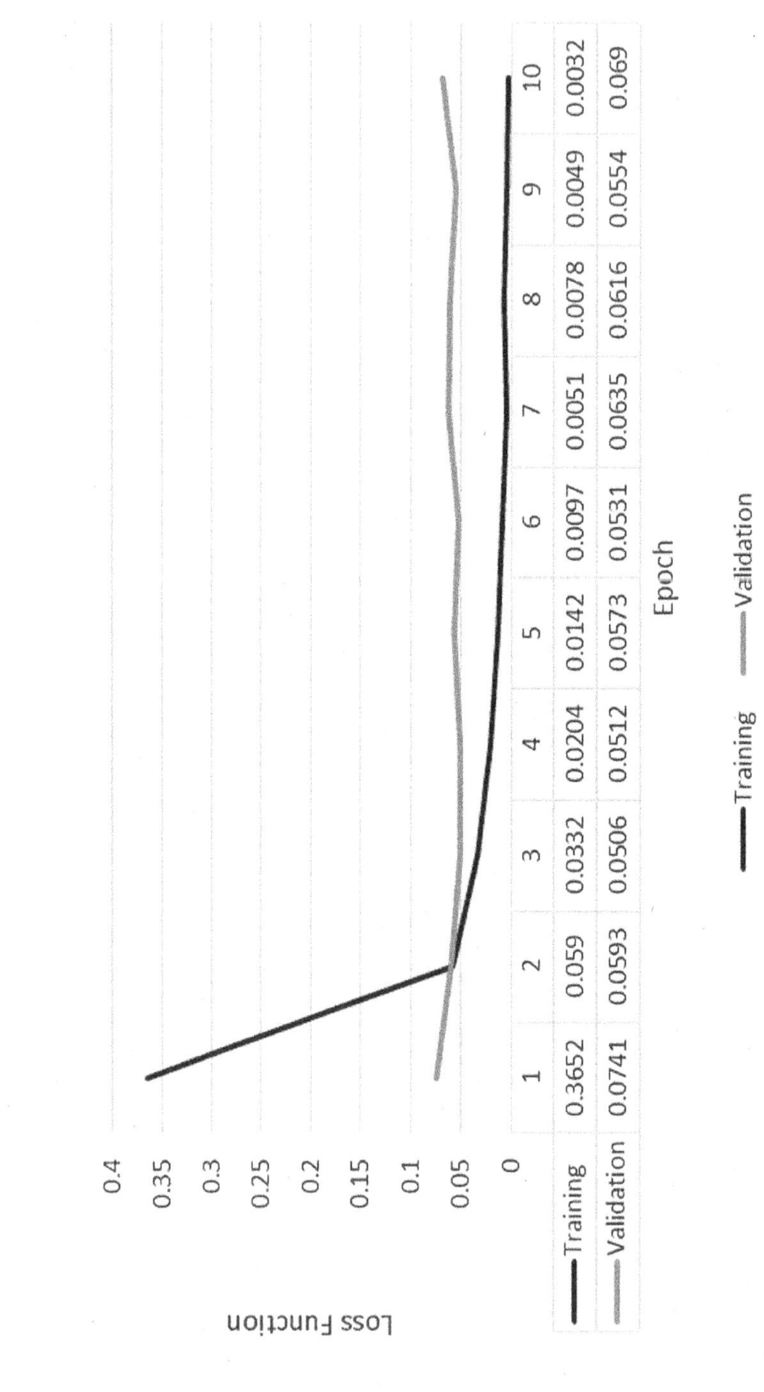

Loss Function
0.4
0.35
0.3
0.25
0.2
0.15
0.1
0.05
0
Training
Validation
1 2 3 4 5 6 7 8 9 10
Training 0.3652 0.059 0.0332 0.0204 0.0142 0.0097 0.0051 0.0078 0.0049 0.0032
Validation 0.0741 0.0593 0.0506 0.0512 0.0573 0.0531 0.0635 0.0616 0.0554 0.069
Epoch
Training
Validation

Figure 8.4 Loss function using 10 epochs

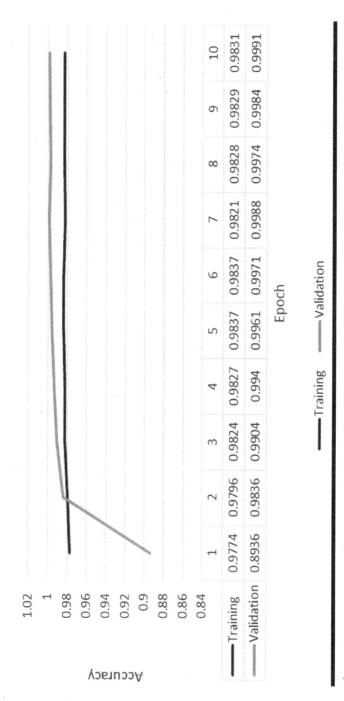

	1	2	3	4	5	6	7	8	9	10
Training	0.9774	0.9796	0.9824	0.9827	0.9837	0.9837	0.9821	0.9828	0.9829	0.9831
Validation	0.8936	0.9836	0.9904	0.994	0.9961	0.9971	0.9988	0.9974	0.9984	0.9991

Figure 8.5   Accuracy using 10 epochs

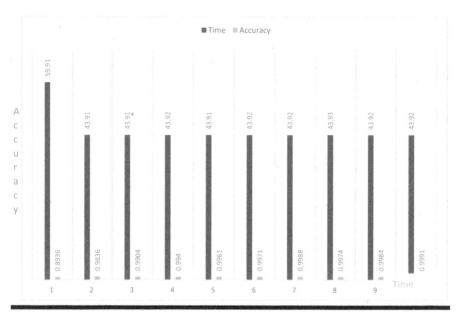

Figure 8.6   Accuracy against time using 10 epochs

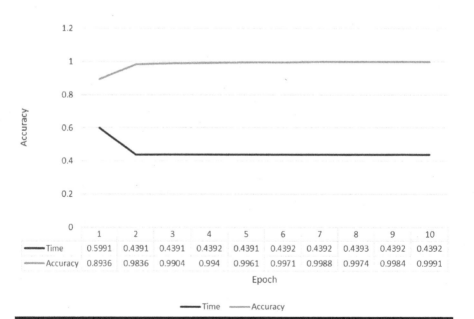

Figure 8.7   Accuracy against time using 10 epochs

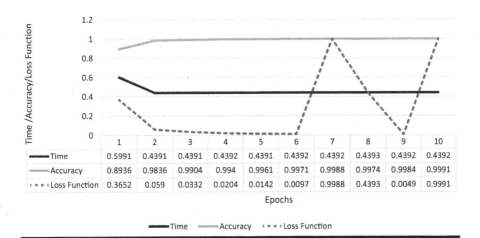

Figure 8.8 Accuracy against loss function and time using 10 epochs

Table 8.2 Number of Epochs, Accuracy, and Timing of the Model

Epoch	Time	Accuracy	Loss function
1	59.91 s	0.8936	0.3652
2	43. 91 s	0.9836	0.059
3	43.91 s	0.9904	0.0332
4	43.92 s	0.994	0.0204
5	43.91 s	0.9961	0.0142
6	43.92 s	0.9971	0.0097
7	43.92 s	0.9988	0.0051
8	43.93 s	0.9974	0.0078
9	43.92 s	0.9984	0.0049
10	43.92 s	0.9991	0.0032

time limit of 43.92 s. At epoch = 8, the accuracy was 99.74% at the same average time. Furthermore, at epochs = 9 and 10, the accuracy was 99.84% and 99.91%, respectively at the same time of 43.92 s.

From Figure 8.8 and Table 8.2, at epoch = 1, it was noticed that the accuracy was 89.36% at 59.91 s. Also, at epoch = 2, the accuracy was 98.36% at 43.91 s. At epoch = 3, there was a slight increase in the accuracy to 99.04% at the same time of 43.91 s. When epoch = 4, the accuracy was 99.4% at a reduced time of 43.92 s. At epoch = 5, the accuracy was 99.61% at 43.91 s. In addition, at epoch = 6, the accuracy was 99.71% at the same time. At epoch = 7, the accuracy was 99.88% with the same time limit of 43.92 s. At epoch = 8, the accuracy was 99.74% at the same average time. Furthermore, at epochs = 9 and 10, the accuracy was 99.84% and 99.91%, respectively at the same time of 43.92 s. The loss function for 10 epochs shows that there were variations from the first epoch and there was consistency in the trained and validation data toward epochs 8–10. Also, as the epochs were increasing, the accuracy increased until knew to stop, which is called early stopping. Also, the validation loss function increase when the epochs were improved, this is overfitting; therefore, to get better accuracy at epoch = 10, we can safely stop the training process. Next, a nonlinear optimized empirical CNN model was built with 25 convolutional layers and 10 hidden layers one input and 10 output. The epoch was finally allocated as10 to train the model and there was a very good accuracy of 99.91%.

Overall, this chapter proved that the CNN model does not require hand-crafted feature extraction and the architectures do not necessarily require the segmentation of tumors or organs by a human expert. Finally, it is more data-hungry because of the millions of learnable parameters for estimations. Thus, it is better for computations and inexpensive and requires graphical processing units for model training (Rikiya et al., 2018). Also, comparing CNNs with other traditional ML techniques requires no preprocessing for characteristic extraction and its performance relatively depends on the existence of large databases (Guimarães et al., 2019).

From Table 8.3, the validation accuracy of the model increased from 97.74% to 98.31% when the epochs were initialized from 1 to 10. In the same vein, from Table 8.3, the accuracy of the model increased from 89.36% to 99.91%, which meant the accuracy increased as the epochs increased. This gave a good accuracy of 99.91% after the epoch was initialized to 10.

Table 8.3   Number of Epochs, Validation_Loss Function and Validation_Accuracy of the Model

Epoch	Validation_Loss function	Validation Accuracy
1	0.0741	0.9774
2	0.0593	0.9796
3	0.0506	0.9824
4	0.0512	0.9827
5	0.0573	0.9837
6	0.0531	0.9837
7	0.0635	0.9821
8	0.0616	0.9828
9	0.0554	0.9829
10	0.069	0.9831

The proposed deep learning algorithm for computational learning techniques alongside an optimization algorithm has shown that accuracy increased as the epochs increased and this complemented the work by Bharati et al. (2021a), which utilized the resize, normalizing, and augmenting of the CO-ResNet with different epochs testing for optimization when detecting COVID-19 and pneumonia with normal healthy lung controls. The accuracy also increased as the epochs increased to 30, and it was noticed that the 10 epochs could not reduce the validation loss. Also, Mondal et al. (2020) highlighted the potential applications of data analytics on pandemics at an accuracy of 91%, which served as an important aspect for mitigating pandemics. The results have shown that ML with a value of 98% can forecast the spread of COVID-19 and predict the need for admissions to ICU units, which agrees with the findings of a study using another method (Podder et al., 2021). A study by Bharati et al. (2020) confirmed that various forms of existing deep learning techniques can be applied for the prediction of lung disease and this has further confirmed that it can be replicated for mitigating pandemics even with an optimization technique. Likewise, it was determined in a review on the application of deep learning models to be an important feature of vaccine discovery that helps when mitigating the pandemic (Bharati et al., 2021b).

8.5 Limitations and Future Scopes

The following are the limitations associated with IOCLT for mitigating pandemics.

1. Imagery dataset was not considered in this chapter, which could have given more elucidating information
2. Datasets are difficult to acquire when thinking about the privacy of patient records besides, they are not readily accessible in large electronic formats for transfer to learning implementation
3. The variations in the outbreaks of pandemics have caused nonconsistency in the research outputs by various researchers, which have led to different variants of COVID-19 vaccines being produced
4. The transparency and rules governing the release of the pandemic test results made the nonavailability of the dataset a problem in real time for timely research

The following could be considered as recommendations for future studies in the pandemic domain.

1. Development of an application for the implementation in the mitigation of pandemics using IOCLT
2. Design of systems with enhanced IUI, which is anchored on the paradigms of IOCLT
3. Utilization of blockchain paradigms for mitigating pandemics alongside IOCLT

8.6 Conclusions

This chapter introduced and described a new term, IOCLT. This new approach showed how best to construct a nonlinear optimized empirical model using a CNN deep learning algorithm for computational learning techniques alongside an optimization algorithm (Adam optimizer) when optimizing the weights of the model. The proposed model was applied to a dataset of 25,266 instances and nine columns from COVID-19 cases and mortality rates. This was carried out in two main phases: training and testing. In the first phase, the data was preprocessed and standardized and was then used to construct a nonlinear optimized empirical model. The optimization techniques were selected, such that the loss function was minimized during the training. Also, the best approach to avoid overfitting could be determined through the process of early stopping (e.g., as soon as the validation error moved up that was when the training process was expected to stop). When the model was overfitted it showed that the model is memorizing the training data, and this will be bad for the model as it was learning then. Then, during the testing phase, the model with the selected parameters was used for mitigation. The performance metrics were used to verify the model. The results demonstrated that the model achieved better performances when the epoch was 10 because the nonlinear optimized empirical model has shown that accuracy increased as the epochs increased, 99.91% after the epoch was initialized to 10. In future work, attention shall be given to other computational learning as well as optimization techniques when considering other deep learning algorithms. Therefore, more examples of the dataset as well as different datasets for efficient comparison will be utilized when following principal component analysis.

References

Abdulrahman, S. A., Khalifa, W., Roushdy, M., & Salem, A. B. M. (2020). Comparative study for 8 computational intelligence algorithms for human identification. *Computer Science Review*, 36, doi.10.1016/j.cosrev.2020.100237

Ahmad, I., & Asad, S. M. (2020). Predictions of coronavirus COVID-19 distinct cases in Pakistan through an artificial neural network. *Epidemiology and Infection*, 148(September), 1–10. doi.10.1017/S0950268820002174

Akinsola, J. E. T., Adeagbo, M. A., & Awoseyi, A. A. (2019). Breast cancer predictive analytics using supervised machine learning techniques. *International Journal of Advanced Trends in Computer Science and Engineering*, 8(6), 3095–3104. doi.10.30534/ijatcse/2019/70862019

Akinsola, J. E. T., Akinseinde, S., Kalesanwo, O., Adeagbo, M., Oladapo, K., Awoseyi, A., & Kasali, F. (2021). Application of artificial intelligence in user interfaces design for cyber security threat modeling. In *Intelligence User Interface* (pp. 1–28). IntechOpen.

Akinsola, J. E. T., Awodele, O., Idowu, S. A., & Kuyoro, S. O. (2020). SQL injection attacks predictive analytics using supervised machine learning techniques. *International*

Journal of Computer Applications Technology and Research, 9(4), 139–149. doi.10.7753/ijcatr0904.1004

Akinsola, J. E. T., Awodele, O., Kuyoro, S. O., & Kasali, F. A. (2019). Performance evaluation of supervised machine learning algorithms using multi-criteria decision making techniques. Paper presented at the International Conference on Information Technology in Education and Development (ITED), 17–34 Retrieved from https://ir.tech-u.edu.ng/416/1/Performance Evaluation of Supervised Machine Learning Algorithms Using Multi-Criteria Decision Making %28MCDM%29 Techniques ITED.pdf

Akinsola, J. E. T., Kuyoro, A., Adeagbo, M. A., & Awoseyi, A. A. (2020). Performance evaluation of software using formal methods. *Global Journal of Computer Science and Technology: C Software & Data Engineering, 20*(1). https://computerresearch.org/index.php/computer/article/view/1930/1914

Alruwaili, M., Shehab, A., & Abd El-Ghany, S. (2021). COVID-19 diagnosis using an enhanced inception-ResNetV2 deep learning model in CXR images. *Journal of Healthcare Engineering,* 1–16. doi.10.1155/2021/6658058

Asraf, A., Islam, M. Z., Haque, M. R., & Islam, M. M. (2020). Deep learning aApplications to combat novel coronavirus (COVID-19) pandemic. *SN Computer Science, 1*(363), 1–7. doi.10.1007/s42979-020-00383-w

Balkhair, A. A. (2020). Covid-19 pandemic: A new chapter in the history of infectious diseases. *Oman Medical Journal, 35*(2), e123. doi.10.5001/OMJ.2020.41

Bansal, A., Padappayil, R. P., Garg, C., Singal, A., Gupta, M., & Klein, A. (2020). Utility of artificial intelligence amidst the COVID 19 Pandemic: A Review. *Journal of Medical Systems, 44*(9). doi.10.1007/s10916-020-01617-3

Bao, H., Zhou, X., Zhang, Y., Li, Y., & Xie, Y. (2020). COVID-GAN: Estimating human mobility responses to COVID-19 pandemic through spatio-temporal conditional generative adversarial networks. Paper presented at the Proceedings of the 28th International Conference on Advances in Geographic Information Systems, 273–282. doi.10.1145/3397536.3422261

Barai, A. K., Singh, A., & Shinde, A. (2020). Modelling and data-based analysis of COVID-19 outbreak in India: A study on impact of social distancing measures. *Medrxiv: Report of the New Medical Research, May,* 1–6. doi.10.1101/2020.05.12.20099184

Bartoszewicz, J. M., Seidel, A., & Renard, B. Y. (2020). Interpretable detection of novel human viruses from genome sequencing data. *NAR Genomics and Bioinformatics, 3*(1), 1–14. doi.10.1101/2020.01.29.92535 4

Bezdek, J. C. (2013). The history, philosophy and development of computational intelligence (how a simple tune became a monster nit). *Encyclopedia of Life Support Systems,* pp. 1–22).

Bharati, S., Podder, P., & Mondal, M. R. H. (2020). Hybrid deep learning for detecting lung diseases from X-ray images. *Informatics in Medicine Unlocked, 20,* 100391. doi.10.1016/j.imu.2020.100391

Bharati, S., Podder, P., Mondal, M. R. H., & Prasath, V. B. S. (2021a). CO-ResNet: Optimized ResNet model for COVID-19 diagnosis from X-ray images. *International Journal of Hybrid Intelligent Systems, 17*(1–2), 71–85. doi.10.3233/his-210008

Bharati, S., Podder, P., Mondal, M. R. H., & Prasath, V. B. S. (2021b). Medical imaging with deep learning for COVID-19 diagnosis: A comprehensive review. *International Journal of Computer Information Systems and Industrial Management Applications, 13,* 1–22.

Brownlee, J. (2021). *Gentle Introduction to the Adam Optimization Algorithm for Deep Learning.* Retrieved from https://machinelearningmastery.com/adam-optimization-algorithm-for-deep-learning/

Carr, J. (2014). An introduction to genetic algorithms. *Senior Project*, 1(40), 7

Chawla, S., & Goswami, N. (2015). Comparative analysis of computational intelligence paradigms in WSN: A review. *IOSR Journal of Computer Engineering Ver. II*, 17(6), 2278–2661. doi.10.9790/0661-17624449

Chen, L., Xu, G., Zhang, S., Yan, W., & Wu, Q. (2020). Health indicator construction of machinery based on end-to-end trainable convolution recurrent neural networks. *Journal of Manufacturing Systems*, 54(1), 1–11. doi.10.1016/j.jmsy.2019.11.008

Creswell, A., White, T., Dumoulin, V., Arulkumaran, K., Sengupta, B., & Bharath, A. A. (2018). Generative adversarial networks: An overview. *IEEE Signal Processing Magazine*, 35(1), 53–65.

Dean, J., Corrado, G. S., Monga, R., Chen, K., Devin, M., & Le, Q. V.(2012). Large scale distributed deep networks Jeffrey. *NIPS 2012: Neural Information Processing Systems*, 1(11).

Duchi, J., Hazan, E., & Singer, Y. (2011). Adaptive subgradient methods for online learning and stochastic optimization. *Journal of Machine Learning Research*, 12, 2121–2159.

Feng, D., Fang, K., & Shen, C. (2020). Enhancing streamflow forecast and extracting insights using long short term memory networks with data integration at continental scales. *Water Resources Research*, 56(9). doi.10.1029/2019WR026793

Ferguson, N., Laydon, D., Nedjati Gilani, G., Imai, N., Ainslie, K., Baguelin, M., ... Ghani, A. (2020). Impact of non-pharmaceutical interventions (NPIs) to reduce COVID-19 mortality and healthcare demand. *Imperial College COVID-19 Response Team.* doi.10.25561/77482

Fouad, M. M., El-Desouky, A. I., Al-Hajj, R., & El-Kenawy, E. S. M. (2020). Dynamic group-based cooperative optimization algorithm. *IEEE Access*, 8, 148378–148403. doi.10.1109/ACCESS.2020.3015892

Gao, R., Tang, Y., Xu, K., Huo, Y., Bao, S., Antic, S. L. ...Landman, B. A. (2020). Time-distanced gates in long short-term memory networks. *Medical Image Analysis*, 65, 101785. doi.10.1016/j.media.2020.101785

Guimarães, M., Costa, F., Paulo, J., Campos, M., & Aquino, G. De. (2019). Evaluating the performance of convolutional neural networks with direct acyclic graph architectures in automatic segmentation of breast lesion in US images. *BMC Medical Imaging*, 19(85), 1–13. doi.10.1186/s12880-019-0389-2

Hao, S., Ge, F. X., Li, Y., & Jiang, J. (2020). Multisensor bearing fault diagnosis based on one-dimensional convolutional long short-term memory networks. *Measurement: Journal of the International Measurement Confederation*, 159, 107802. doi.10.1016/j.measurement.2020.107802

Hassan, A., Shahin, I., & Alsabek, M. B. (2020). COVID-19 detection system using recurrent neural networks. Paper presented at the 2020 International Conference on communications, computing, cybersecurity, and informatics (CCCI) IEEE Xplore, December, 6–10. doi.10.1109/CCCI49893.2020.9256562

IBM Cloud Education. (2020). *Convolutional Neural Networks.* IBM Cloud Learn Hub.

Joynt, G. M., & Wu, W. K. (2020). Understanding COVID-19: what does viral RNA load really mean? *The Lancet Infectious Diseases*, 20(6), 635–636. doi.10.1016/S1473-3099(20)30237-1

Khalifa, N. E. M., Taha, M. H. N., Hassanien, A. E., & Elghamrawy, S. (2020). Detection of Coronavirus (COVID-19) associated pneumonia based on generative adversarial networks and a fine-tuned deep transfer learning model using chest X-ray dataset. *arXiv preprint arXiv:2004.01184*. 1–15.

Khan, A. H., Cao, X., Li, S., Katsikis, V. N., & Liao, L. (2020). BAS-ADAM: An ADAM based approach to improve the performance of beetle antennae search optimizer. *IEEE/CAA Journal of Automatica Sinica*, *7*(2), 461–471. doi.10.1109/JAS.2020.1003048

Khan, A. I., Shah, J. L., & Bhat, M. M. (2020). CoroNet: A deep neural network for detection and diagnosis of COVID-19 from chest X-ray images. *Computer Methods and Programs in Biomedicine*, *196*, 105581, 1–9. doi.10.1016/j.cmpb.2020.105581

Kritikos, M. (2020). Ten technologies to fight coronavirus. *European Parliamentary Research Service*. Retrieved from https://policycommons.net/artifacts/1337141/ten-technologies-to-fight-coronavirus/1944801/

Lan, L., You, L., Zhang, Z., Fan, Z., Zhao, W., Zeng, N., … Zhou, X. (2020). Generative adversarial networks and its applications in biomedical informatics. *Frontiers in Public Health*, *8*(May), 1–14. doi.10.3389/fpubh.2020.00164

Liu, D., Wu, Y. L., Li, X., & Qi, L. (2020). Medi-Care AI: Predicting medications from billing codes via robust recurrent neural networks. *Neural Networks*, *124*, 109–116. doi.10.1016/j.neunet.2020.01.001

Madhav, N., Oppenheim, B., Gallivan, M., Mulembakani, P., Rubin, E., & Wolfe., N. (2017). *Pandemics: Risks, Impacts, and Mitigation – Disease Control Priorities: Improving Health and Reducing Poverty – NCBI Bookshelf*.

Marks, R. (1993). Intelligence: Computational versus artificial. *IEEE Transactions on Neural Networks*, *4*(5), 1–3.

Mitchell, M. (1999). An Introduction to genetic algorithms. In *A Bradford Book the MIT Press* (fifth). Massachusetts Institute of Technology.

Mondal, M. R. H., Bharati, S., & Podder, P. (2021) CO-IRv2: Optimized InceptionResNetV2 for COVID-19 detection from chest CT images. *PLoS One*, *16*(10): e0259179. doi.10.1371/journal.pone.0259179

Mondal, M. R. H., Bharati, S., Podder, P., & Podder, P. (2020). Data analytics for novel coronavirus disease. *Informatics in Medicine Unlocked*, *20*. doi.10.1016/j.imu.2020.100374

Newhagen, J. E., & Bucy, E. P. (2020). *Overcoming resistance to COVID-19 vaccine adoption: How affective dispositions shape views of science and medicine.* Harvard Kennedy School Misinformation Review. doi.10.37016/mr-2020-44

Nguyen, T. T., Nguyen, Q. V. H., Nguyen, D. T., Hsu, E. B., Yang, S., & Eklund, P. (2020). Artificial intelligence in the battle against Coronavirus (COVID-19): A survey and future research directions. *Arxiv*, 1–14.

Oladapo K.A., Ayankoya F.Y., Adekunle, F.A., & Idowu, S.A. (2021). Detection and prediction of pluvial flood using machine learning techniques. *Journal of Computer Science and Its Application 27*(2),139–145.

Olyaie, E., Zare Abyaneh, H., & Danandeh Mehr, A. (2017). A comparative analysis among computational intelligence techniques for dissolved oxygen prediction in Delaware River. *Geoscience Frontiers*, *8*(3), 517–527. doi.10.1016/j.gsf.2016.04.007

Osisanwo, F. Y., Akinsola, J. E. T., Awodele, O., Hinmikaiye, J. O., Olakanmi, O., & Akinjobi, J. (2017). Supervised machine learning algorithms: Classification and comparison. *International Journal of Computer Trends and Technology 48*(3), 128–138.

Pennington, J., Socher, R., & Manning, C. D. (2014). GloVe: Global vectors for word representation. Paper presented at the Proceedings of the 2014 Conference on Empirical Methods in Natural Language Processing 1532–1543. doi.10.3115/v1/D14-1162

Plagianakos, V. P., Magoulas, G. D., & Vrahatis, N. M. (2013). Learning rate adaptation in stochastic gradient descent. In Hadjisavvas, Nicolas, Pardalos, & Panos (Eds.), *Advances in convex analysis and global optimization: Honoring the memory of C. Caratheodory (1873–1950)* (54). doi.10.1007/978-1-4613-0279-7_27

Podder, P., Khamparia, A., Rubaiyat Hossain Mondal, M., Rahman, M. A., & Bharati, S. (2021). Forecasting the spread of COVID-19 and ICU requirements. *International Journal of Online and Biomedical Engineering, 17*(5), 81–99. doi.10.3991/ijoe. v17i05.20009

Punia, S., Nikolopoulos, K., Singh, S. P., Madaan, J. K., & Litsiou, K. (2020). Deep learning with long short-term memory networks and random forests for demand forecasting in multi-channel retail. *International Journal of Production Research, 58*(16), 4964–4979. doi.10.1080/00207543.2020.1735666

Rikiya, Y., Mizuho, N., Richard, K., Do, G., & Kaori, T. (2018). Convolutional neural networks: an overview and application in radiology. *Insights Imaging, 9*, 611–629. doi.10.1007/s13244-018-0639-9

Roy, D., Panda, P., & Roy, K. (2019). Tree-CNN: A hierarchical deep convolutional neural network for incremental learning. *Neural Networks, 121*, 148–160. doi.10.1016/j.neunet.2019.09.010

Ruder, S. (2020). An overview of gradient descent optimization algorithms. *ArXiv, abs/1609.04747.*

Saeed, A. Q., Norul, S., Sheikh, H., & Che-hamzah, J. (2021). Accuracy of using generative adversarial networks for glaucoma detection during the COVID-19 pandemic: A systematic review and bibliometric analysis. *National Library of Medicine,* 1–2. doi.10.2196/27414

Salgotra, R., Gandomi, M., & Gandomi, A. H. (2020). Time series analysis and forecast of the COVID-19 pandemic in India using genetic programming. *Chaos, Solitons and Fractals, 138*, 109945. doi.10.1016/j.chaos.2020.109945

Saxena, S. (2021). Introduction to long short term memory (LSTM). *Analytics Vidhya.* www. analyticsvidhya.com/blog/2021/03/introduction-to-long-short-term-memory-lstm/.

Shams, M. Y., Elzeki, O. M., Abd Elfattah, M., Medhat, T., & Hassanien, A. E. (2020). *Why Are Generative Adversarial Networks Vital for Deep Neural Networks? A Case Study on COVID-19 Chest X-ray Images.* Springer International Publishing. doi.10.1007/978-3-030-55258-9_9

Sharma, E., Deo, R. C., Prasad, R., Parisi, A. V., & Raj, N. (2020). Deep air quality forecasts: Suspended particulate matter modeling with convolutional neural and long short-term memory networks. *IEEE Access, 8*, 209503–209516. doi.10.1109/ACCESS.2020.3039002

Somu, N., Guathama Raman M.R., & Ramamritham, K. (2020). A hybrid model for building energy consumption forecasting using long short-term memory networks. *Applied Energy, 261*(November), 114131. doi.10.1016/j.apenergy.2019.114131

Tayarani, M. (2021). Applications of artificial intelligence in battling against COVID-19: A literature review. *Chaos, Solitons and Fractals.* 142:110338. doi. 10.1016/j.chaos.2020.110338.

Tseng, V. S., Ying, J., Wong, S. T. C., Cook, D. J., & Liu, J. (2020). Computational intelligence techniques for combating COVID-19: A survey. *IEEE Computational Intelligence Magazine, 15*(4), 10–22. doi.10.1109/MCI.2020.3019873

Vaishya, R., Haleem, A., Vaish, A., & Javaid, M. (2020). Emerging technologies to combat the COVID-19 pandemic. *Journal of Clinical and Experimental Hepatology, 10*(4), 409–411.

Venter, G. (2010). Review of optimization techniques. *Encyclopedia of aerospace engineering,* 1–12. doi.10.1002/9780470686652.eae495

Waheed, A., Goyal, M., Gupta, D., Khanna, A., Al-Turjman, F., & Pinheiro, P. R. (2020). CovidGAN: Data augmentation using auxiliary classifier GAN for improved Covid-19 detection. *IEEE Access, 8,* 91916–91923. doi.10.1109/ACCESS.2020.2994762

Wang, Y., Hu, M., Li, Q., Zhang, X.-P., Zha, G., & Yao, N. (2020). Abnormal Respiratory Patterns Classifier May Contribute to large-Scale Screening of People Infected with Covid-19 in an Accurate and Unobtrusive Manner. arXiv preprint arXiv:2002.05534

Wang, Y., & Lin, G. (2019). Efficient deep learning techniques for multiphase flow simulation in heterogeneous porous media. *Journal of computational physics, 401,* 1–30. doi.10.1016/j.jcp.2019.108968

Whitelaw, S., Mamas, M. A., Topol, E., & Spall, H. G. C. Van. (2020). Viewpoint applications of digital technology in COVID-19 pandemic planning and response. *The Lancet Digital Health, 2*(8), 1–6. doi.10.1016/S2589-7500(20)30142-4

WHO. (2020). Epidemic and pandemic diseases. *WHO EMRO | MERS Situation Update,* 58–65.

Wu, X., Hui, H., Niu, M., Li, L., Wang, L., He, B., …Zha, Y. (2020). Deep learning-based multi-view fusion model for screening 2019 novel coronavirus pneumonia: A multicentre study. *European Journal of Radiology, 128*(March), 1–9. doi.10.1016/j.ejrad.2020.109041

Ye, X., Zeng, Q. T., Facelli, J. C., Brixner, D. I., Conway, M., & Bray, B. E. (2020). Predicting optimal hypertension treatment pathways using recurrent neural networks. *International Journal of Medical Informatics, 139*(November), 104122. doi.10.1016/j.ijmedinf.2020.104122

Zhavoronkov, A., Aladinskiy, V. A., Zhebrak, A., Zagribelnyy, B., Terentiev, V., Bezrukov, D. S., … Ivanenkov, Y. A. (2020). Potential 2019-nCoV 3C-like protease inhibitors designed using generative deep learning approaches. *Insilico Medicine.* doi.10.26434/chemrxiv.11829102.v2

Zhou, D. X. (2020). Universality of deep convolutional neural networks. *Applied and Computational Harmonic Analysis, 48*(2), 787–794. doi.10.1016/j.acha.2019.06.004

Zhou, Y., Zhang, M., Zhu, J., Zheng, R., & Wu, Q. (2020). A randomized block-coordinate Adam online learning optimization algorithm. *Neural Computing and Applications, 32*(16), 12671–12684. doi.10.1007/s00521-020-04718-9

Zokaeinikoo, M., Kazemian, P., Mitra, P., & Kumara, S. (2020). AIDCOV: An interpretable artificial intelligence model for detection of COVID-19 from chest radiography images. *Medrxiv: Report of New Medical Research,* 1–8. doi.10.1101/2020.05.24.20111922

Chapter 9

Various Deep Learning Methodologies for COVID-19 Diagnosis

K. Patel, B. Patel, and M. Bohara
Computer Science and Engineering, Devang Patel Institute of Advance Technology and Research, CHARUSAT, India

D. Patel
Computer Engineering, Chandubhai S. Patel Institute of Technology, CHARUSAT, India

A. Ganatra
Devang Patel Institute of Advance Technology and Research, CHARUSAT, India

Contents

DOI: 10.1201/9781003324447-9

9.1 Introduction: Background and AI in COVID-19

A novel coronavirus (SARS-CoV-2,) appeared in late December 2019, which was the start of the pandemic. This illness in a respiratory pandemic, also known as coronavirus, has been a difficult issue that can present in a number of different forms and severities, varying between minor to serious, with the possibility of organ failure and death of the patient. Symptoms range from multiorgan failure, moderate and severe progressive pneumonia, and self-limiting respiratory infections, to death. There are significant reasons to be concerned about the virus' implications as the pandemic progresses, with an increasing number of COVID-19 confirmed cases and individuals suffering from severe respiratory failure and cardiovascular issues (Jamshidi, 2020). The significance of defining suitable strategies to address COVID-19–related difficulties has attracted a lot of attention. There are many other problems that researchers face today, such as the increasing amounts of data, which is termed big data, in the fight against COVID-19. This demonstrates the need for artificial intelligence (AI), and how it could be critical in the development and improvements in the worldwide health care systems. AI has recently received increased research in a variety of domains, including medicine, psychology, engineering, and economics (Bharati, 2021a). As a result, in a difficult condition like this, it's critical to mobilize and save medical, logistical, and resources that humans rely on. Therefore, AI is the solution that could help with that and save a lot of time in a pandemic situation where 1 h saved could help to save the lives of others where coronavirus is taking the lives of people. With AI's growing popularity in healthcare settings, it can help to reduce the number of irrelevant data unwanted removals while also improving productivity and efficiency in large-scale research, and greater prediction and diagnosis accuracy is needed. In addition, research on modeling viral activity in any country could be facilitated with the use of big data. Health care policymakers could use the outcomes analysis to prepare their country for a disease outbreak and make well-informed decisions. For example, medical diagnosis based on images, which can provide a quick and precise diagnosis of COVID-19 and save lives, is one field that could benefit from AI's beneficial input. The different techniques in AI could be helpful to address coronavirus-related concerns, filling the gap between medical techniques and therapies and AI solutions and medical approaches and therapies. The AI experts use an AI platform, which assists in creating collaborations between different aspects and speeds up procedures to achieve an optimal outcome. The most recent research emphasized COVID-19, and its numerous issues are used in this chapter to generalize and recommend a number of techniques that are relevant to radiology, epidemiology, high-risk groups, and other topics. The chapter analyzes and shows the possibilities of AI-based deep learning (DL) techniques to address COVID-19–related difficulties as it progresses.

9.1.1 AI and COVID-19

This section discusses the different AI-based DL approaches that can supplement the COVID-19–related techniques in healthcare organizations around the globe. The formulation of these strategies and approaches are from the latest publications on COVID-19 medical updates related to AI-based technology, which aims to provide improved effectiveness in these approaches and methodologies or strategies. Hence, this section provides ways that can help to enhance and accelerate the acquisition of approaches that are based on artificial neural networks (ANNs), which can help to upgrade the methods used for the treatment, management of health, detection, and diagnosis. However, the adaptive performance of technologies in different AI algorithms during the pandemic depends on the level of human participation and collaboration at various levels. Data scientists, on the other hand, have a unique understanding of AI's potential and limits as data scientists write the code when developing AI systems.

The flowchart in Figure 9.1 shows the processes in the implementation of AI-based solutions to tackle COVID-19 issues. The first stage is to collect and prepare the data for data mining, which is essential for data interpretation, preprocessing of data, handling big large amounts of data and medical records, such as pathology reports, past health records, X-rays or computed tomography (CT) images, and remaining health-related information are the different forms of input data that machines can read, interpret, and understand (Bharati, 2020). The objectives, such as the volume of data, different attributes of data, and characteristics of the attribute can summarize the data. Preprocessing of data is the step that must be initiated before the analysis and processing steps take place. In the preprocessing of the data, the raw data are refined and converted into a form that the machine can understand and process further. Data preparation, or the process of refining and converting raw data, comes before processing and analysis. The collection of data, analysis of data, and utilizing data, for example, physical and clinical records, and patient data are defined as big data. Here, researchers explore and evaluate the data as part of the machine learning (ML) approaches for extracting meaningful data from the patterns, characteristics, and structure.

ML or DL algorithms can handle a large amount of data with the help of programming software and humans. Furthermore, the approaches in DL can be used in situations where massive or sophisticated processing of data challenges ML, or the standard techniques in the data processing. As shown in Figure 9.2, DL approaches do not require human interaction. DL is a subtype of ML that is composed of multiple levels, which provide alternative interpretations of the input. DL, on the other hand, differs from ML in that its representation of data is different in the system. ML techniques are typically dependent on structured data, whereas DL techniques use different ANN layers (Bharati, 2020). Unsupervised learning, in contrast to supervised learning, is a technique where mapping of the input function to output is based on a predefined input–output pair, which requires less supervision from

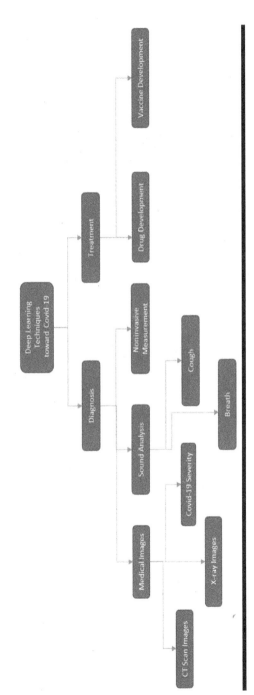

Figure 9.1   DL and ML methodologies survey for the diagnosis and detection of COVID-19

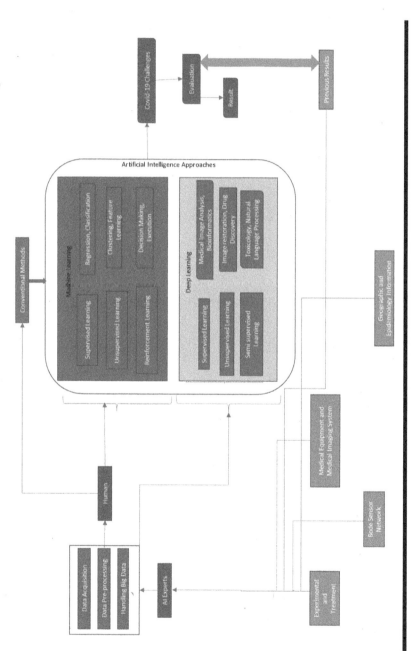

Figure 9.2 Using AI-based methodology to overcome the difficulties related to COVID-19

Source: Jamshidi (2017)

humans and is known as an algorithm of ML type where the unknown pattern is searched within the dataset with no previously defined label (Bharati, 2021b). The healthcare workers, such as therapists, nurses, pharmacists, the doctors use radiation, drugs, or surgery to treat illnesses and try to eliminate the primary symptoms in conventional medicine, which is also known as orthodox medicine, western medicine, and allopathic medicine, mainstream medicine, or biomedicine. Based on the assumption that AI might be applied significantly for COVID-19, this chapter aims to identify the best, most effective, and efficient solutions to the issues related to coronavirus that have created massive challenges for healthcare organizations. These methodologies are divided into three categories: (1) classification; (2) diagnosis and detection; and (3) control an epidemic. Figure 9.3 shows the different ANN techniques that are used for tracking symptoms and diagnosis. Even though the procedure was created primarily for the issues related to COVID-19, it can also be used for examining other medical images for different diseases. The input layer is the first layer that is used for accessing the database (Mondal, 2020). This input layer can be connected to the main front-end computer using the high-speed channel. The main central processing unit is tied to the database machine and the network is used to loosely couple with the database server.

The large packets of information are transferred to the mainframe by a database machine that combines database software with many microprocessors. The next layer the flowchart, which was developed by an intelligent selector based on ANN, has the responsibility of choosing the feasible techniques for imaging based on the system's previous knowledge. If the decisions made by this layer are confirmed by physicians, the third layer's proposed approaches take the appropriate images (Mondal, 2021). As a result of the previously acquired results, one or more imaging approaches might be suggested. Images of CT scans, optical and digital microscopic imaging, magnetic resonance imaging, and positron emission tomography (PET) are all used to evaluate patients. Pathology techniques and applications, as well as X-rays, are examples of methods that could also be employed (Taresh et al. 2020). The optical microscope is the standard instrument that is used in pathological examinations. The image scan from PET is a useful test for determining the body tissue's quality and extent and functioning of an organ. In some scenarios, before the imaging test reveals the disease, the PET scan can detect the disease. A radioactive substance (tracer) is used in the PET scan to explore the procedures.

The next layer is responsible for image enhancement and optimization. To extract the feature conventional ResNet was used and techniques of DL were employed for the structure of the ANN, and both techniques were used to make a classification network that differentiated influenza A, viral pneumonia and COVID-19 (Podder, 2021). The last layer uses the information saved in the system for the final diagnosis, and in this layer, the learning techniques should be employed ANNs. To reach these goals, among all the DL methods, convolutional neural networks (CNNs) are the best (Ghaderzadeh et al. 2021). Forming this type of network could be best suited

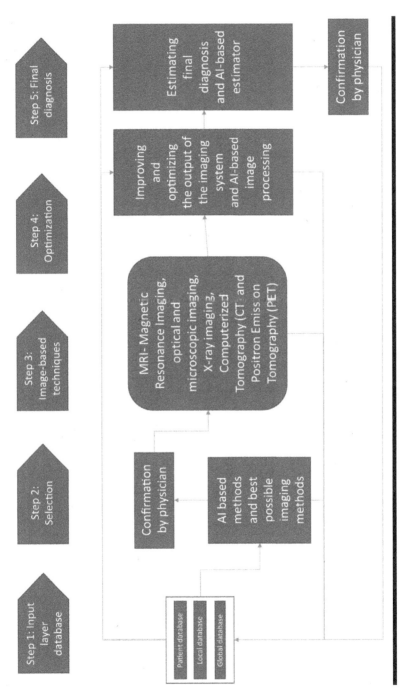

Figure 9.3   Using AI-based methodology for improvising, analyzing, and classifying approaches to medical imaging

Source: Jamshidi (2017)

for nonlinear modeling and has been applied in numerous medical imaging diagnoses and processes.

The objectives of this chapter are to discuss the following.

1. AI-based ML or DL methodologies to improve the analysis and classification of the diagnosis with the help of chest CT scan images or chest X-ray (CXR) images of the patient
2. Different techniques used for the extraction of data
3. Methodologies of ML or DL for the development of vaccines and drugs
4. Challenges faced when incorporating ML or DL methodologies
5. Some of the future directions

9.2 Materials and Diagnosis Methodologies for COVID-19

9.2.1 DL

DL is one type of ML that uses an ANN with any number of hidden layers, which enhances the learning potential of features. These methods can improve the classification accuracy of various sorts of data (Bohara, 2021). One of the most important and significant algorithms for detecting anomalies and pathologies from chest CT images is the DL-based CNN (Tayarani, 2021). These researchers focused on different DL algorithms and structures used for detecting and diagnosing COVID-19. All these algorithm studies are extensively evaluated in this chapter. A structured review strategy was used to find similar studies related to the detection and diagnosis of COVID-19. Using previous studies and the authors' opinions, a systematic search approach was established.

9.2.2 Prerequisites for a Search to Diagnose COVID-19

The following are the prerequisites for a search for COVID-19 diagnosis.

1. Has the use of DL improved the usual procedures FOR diagnosing COVID-19 to any extent
2. What modalities can be utilized in association with DL that help with the diagnosis and detection of COVID-19
3. Have methodologies for DL been able to compensate for diagnostic methods' flaws
4. How effective are the various DL algorithms and their frameworks that could help with coronavirus diagnosis comparison with one another

The researchers looked through different electronic databases available to find the different learning that was carried out on drugs and computer science and discovered that Scopus, Web of Science, and PubMed had the most papers connected to the topic. From November 1, 2019, to July 20, 2020, the different keywords utilized to search were: "COVID-19," "diagnosis," "detection," "deep learning," and associated published articles were extracted from the databases. From the search domain, two different databases, such as Embase and the Institute of Electrical and Electronics Engineers (IEEE) were removed due to the homogeneity of their articles.

9.2.3 Extraction of Data

In the data extraction phase related research, descriptions of the procedures, and their outcomes were noted. The primary details of the techniques, as well as their outcome received, were stored in the extraction sheet of data that identified which of the DL techniques and algorithms were used (Ghaderzadeh, 2021). The data was extracted, and differences between the investigators were resolved through conversations. The year of publication, modality, name of the study, assessment methods, data used, country, DL techniques, research population, and outcomes were among the extracted data items.

9.3 COVID-19 Detection Using AI-Based ML and DL for Medical Image Inception

The SARS-CoV-2 outbreak is growing across India and the world. The different medical imaging techniques, such as medical imaging, images of CT scans, and X-rays play a significant part in the global fight against coronavirus, for example, and recent AI breakthroughs with improvements in the capability of medical imaging instruments, make the doctors and health worker's lives easier. Clinicians frequently employ medical imaging studies to determine the presence of COVID-19. COVID-19 clinical imaging trials primarily use two types of medical image samples: CT scans of the lungs and CXRs. Figure 9.4 (a) shows the different aspects in which the ML and DL techniques are used.

In the testing of medical imaging, AI is an important technology. It has obtained incredible results in picture and organ recognition, regional infection categorization, and classification of diseases. These results not only reduce the radiologist's time for diagnosing a medical image but the diagnosis' precision and accuracy are also improved. As follows, techniques of AI can improve the efficiency of work by enhancing the precision of diagnostic from CT and X-ray imaging, making it less difficult to evaluate. Radiologists can use networks that are computer-aided to make clinical choices, such as illness detection, monitoring, and prognosis. The following are the details about the latest AI techniques, such as CT imaging and CRXs used for the diagnosis and treatment of COVID-19. Figure 9.4(b) shows the different AI-based ML and DL methods used for the detection of COVID-19.

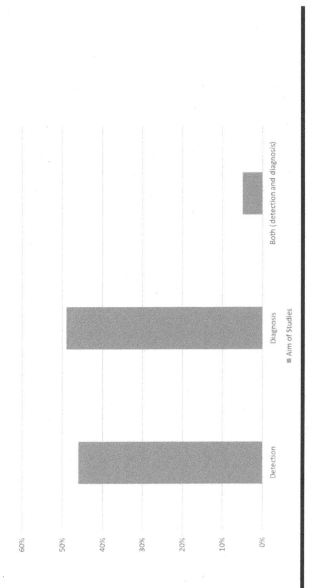

Figure 9.4   Showing: (a) aim of the research is to use DL to process COVID-19 radiological modalities   (Continued)

Source: Ghaderzadeh (2021)

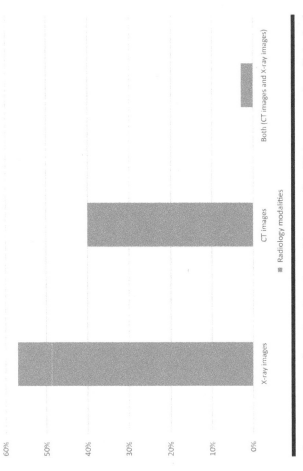

Figure 9.4 (Continued) Showing: (b) rate of utilizing several radiological modalities in the DL analysis of COVID-19 (Continued)

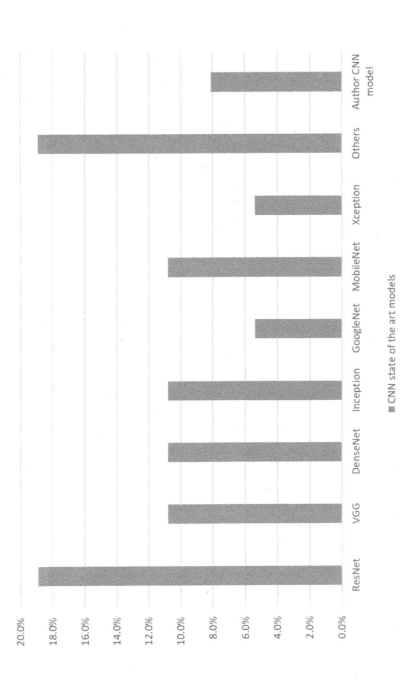

Figure 9.4 (Continued) Showing: (c) COVID-19 radiological modality images are processed using a high rate of CNN architectures

9.3.1 Detection from Chest CT Images

The chest CT image is an important part of the evaluation of individuals with a suspected COVID-19 infection. Using SARS-CoV-2 infection imaging for treatment and diagnosis is gaining popularity. The infection causes a wide range of CT imaging results, the most common of which are peripheral consolidations of the lungs and ground glass opacities. The sensitivity of CT images of chests to identify SARS-CoV-2 infection has been discovered to be substantially greater, this can happen before a laboratory test for the virus. As a result, in epidemic areas when the basic healthcare system is under strain, the healthcare system admits a high number of patients with suspected COVID-19 infection using CT images for rapid emergency treatment of patients. The chest CT scan images require the evaluation of SARS-CoV-2 infected patients who have severe and complicated respiratory symptoms. It is possible to evaluate how much the lungs are damaged and how the individual's condition advances using scans, which are useful in making treatment decisions. The rapid occurrence of COVID-19-induced lung abnormalities in CT scans that were performed for other types of medical causes, such as CT scans of the abdomen for bowel disease or for those patients who do not have any respiratory symptoms, is becoming better understood (Chauhan, Palivela & Tiwari, 2021). The evaluation by AI could be a key element used in this pandemic, which minimizes the pressure on clinicians. The interpretation of CT scan images manually could take ≤15 min to complete; however, AI can analyze the pictures in 10 s. As a result, AI technology combined with an ANN for image processing has the potential to dramatically enhance the usefulness of CT scans for the diagnosis of coronavirus, which could allow a large number of infected patients to be quickly and accurately diagnosed with the disease. The following phases are commonly included in CT imaging by applying AI techniques; identification of regional infection, region of interest (ROI) for regional division, classification of COVID-19 results, and removal of lung tissue.

In CT scan imaging of bronchopulmonary segments, lung lobes, regions with infection or ulcers, and lungs, ROI has been proven for additional testing and analysis. A few DL network types, such as VB-Net, VNET-IRRPN, U-Net, and V-Net have been employed for CT image categorization. In total, 419 cases were confirmed with SARS-CoV-2 using an AI device that had been tested with the two types of reverse transcription–polymerase chain reaction (RT-PCR) test, such as real-time RT-PCR and next-generation RT-PCR (Sakib, 2020). For the initial CT scan, the AI technique uses deep CNNs that analyze the image features and properties of people who are infected with SARS-CoV-2. Random forest (RF), support vector machine (SVM), and multilayer perceptron (MLP) classifiers were then utilized, which recognize a patient based on clinical knowledge. To predict COVID-19 status, the AI system uses medical parameters and radiological data. Furthermore, the AI approach was improved to detect and diagnose the patients with SARS-CoV-2 who had presented conventional images of CT scans, successfully classifying 17 out of 25 cases (68%) and marking all cases as COVID-19 negative by radiologists.

In total, 71 images of CT scans from 52 COVID-19 infected people from five hospitals were acquired. They extracted 1,218 features from each CT using the Pyradiomics technique. CT radiomics models focus on logistic regression and RF algorithms. During training and interactions, they were developed using pneumonia lesion extracts (Mondal, 2021). The experimental database also assessed prediction efficacy at the lung lobe and patient levels. With a 97% area under the curve (AUC) and 92% LR and RF, they were able to distinguish between SARS-CoV-2-related pneumonia in long- and short-term stay patients in a hospital. The LR model had specificity and sensitivity of 89% and 100%, respectively, and the RF model had a 75% sensitivity and 100% specificity, respectively. A short-term stay in the hospital lasts <10 days, whereas a long-term duration in the hospital lasts >10 days.

9.3.2 Using CXR Images for Detection

For evaluating and testing SARS-CoV-2 patients, CXRs have been presented as a very useful tool.

CXRs are easier to obtain than CT images in clinical radiology. Various studies have used CXRs to diagnose COVID-19. The AI-based CXR methodologies mostly consider parameters like COVID-19 segmentation, input data rectification, and model training. Several DL approaches, such as U-Net++, CNN, and nCOVnet are applied for the optimal and faster detection of COVID-19 on CXRs. X-ray machines in medical facilities and hospitals provide less expensive and faster results when scanning various human organs. Radiologists often carry out manual interpretation of a large number of X-ray images. Only 69% of COVID-19 cases were detected by radiologists on X-rays. COVID-19 detection was made easier and faster thanks to pretrained models. A few researchers employed a dataset of SARS-CoV-2 positive cases, stable patients' cases with no COVID-19 infection, and regular bacterial infections of pneumonia, and. To demonstrate the importance of segments and conduct categorization, the scientists used the VGG-16 pretrained model. The examiner achieved 96% and 92.5% accuracy in two and three production class instances, respectively. The medical community could use CXR images as a feasible strategy for the instant and quick detection of COVID-19, based on these findings, to enhance current diagnostic and symptomatic approaches. There has been a misdiagnosis of pneumonia and the subsequent phases of the disease. In order to study COVID-19, the majority of research papers employed a variety of methodologies. A deep neural network model CovidAID was built to give patients a proper evaluation using the publicly accessible covid-CXR dataset. According to a researcher, they demonstrated the viability of using the proposed Truncated Inception Net as a screening approach and outperformed all current tools. COVID-19 prediction from X-rays is the subject of research, and a paper employed transfer learning. There are four common deep-trained networks, such as ResNet18, ResNet50,

SqueezeNet, and other CNNs. The results of DenseNet-161 were compared with the predictions. COVID-19 and non-COVID were used. In total,14 subclasses composed of normal ChexPert data were used to train the four models on images from the dataset. The models had an average 80% sensitivity rate and a 90% of specificity rate. This strongly suggests that COVID-19 could be distinguished from normal lung diseases and other infections using CXR imaging. In a study diagnosing COVID-19 in CXR images from the dataset of CXR with deep transfer learning, a generative adversarial network was proposed. In total, 307 pictures were collected for four separate class groups: normal, viral pneumonia, bacterial pneumonia, and COVID-19. Three deep transfer models were chosen for the operation: AlexNet, GoogLeNet, and ResNet18. Three case situations were investigated in this study: the first model had four classes in the database, the second model had three classes in the database, and the third model had two classes in the database. Under all circumstances, the COVID-19 class was required.

9.3.3 Various Severity Levels of COVID-19 Classification Using DL and CXR Images

CXRs with AI allow us to learn more, especially when utilizing AI approaches of ML and DL. The effective application of DL in computer vision in the biomedical area has prompted researchers to investigate AI-based solutions for COVID-19 identification using CXR and CT scan pictures. To acquire the features of CXR images from the large X-ray images dataset, a pretrained ANN (DenseNet) was used. The severity level of COVID-19 prediction was studied using 94 images from COVID-19 certified patients using DL. A score-based approach was used, with two types of scores.

The ground glass ambiguity shows the degree of involvement of the lungs and the unification degree was graded for each lung. On the right and left lungs, the overall degree and ambiguity scores varied from zero to eight and zero to six, respectively. The score can be used to determine the severity of an illness, which is used to determine whether care should be increased or decreased, along with the ability to track the therapy effectiveness for the patient, particularly for those who are in the intensive care unit (ICU). Table 9.1 demonstrates the severity level and ambiguity

Table 9.1 Disease Severity Levels by Displaying the Lung Involvement Level and the Amount of Ambiguity in a Single X-Ray Image

Parameters	Score of Severity				
	0	1	2	3	4
Involvement of lungs	No	<25%	Between 25% and 50%	Between 50& and 75%	>75%
Ambiguity	No	Ground glass ambiguity	Unification	White-Out	–

found in the individual X-ray images. AI is also used in mobile app development to monitor the different severity levels of COVID-19 in the game. Researchers from the New York University College of Dentistry, New York, US developed a smartphone app based on a collection of 160 photos of COVID-19 patients from China. The various biomarkers found in the blood that identify SARS-CoV-2 patient severity levels ranged from low to severe utilizing the mobile app (extreme). On all the test sets, the researchers discovered that patients who were intubated or died had a higher median pulmonary X-ray severity (PXS) score (PXS score = 7.9) than those who were not intubated (PXS score = 3.2). There was a statistically significant variance ($p = 0.001$). Figure 9.4 (c) shows the various ML and DL-based algorithms used for COVID-19 detection and diagnosis.

9.4 Vaccine and Drug Development using ML and DL Techniques for the Treatment of COVID-19

The ability to automatically abstract component learning, when combined with a vast quantity of data, has had a significant impact on the efficacy of ML. ML provides reaction predictions, ligand–protein interactions, and behavior predictions, and that are combined in two high-profile fields: drug discovery and vaccination. Proteomics and genome investigations have been suggested as a focus for SARS-CoV-2 therapeutic development programs and vaccines. For the development of new medical care and medication, using ML and DL is important and they play a key element in the fight against the COVID-19 pandemic.

9.4.1 Vaccine Development using ML and DL

In vaccine development, ML and DL perform two important roles: distributing components of the vaccine by analyzing viral protein structure and assisting healthcare practitioners when quickly assessing a high number of important research papers.

Understanding a protein's composition is crucial when determining how it operates. Once the problem is solved, researchers can develop medications that operate in a variety of protein configurations. However, determining the unique three-dimensional (3D) structure of any protein requires a long time. AI systems based on DL can make the analysis of protein structures and genetic sequences easier.

In January, Google DeepMind unveiled AlphaFold, a sophisticated and specialized algorithm that predicts the synthesis of 3D proteins based on their genetic sequence. The method was put to the test in COVID-19 at the beginning of March 2020. They are presently pursuing this goal by developing novel proteins to reduce coronavirus. In theory, these proteins will respond with a protein spike,

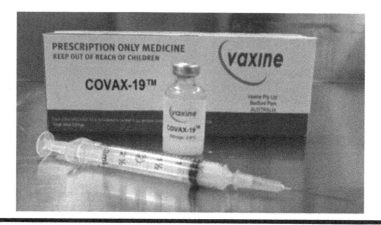

Figure 9.5 Covax-19TM is a COVID-19 vaccine developed in Australia and modeled using AI-based technology

protecting healthy cells from virus particles. Researchers combined AI and cloud computing to prevent the protein spike from attaching to the ACE2 receptor in human cells and develop a potential COVID-19 vaccine. Researchers from Flinders University, Bedford Park, SA, Australia examined the symptoms of COVID-19 and used their findings to develop a vaccine (Covax-19), shown in Figure 9.5.

Then, they attempted to develop a vaccination that would block this mechanism. To speed up vaccine production, the researchers deployed cutting-edge AI and powerful cloud computing technology. The COVD-19 protein sequence was identified in GenBank and used the multiple sequence alignment technique to identify and sequence the peptides in the nucleocapsid phosphoprotein structure. It also suggests that a peptide vaccine based on CD8 + T cell immunity is relevant and viable for Ebola virus (West African Epidemic 2013–2016) survivors. The OptiVax design program combines methods for creating new peptide medications, analyzing current vaccinations, and enhancing the composition of existing vaccines.

Podder et al. (2022) used immune informatics and relative approaches to create an antipeptide vaccine for SARS-CoV-2 made up of three proteins: membrane epitopes (M), envelope (E), and spike (S). Furthermore, using the ElliPro antibody epitope predicting system to anticipate epitopes in S-proteins. Ellipro employs many ML approaches, which are used to predict and visualize a certain epitope B-cell or sequence of a protein in a structure. Vaccines are designed based on epitopes to cure COVID-19. To predict the toxicity of selected epitopes, they used an SVM approach. It uses 19 combined epitope-human leukocyte antigens methods to predict and validate 174 SARS-CoV-2 epitopes, including the position-specific scoring matrix, and immune epitope database (IEDB), and ANN algorithms.

9.4.2 Drug Development

A DL-based AI system provided a learning model to precisely predict the evaluation. With a drug discovery procedure, AI algorithms can readily categorize medications that help to fight against COVID-19. Drug development is a risky, time-consuming, and expensive process. According to the Eastern Research Group (ERG), opening a new molecular company takes 10–15 years and the success rate is 2.01% (Xue et al., 2018).

Drug repurposing is a concept that repurposes existing medications for a previously unconsidered medicinal purpose. It's an investigational method for finding preapproved, discontinued, shelved, and experimental drugs that have been approved for use in the treatment of other diseases. There are five processes in the development of conventional pharmaceuticals.

1. Development and discovery of drugs
2. Preclinical drug research
3. Clinical drug research
4. Drug review by FDA
5. Drug safety and after-market monitoring and development are overseen by the FDA

Drug repurposing; however, has four processes.

1. Identify compounds
2. Purchase a compound
3. After-market drug safety monitoring and development are overseen by the FDA
4. Drug clinical research

The process of discovering and developing novel particles in molecular structures is slow, time-consuming, and costly. As a result, repurposing authorized medications for SARS-CoV-2 therapy is the best option. For a normal viral infection, the hydroxyl analogs hydroxychloroquine and chloroquine are recognized as the most effective. Such medications are effective against malaria and have cured COVID-19.

AI places emphasis on finding new medication-like molecules at the molecular level. The 3D crystal structures with target proteins are categorized using the sequences of amino acids and strings of the simplified molecular-input line-entry system (SMILES). The findings revealed that when treating and preventing HIV with atazanavir, an antiretroviral drug, it could be the most effective chemical compound against 3C-like SARS-CoV-2 proteinase, with a content of Kd = 94.94 nM, which was followed by efavirenz (199.17 nM), ritonavir (204.05 nM), remdesivir (113.13 nM), and dolutegravir (204.05 n (336.91 nM).

The authors used the BindingDB databases, National Center for Biotechnology Information, and Drug Target Center, to compile the amino acid sequences of 3C-like proteases and the associated antiviral medications and drug targets. Furthermore, AutoDock Vina was used to estimate the affinity of binding between SARS-CoV-2 and the 3CL protease (3CLpro) enzyme and 3,410 medicines. Experiments with six different drugs, including dolutegravir, atazanavir, ritonavir, Kaletra, remdesivir, and efavirenz, yielded positive results. The drug remdesivir seemed to be effective in a clinical experiment.

KronRLS and SimBoost are the two similarity-based algorithms that have been presented that used effective ML techniques. This matrix; however, has two disadvantages. First, the feature representation is reduced, causing the forecast to be inaccurate. Second, it entails estimating the matrix of similarity, which will limit the maximum number of molecules in the training phase. DeepDTA, which is a deep learning-based model, was developed to address these constraints. It's a model based on CNN that doesn't require any feature engineering.

The software automatically detects valuable features from a raw molecule and protein sequence. SimBoost and KronRLS, two publicly available drug–target interaction benchmarks, demonstrated the performance. They utilized blocks of CNNs to combine these representations of features and input them into a deep CNN, which they named DeepDTA, which was used to extract features from raw sequences of proteins and SMILES strings and to train it. The Smith–Waterman and PubChem similarity algorithms were used to process the pair-wise similarities between proteins and ligands. Three different combinations used this information as input knowledge to the DeepDTA model that was improved and proposed when training the data patterns.

This model can be trained in three different ways.

1. Train representations of the compound
2. Train sequences of protein representations
3. Train representations of compound and protein

Combining all models has become the final approach. Many studies have employed an integrated model for the repurposing of medication against COVID-19.

Researchers developed deepDR, a DL approach based on different integrated networks that were used for drug repurposing in silico. The deepDR, specifically, interprets high-stage medication properties from the different networks with the help of a deep autoencoder. The learned low-dimensional feature representations of pharmaceuticals are then merged with clinically reported drug–disease combinations and encoded and decoded by a variational autoencoder to develop applications for licensed medications that were not previously allowed. The deepDR outperformed other methods based on CNN and ML, with an AUC of 90.8% (Kothadiya et al, 2021). Some of the additional methodologies, such as kGCN, D3Targets-2019-nCoV, DeepPurpose, and DeepChem are based on DL drug testing, repurposing, and discovery methodologies for COVID-19.

The advances in recent SARS-CoV-2 3CLpro chemical structure were investigated by Bung et al. (2021) using DL. They developed an RL-based RNN model for protease inhibitor drugs and uncovered a small group of molecules. Finally, 2,515 SMILES format protease inhibitor compounds from the database ChEMBL were used for the training, with every SMILES sequence as well as the location and symbol regarded as a time series.

9.5 Limitations and Future Direction

In this section, the difficulties encountered when utilizing ML and DL to solve the COVID-19 problem will be discussed. Furthermore, how DL can be used in the fight against COVID-19 in the future will be demonstrated.

9.5.1 Limitations

9.5.1.1 Regulations

Due to the widespread coronavirus and the rise in the number of COVID-19 confirmed cases and deaths, several measures, such as a few days of lockdown and social distancing, have been proposed by state and district authorities to control the outbreak. The authorities play a vital role in deciding the new rules and legislation that can ensure that individuals, company owners, big enterprises, researchers, medical centers, technology giants, and scientists contribute to the prevention of COVID-19 during a pandemic.

9.5.1.2 Large-Scale Training Data is Scarce and Unavailable

Most of the DL approaches rely on training data on a large-scale, such as images of medical examinations and various environmental variables. However, because of the quick spread of coronavirus, there are not enough datasets for AI. This means that it might take more time to evaluate samples for training samples in practice and might require assistance from medical personnel.

9.5.1.3 Data That Is Noisy, as Well as Fake Rumors

A few difficulties might arise when relying on online internet news; vast amounts of prerecorded audio data and misleading documents regarding COVID-19 exist on various news channels without any substantial modifications. However, algorithms for DL appear to be less accurate when deciding and filtering audio and error-prone data. Furthermore, the outputs from ML and DL algorithms become skewed when noisy data is used. This issue minimizes the usefulness and execution of methods that are based on AI, mainly in pandemic forecasting as well as spread analyses.

9.5.1.4 There is a Gap between Medicine and Computer Science

Almost all the researchers in DL have a background in computer science; however, substantial competence in virology, other relevant domains, medical imaging, and bioinformatics is essential to incorporate other information related to the medical field in the COVID-19 battle. When fighting COVID-19, it is necessary to form a team of experts from different sectors where multiple studies can be included in the data.

9.5.1.5 Data Security and Privacy

Obtaining personal private data is fairly inexpensive in the era of big data and AI. When dealing with public health issues, such as COVID-19, many ministry authorities try to accumulate a variety of individuals' information, such as identification numbers, mailing addresses, mobile numbers, and medical history. During AI-based discovery and processing, an unaddressed issue is how to properly maintain individual personal information and their human rights.

9.5.1.6 Early Detection of COVID-19 through CXRs and CT Scans

Working with datasets that are not properly balanced as a result of insufficient medical imaging and extensive training periods, cannot describe the challenges to the findings.

9.5.1.7 Structurally Incorrect Data and Data that is not Structurally Correct (e.g., image, text, and numerical data)

Difficulties arise when working with data that is erroneous and confusingly written in the text descriptions. Large amounts of data from several sources can be erroneous. Furthermore, extracting valuable information from large amounts of data is impossible.

9.5.1.8 Patients are Screened and Triaged, Functional Therapy and Cures are Sought, and Risk Assessments are Conducted

Predictions of survival, medical assets, and health wellness care are analyzed and could help to accumulate data from the patients for their physical characteristics. Another challenge is dealing with data that is low-quality, which can lead to incorrect evaluation and predictions.

9.5.2 Future Research Direction

DL algorithms can contribute to combating COVID-19 in the following research directions.

9.5.2.1 Contactless Detection of Diseases During a Pandemic

The automatic image classification of X-ray and CT scan images reduce the transmission of diseases from patients to radiologists. The DL techniques can classify patients with the help of imaging techniques, such as X-rays and CT scans.

9.5.2.2 Video Diagnostics and Consultations via the Internet

It is conceivable to construct robot systems and video diagnostic programs operated remotely by combining natural language processing tools and AI in to conduct COVID-19 diagnosis.

9.5.2.3 Research in Biological Field

In the biological field, DL algorithms may be helpful to accurately analyze biomedical knowledge, for example, the major structure of proteins, sequences of genes, and viral routes to determine protein composition and viral components.

9.5.2.4 Vaccination and Drug Development

DL algorithms are used not only to find promising vaccines and medications but may imitate vaccine–receptor and drug–protein interactions, allowing for the future prediction of vaccine and drug reactions in patients affected with COVID-19.

9.5.2.5 Fake Information is Identified and Screened

In order to give genuine, correct studies on the COVID-19 pandemic, DL algorithms are helpful to place limits and remove misleading audio data on COVID-19 and information from online platforms.

9.5.5.6 Assessment and Evaluation of the Impact

Different types of simulations using DL approaches may be used to inspect the influence of various techniques on the transmission of the disease. Further, it could help to evaluate scientific and the most definitive methods to control the spread of disease and prevention in the general public.

9.5.2.7 COVID-19 Patient Tracking

By establishing online communities and statistical models, DL techniques can track and monitor the attributes of people living in immediate contact with coronavirus patients and accurately track and forecast the disease's probable spread.

9.5.2.8 AI Robots

Smart robots need to be used in programs, for example, product delivery, cleanliness of public areas, and hospital care that do not necessitate any form of assistance from humans. This will slow down or could stop the increase in COVID-19.

9.5.2.9 More Research Work on Descriptive AI-Based DL Algorithms in the Future

It is necessary to determine the overall performance of DL models and diagrammatical features representation that helps distinguish other types of pneumonia from COVID-19. This might support radiologists and medical practitioners to be more aware of the virus and analyze the probable COVID-19 effects from X rays and CT scans.

9.5.2.10 What is the Significant Aspect of COVID-19 Diagnosis and Treatment?

Diagnosis and treatment are necessary; however, finding a viable solution to cure COVID-19 is vital. This chapter discovered that the majority of readily available techniques used by DL mainly focused on detecting COVID-19 patients from the available literature. Future research that considers ML and DL as core parts are required in order to find a COVID-19 therapy.

9.6 Conclusions

In this chapter, the different platforms and structures were presented, which are the recent research fields that used AI-based techniques, which could be helpful when dealing with COCID-19. For COVID-19 diagnosis and treatment, different AI-based ML and DL techniques were explained. In addition, this chapter summarized the available datasets for COVID-19 and the tools used for diagnosis and treatment. It also explained the state-of-the-art techniques used against COVID-19, which could help healthcare professionals to deal with the outbreak of coronavirus. Vaccine and drug developments in different countries to cure COVID-19 were presented. The chapter included future work and constraints when exploring the different AI-based ML and DL techniques.

References

Bharati, S., & Mondal, M. R. H. (2021) 12 Applications and challenges of AI-driven IoHT for combating pandemics: A review. *Intelligence for Managing Pandemics, 213.*

Bharati, S., Podder, P., & Mondal, M. R. H. (2020). Hybrid deep learning for detecting lung diseases from X-ray images. *Informatics in Medicine Unlocked, 20,* 100391.

Bharati, S., Podder, P., Mondal, M., & Prasath, V. B. (2021a). CO-ResNet: Optimized ResNet model for COVID-19 diagnosis from X-ray images. *International Journal of Hybrid Intelligent Systems, 17*(1–2), 71–85.

Bharati, S., Podder, P., Mondal, M., & Prasath, V. B. S. (2021b). Medical imaging with deep learning for COVID-19 diagnosis: A comprehensive review. *International Journal of Computer Information Systems and Industrial Management Applications, 13*

Bohara, M., Patel, K., Patel, B., & Desai, J. (2021). An AI based web portal for cotton price analysis and prediction. In 3rd International Conference on Integrated Intelligent Computing Communication & Security (ICIIC 2021) (pp. 33–39). Netherlands: Atlantis Press.

Bung, N., Krishnan, S. R., Bulusu, G., & Roy, A. (2021). De novo design of new chemical entities for SARS-CoV-2 using artificial intelligence. *Future Medicinal Chemistry,* 13(06), 575–585.

Chauhan, T., Palivela, H., & Tiwari, S. (2021). Optimization and fine-tuning of DenseNet model for classification of Covid-19 cases in medical imaging. *International Journal of Information Management Data Insights, 1*(2) 100020.

Ghaderzadeh, M., & Asadi, F. (2021). Deep learning in the detection and diagnosis of COVID-19 using radiology modalities: a systematic review. *Journal of Healthcare Engineering.* doi.10.1155/2021/6677314

Ghaderzadeh, M., Asadi, F., Hosseini, A., Bashash, D., Abolghasemi, H., & Roshanpour, A. (2021). Machine learning in detection and classification of leukemia using smear blood images: A systematic review. *Scientific Programming.* doi.10.1155/2021/9933481

Jamshidi, M., Lalbakhsh, A., Talla, J., Peroutka, Z., Hadjilooei, F., Lalbakhsh, P., & Mohyuddin, W. (2020). Artificial intelligence and COVID-19: deep learning approaches for diagnosis and treatment. *IEEE Access, 8,* 109581–109595.

Kothadiya, D., Chaudhari, A., Macwan, R., Patel, K., & Bhatt, C. (2021). The convergence of deep learning and computer vision: Smart city applications and research challenges. Paper presented at the 3rd International Conference on Integrated Intelligent Computing Communication & Security (ICIIC 2021) (pp. 14–22). India: Atlantis Press.

Mondal, M. R. H., Bharati, S., Podder, P., & Podder, P. (2020). Data analytics for novel coronavirus disease. *Informatics in Medicine Unlocked, 20,* 100374.

Mondal, M. R. H., Bharati, S., & Podder, P. (2021). Diagnosis of COVID-19 using machine learning and deep learning: A Review. *Current Medical Imaging, 17*(12), 1403–1418.

Mondal MRH, Bharati, S., & Podder, P. (2021) CO-IRv2: Optimized Inception ResNetV2 for COVID-19 detection from chest CT images. *PLoS ONE, 16*(10): e0259179. doi.10.1371/journal.pone.0259179

Paul, P., Bharati, S., Podder, P., & Mondal, M. R. H. (2021) 10 The role of IoMT during pandemics. Intelligence for managing pandemics. In A. Khamparia, R. Hossain

Mondal, P. Podder, B. Bhushan, V. Albuquerque, & S, Kumar (Eds.) *Computational Intelligence for Managing Pandemics* (pp. 169–186) Berlin, Boston: De Gruyter.

Podder, P., Bharati, S., Mondal, M. R. H., & Kose, U. (2021). Application of machine learning for the diagnosis of COVID-19. In *Data Science for COVID-19* (pp. 175–194). Academic Press. doi.org/10.1016/B978-0-12-824536-1.00008-3

Podder, P., Khamparia, A., Mondal, M. R. H., Rahman, M. A., & Bharati, S. (2022). Forecasting the spread of COVID-19 and ICU requirements. *International Journal of Online and Biomedical Engineering*, 17(05), 81–99. doi.10.3991/ijoe.v17i05.20009

Raza, K. (2020). Computational intelligence methods in COVID-19: Surveillance, prevention, prediction and diagnosis. *Nature, 923*.

Sakib, S., Tazrin, T., Fouda, M. M., Fadlullah, Z. M., & Guizani, M. (2020). DL-CRC: Deep learning-based chest radiograph classification for COVID-19 detection: a novel approach. *IEEE Access, 8*, 171575–171589.

Taresh, M. M., Zhu, N., Ali, T. A. A., Hameed, A. S., & Mutar, M. L. (2020). Transfer learning to detect COVID-19 automatically from X-ray images using convolutional neural networks. *International Journal of Biomedical Imaging, 2021*.

Tayarani-N, M. H. (2020). Applications of artificial intelligence in battling against covid-19: A literature review. *Chaos, Solitons & Fractals* doi.10.1016/j.chaos.2020.110338

Xue, H., Li, J., Xie, H., & Wang, Y. (2018). Review of drug repositioning approaches and resources. *International Journal of Biological Sciences*, 14(10), 1232.

Chapter 10

Hybridization of Decision Tree Algorithm Using Sequencing Predictive Model for COVID-19

A. A. Awoseyi, Jide Ebenezer Taiwo Akinsola, O. M. Oladoja, and Moruf Adeagbo
Mathematics and Computer Sciences Department,
First Technical University, Ibadan, Nigeria

O. O. Adebowale
Veterinary Public Health and Preventive Medicine Department,
Federal University of Agriculture, Abeokuta, Nigeria

Contents

DOI: 10.1201/9781003324447-10

10.1 Introduction

The first identified case of the highly infectious severe acute respiratory syndrome coronavirus-2 (SARS-CoV-2) virus was in Wuhan, China in January 2020, when people started becoming sick with pneumonia-like symptoms. It was the seventh identified human coronavirus (Ciotti et al., 2020; Mondal et al., 2020). It soon spread around the world and the world health organization (WHO) declared the disease a global pandemic on March 12, 2020. Since this outbreak, COVID-19 has affected different sectors of human life, with countries declaring lockdowns and many businesses implementing a work-from-home policy. The medical and public health sectors rapidly deployed innovative alternative and complementary methods to traditional clinical methods. Concepts like machine learning (ML), big data, blockchain technology, the internet of things, and artificial intelligence (AI) are rapidly being employed and deployed to complement existing diagnosis and monitoring techniques. In this chapter, the use of decision tree (DT)-based ML techniques on the COVID-19 dataset is compared. The highlights of this chapter are.

1. Discussion of coronavirus phylogenetics to understand the diagnosis and monitoring approaches
2. Elucidation of three main COVID-19 diagnostic techniques
3. Implementation of different DT techniques for COVID-19 prediction
4. Performance comparison of hybridized DT-based techniques

The contribution of this chapter is in relation to the hybridization of DT algorithms, such as bagging (Bag), random forest, BART, and boosting for fitting an optimal regression line when predicting the COVID-19 pandemic.

10.2 COVID-19 Virus

The phylogenetic study of the COVID-19 virus showed that it belongs to the Nidovirale order, which is made up of three families: Arteriviridae, Roniviridae, and Coronaviridae. The Coronaviridae has two subfamilies, Torovirinae and Coronavirinae. The Coronavirinae coronavirus subfamily further divides into four groups: alpha, beta, gamma, and delta (Berekaa, 2021; Gorbalenya et al., 2020). Seven known coronaviruses cause infections in humans. Three out of these seven cause severe respiratory infections and are dangerous to humans, these are: MERS-CoV, SARS-CoV, and SARS-CoV-2. There are insinuations that the COVID-19 virus was created in a laboratory; however, according to Ciotti et al. (2020), this hypothesis is not supported by genetic data. The genetic data shows that the virus was not derived from a previously known virus backbone. The COVID-19 virus seems to have evolved naturally, showing similarities with the RaGT13 coronavirus found in bats and bats are thought to serve as COVID-19 virus reservoirs. It spread from bats to pangolins to humans and finally human to human transmission via direct contact, respiratory secretions, and droplets. The virus transmission is through the major viral entry routes to the body, for example, the nose, mouth, and eyes when they are in contact with contaminated media.

10.3 Detection and Diagnosis of COVID-19 Infection

The WHO website as of July 24, 2021, reported that more than 192 million COVID-19 cases were confirmed with more than 4 million deaths caused by the virus (WHO, 2021). Hence, detection and prompt diagnosis of the infection are essential. According to Berekaa (2021), there are three ways of detecting the SARS-CoV-2 virus in infected patients: symptomatic, molecular, and, medical imagery detection.

10.3.1 Molecular Detection

COVID-19 can be detected at the molecular level; this allows scientists to develop primers for detecting the virus molecules. Studies showed that it takes approximately 3 hours to detect the COVID-19 virus using reverse transcription-polymerase chain (RT-PCR) reactions, with a complete sequencing of the gnome in 11 hours and isolation of the culture in 72 hours (Bharati et al., 2021b; Colson et al., 2020). Currently, RT-PCR is one of the most effective methods of detecting the virus. However, it only works when the virus or infection is present in the person.

10.3.2 Medical Imagery Detection

The main target of the coronavirus is the lower respiratory system; this makes it possible to detect the presence of the virus through computerized tomography (CT) chest scans. The most common symptom in the image is the appearance of mutual-sided ground glass opacities, as shown in Figure 10.1 (Berekaa, 2021; Hani et al., 2020). This makes it possible to identify the presence of the infection in the patient by taking a CT scan of the chest region (Bharati et al., 2020, 2021a, 2021b).

10.3.3 Symptomatic Detection

The three leading symptoms of the infection are fever, cough, and shortness of breath, other symptoms include vomiting, diarrhea, and nausea, with some patients showing a combination of major and other symptoms (Bharati et al., 2021a; Kumar

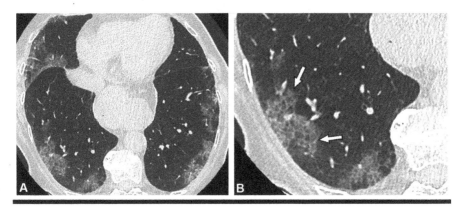

Figure 10.1 CT image of COVID-19 pneumonia (belonging to an 86-year-old woman): (A) CT image after 4 d of symptom (e.g., cough and chest pain); (B) arrows show peripheral ground glass opacities with intralobular reticulation superimposition

Source: Hani et al. (2020)

et al., 2021). However, the disease is asymptomatic in a large portion of infected people. Nevertheless, symptomatic detection seems to be a common approach to identifying infected people, especially for non medics. ML techniques are also used in this approach.

10.4 The Role of ML

The medical sector has explored new approaches to speed up COVID-19 diagnosis, detection, prediction, and vaccinations in response to the pandemic. This brought about the application of ML in various health sectors. ML will be discussed in the following section.

10.5 ML

Arthur Samuel came up with the term "machine learning" to show how a computing device might become usable to take on checker games in a way characterized as learning processes "whether being executed by humans or by animals" (Samuel, 1959). ML is a specialty of AI that allows computing systems data automation on how to carry out the required task (Ali et al., 2016). ML is meant to assist computers to learn about the past or present and predict or forecast what will happen in unknown circumstances in the future (Akinsola et al., 2019) as evident from the study conducted by these researchers on the application of supervised ML for breast cancer prediction. A fresh approach to combat a recent coronavirus outbreak encouraged researchers to use ML applications in addition to AI on the previous pandemics (Lalmuanawma et al., 2020). ML analytics approaches are now being employed in many fields (Akinsola et al., 2019), and are a prominent application in the recent COVID-19 pandemic. ML approaches are extensively employed in medical fields. ML-enabled diagnostic devices that track, forecast, and screen the spread of COVID-19 are currently significantly needed as well as discovering the required treatments for it (Shahid et al., 2021).

AI is not deployed as a replacement for human involvement; however, it is used to enhance the decision-making processes of physicians (Phillips-Wren et al., 2008). AI and ML technologies are utilized for the prediction of infectious and noninfectious diseases more accurately. Predictive analytics uses a variety of techniques to analyze current data for forecasts including data mining, ML, modeling, and simulation that includes AI (Idowu et al., 2020). According to recent research, healthcare providers who use ML and AI see an increase in processing capacity, speed, and reliability in their activities (Davenport & Kalakota, 2019). AI, which is a disruptive technology (Hinmikaiye et al., 2021) has touched every area of the economy. This technology became a phenomenon with the advent of the internet and with the creation of a pioneer expert system termed MYCIN in the health industry for treating bacterial infection by predicting antibiotics for patients. ML techniques and AI paradigms are being utilized to combat various pandemic outbreaks, including communicable and noncommunicable diseases. The significance of pattern-driven datasets on supervised ML helps AI achieve its disruptiveness (Akinsola et al., 2020).

Researchers have suggested numerous theories to better explain the dynamics of COVID-19. Krishna & Prakash, (2020) suggested a mathematical model that included infected patients, the sanitization of hospitalized cases, and a proportion of identified cases. According to Adewole et al. (2021), a mathematical model that incorporated the key parameters of COVID-19 in Nigeria has been formulated. This model is calibrated using data obtained from the Nigeria Centre for Disease Control and key parameters of the model are estimated. Nonetheless, formal approaches for performance assessment compared with conventional methodologies have been demonstrated to be profound (Akinsola et al., 2020). Vaishya et al. (2020) thought that early disease identification, whether infectious or noninfectious, was a vital task when saving additional lives during early treatment, as supported by Ai et al. (2019) in which ML has been largely successful, especially regarding COVID-19 screening and treatment, contact tracing, in addition to prediction and forecasting.

Health professionals can utilize radiation images as everyday instruments to increase conventional diagnosis with screening like X-ray or CT scans. However, with the large SARS-CoV-2 pandemic outbreak, these devices' performance is modest. Ardakani et al. (2020) demonstrated ML and AI capabilities through the proposition of a fast novel model as well as an effective technique (deep convolutional network diagnosis) against SARS-CoV-2. Thus, validating the reliability of ML compared with the traditional approaches for predicting and treatment of COVID-19. However, most of the studies utilized more than one ML algorithm for classification with single data. Therefore, a hybrid classification method should be developed that applies more potential hybrid databases or multi-database composed of demographic, mammographic, and clinical data using algorithms with sequencing predictive analytic capabilities, since every data type has a major feature that may signify a real disease-ridden patients' identity that can be applied in real time. The model built from such algorithms must take into consideration an intelligent user interface (Akinsola et al., 2021). Several contact tracing applications have been developed using ML and AI-based graphical theory to enhance the efficacy of the standard healthcare diagnosis methods. However, issues, such as privacy, data control, and even data security breaches are still limited, and these challenges have to be resolved to combat the current pandemic holistically.

ML has been used to construct a model that predicts cumulative positive COVID-19 cases in advance using a stacking (STA) ensemble and support vector regression (Ribeiro et al., 2020). Several supervised learning algorithms can determine the most efficient technique in relation to the dataset, the number of occurrences, and the variables involved (Osisanwo et al., 2017). The application of ML on two datasets using 80 existing drugs suggested the best drugs and vaccinations for COVID-19, which included eight drugs, such as bedaquiline, gemcitabine, brequinar, clofazimine, vismodegib, celecoxib, conivaptan, and tolcapone. Another five drugs were found to be useful for curing the disease, such as chloroquine, salinomycin, tilorone, boceprevir, and homoharringtonine from the AI experimentation for drug administration and vaccines development. Therefore, the application of ML and AI technologies have been playing significant roles in the detection and prevention of COVID-19 spread across the globe.

10.5.1 Types of ML

Learning in ML is divided broadly into four types, such as statistical inference, learning techniques, learning problems, and hybrid learning (Brownlee, 2019). Deep learning (DL) and evolutionary learning have evolved as other classes of learning in ML in addition to the four categories previously mentioned, which makes six learning types in the classification. Each of these major groups has the following subdivisions.

10.5.2 Statistical Inference

Statistical inference denotes the method through which inferences are drawn from the model estimate. The inference is the attainment of a conclusion or choice. In ML both forms of inference are used to fit a model and predict. Inferences may be used as a foundation for understanding how certain ML algorithms function or how certain learning issues can be dealt with.

The examples of learning under this category are transductive learning, in addition to inductive learning and deductive inference.

10.5.3 Learning Techniques

Many approaches are classified as learning techniques. Active, ensemble, online, transfer, and multitask learning are ML groups referred to as learning techniques.

10.5.4 Learning Problems

There are three basic categories of learning problems in ML. These can be classified under these three types, supervised learning, reinforcement, and unsupervised learning

10.5.5 Hybrid Learning Problems

The boundaries between supervised and unsupervised learning are blurred, and numerous hybrid techniques have been derived from every field of research. Hybrid learning includes self-supervised, semi-supervised, and multi-instance learning.

10.5.6 DL

DL is an ML variant that is extremely sophisticated and uses more advanced approaches to solve tough issues. Mondal et al. (2021) applied DL techniques to diagnose COVID-19 disease, the study introduced the use of optimized Inception ResNetV2. According to Anirudh, (2019), DL is decisive. DL includes neural networks (NN), a sort of algorithm patterned on the physical nature of the human brain. NNs appear as the fundamentally profound aspect of AI inquiry because they offer a far more accurate human brain simulation, which is better than before. DL designs can reach better accuracy, specificity, and possibly higher performance compared with human beings. The use of a complete range of labeled data in addition to multifaceted NN architecture is trained for these approaches.

10.5.7 Evolutionary Learning

Evolutionary algorithms are applied to tackle optimization problems, leading to positive results in many areas (Vikhar, 2016). Due to the heuristic character of the optimization of evolution; however, most of the results to date were experiential and without theoretical inclination. Evolutionary learning is highly regarded in the community of ML due to its weakness, which promotes sound theoretical methods (Zhou et al., 2019). The evolutionary computation field involves the following major algorithms: genetic (GA), differential evolution, evolution strategy, genetic programming, and evolutionary programming (Slowik & Kwasnicka, 2020).

10.6 DT Algorithm

DTs are applied to two types of problems: regression and classification. Tree-based methods are easy and important in analysis. However, when used in their basic form, they perform worse than other supervised learning approaches. Regression trees use continuous dependent variables, whereas classification trees are used when the dependent variable is categorical.

10.6.1 Regression Tree Modeling

Building a regression tree model consists of two basic approaches.

1. Dividing the predictor or feature space into possible set values for $x_1, x_2, \ldots, x_n$ into J nonoverlapping and distinct subspaces or regions, $R_1, R_2, R_3, \ldots, R_J$
2. After training, if an observation is within an R_j region, then the observation is given the same prediction as the mean response values corresponding to that region

To find the regions $R_1, R_2, R_3, \ldots, R_J$ a recursive binary splitting (RBS) technique is used to minimizes the residual sum of squares (RSS), RSS is given by

$$\sum_{j=1}^{J} \sum_{i \in R_j} (y_i - \widehat{y_{R_j}})^2 \tag{10.1}$$

where:

$\widehat{y_{R_j}}$ = mean response value of each jth region for the training observations.

RBS grows a large tree by training on data, starting from the top, RBD splits the tree into two branches. This creates a two-space partition; multiple instances of this split use different features. It stops when each terminal node has less than some minimum observations. However, reducing the tree to a smaller size with fewer splits can lead to lower variance and better interpretation with little bias.

A number of training sets are taken from a population, for which separate models are built for each set, and then aggregate their predictions as a way of improving accuracy and reducing variance. Generating different bootstrapped training data sets and averaging all the predictions to obtain Bag in the following form

$$f_{bag}(x) = \frac{1}{B} \sum_{b=1}^{B} f^{*b}(x) \tag{10.2}$$

Bag is useful for DTs as it improves prediction. To apply Bag, B instances of regression trees were constructed with B instances of bootstrapped training sets. The resulting trees were deep and unpruned.

Boosting and Bag work similarly except for, in boosting trees are grown sequentially. However, boosting has a danger of overfitting especially when B is too large. Because of boosting overfitting, cross-validation is used to select B with the help of a shrinkage parameter λ, it controls boosting the learning rate.

$$f(x) = \frac{1}{B} \sum_{b=1}^{B} \lambda f^b(x) \tag{10.3}$$

10.6.2 Classification Trees

Growing a classification tree employs a similar approach to growing a regression tree, using a Gini index defined by

$$G = \sum_{k=1}^{K} p_{mk}(1 - p_{mk}) \tag{10.4}$$

This is a measure of total variance across the *K* classes. The observed proportion of training set (p_{mk}) was found in the *m*th region belonging to the *k*th class.

10.6.3 BART

For *p*-dimension, vectors x_i and Y_i ($1 \leq i \leq n$) represent the predictors and response in a BART model posit.

$$Y_i = f(x_i) + \epsilon_i \qquad (10.5)$$

The error term is normally distributed with a mean of zero and variance, σ^2. where: *f* = the sum of many regression trees.

The regression tree makes up the basic building block for BART. A BART original formula for the sum-of-trees model by Chipman et al., (2012), defines the sum of the fit of many trees, *f*, as:

$$f(x) = g(x, T_1, M_1) + g(x, T_2, M_2) + \ldots + g(x, T_m, M_m) \qquad (10.6)$$

Here each (T_m, M_m) corresponds to a single subtree model. To avoid overfitting, the trees must be small, and the parameters reduced toward zero, so that each tree–parameter pair constitutes a weak learner.

10.7 DT Hybridized Ensembles

DT is a common method in ML. DT resolves the ML challenges when converting the information into a tree likeness. The DT algorithm belongs to the supervised learning algorithm family. The DT approach may also be used to resolve regression and classification difficulties, unlike other supervised learning techniques (Chauhan, 2021). An attribute is indicated in each internal node and each node in the leaf represents a class label. To fix regression and classification problems, a DT technique might be employed (Dhiraj, 2019).

DT may be categorized by target variable type. The two forms are, therefore, categorical DT and continuous DT variables. The algorithms used in the DT according to target variables are: (1) multivariate adaptive regression splines (MARS); (2) J48, which is produced by C4.5 (ID3 extension); (3) C4.5 (replacement of ID3): (4) Chi-squared automatic interaction detection (CHAID); CHAID is used to perform multilevel splits when computing classification trees to generate a decision; (5) classification and regression tree; and (6) ID3 (extension of D3) (Chauhan, 2021).

Ensemble learning (EL) is an approach in which two or more modes are adapted to the same data and predictions are combined from each model (Brownlee, 2019). There are four types of EL, which are STA, bootstrap aggregation (Bag), random subspace (RS), and boosting (Shin, 2020). A hybridized DT ensemble is a combination of an RS–DT ensemble and an instance-based DT ensemble technique. Ho (1995; 1998) proposed the RS approach to enhance prediction precision by combining the strength of many classifiers with different methods of ensembles. The RS technique usually resembles Bag. Nevertheless, RS changes the data set used for training in creating attribute subdatasets rather than instance subdatasets (Ho, 1995; 1998). DT-based ensembles possess virtually all DT benefits and their imprecision is overcome (Chou et al., 2010).

10.8 DT Hybridized Ensemble Modeling

Ensemble modeling can be carried out with DTs using three approaches, such as a single DT ensemble, a multilevel DT ensemble (two-, three-, or more level DT ensemble), and a hybrid DT ensemble.

10.8.1 Single DT Ensemble

Single DT (SDT) ensembles involve the use of one ensemble of the DT when building models. The fundamental and most popular model that aggregates basic learner strength with the ensemble technique is the single ensemble approach. Examples of SDT are RS–DT, which is an attribute-based EL approach, and instance-based EL approach, such as Bag–DT as well as stochastic gradient boosting (SGB–DT), and STA–DT.

10.8.2 Multilevel DT Ensemble

A multilevel (poly-) ensemble approach can be enhanced, in which the principal concept is to combine predictors across a sequence of resamplings (Erdal, 2013). The series of resamplings can be subsequently repeated multiple times to achieve multilevel ensembles. The justification for a multilevel ensemble technique is that it reduces forecast error. The multilevel could be two-, three-, or more levels. For example, SGB–SGB–SGB–DT.

10.8.3 Two-Level DT Ensemble

The two-level DT (TLDT) ensemble technique utilizes a similar ensemble procedure twofold for the construction of ensemble models. Some examples of two-level ensembles are Bag–Bag–DT, RS– RS–DT in addition to SGB–SGB–DT.

10.8.4 Hybrid DT Ensemble

The hybrid DT (HDT) ensemble approach to the ensemble is the merging of RS along with an instance-based ensemble methodology, such as SGB, STA in addition to Bag, for example, RS–SBG–DT, RS–BAG–DT, RS–STA–DT or any other combination.

10.9 HDT Disease Detection

In order to determine quickly and to predict infected people at the most danger, the decision rules prediction model was implemented by various researchers to curtail the spread of coronavirus. Holdout and cross-validation techniques have been applied for the prediction as well as forecasting of SARS-CoV-2 using various ML and AI approaches, including STA ensembles, XGBoost classifier, support vector, and DL using regression tree, hybrid wavelet autoregressive integrated moving (AIMV) average model including a long-short-term-memory network.

Moreover, according to Lalmuanawma et al. (2020), a key element in the classification of most medical care-intensive patients with high lactic acid dehydrogenase(LDH) levels might experience respiratory illnesses, such as bronchitis, pneumonia, and asthma.

The results show that the DT ensembles created, achieved better outcomes than traditional DT ensembles for unbalanced data sets. The research implied that the classification techniques should be selected based on data characteristics. The results showed that it can also enhance prediction performance if the age variable is combined with other laboratory tests (Ahmad et al., 2021). Yoo et al. (2020) explored the possible use of a DL–DT classification to detect COVID-19 through chest X-ray pictures by implementing three binary DT algorithms with an accuracy of 98% from the optimized data with three levels of ensemble modeling.

J48 and Hoeffding trees were the DTs utilized in research by Rochmawati et al. (2020). J48 and the Hoeffding trees can create unambiguous guidelines as to whether somebody is subjected to mild, moderate, and severe COVID or not. Nonetheless, the Hoeffding Tree is easy and simple to construct compared with a J48 that has a greater number of nodes. The results from J48 were better than that of Hoeffding trees.

According to Ardakani et al. (2020), 10 COVID-19 infections were separated from non-COVID-19 groups using 10 CNNs. The best performance of ResNet-101 with Xception was 0.994 area under the curve (AUC). Hence, DL can be utilized as a diagnostic tool for COVID-19.

10.10 Results and Discussion

10.10.1 Fitting Classification Trees

Classification trees were used to analyze the COVID-19 data set. From the data, the number of deaths was used to explain other variables. The actual variables (internal nodes) in the data were the number of cases of COVID-19 as displayed in

Table 10.1   Table of Classification Tree

Variable	Cases
Number of terminal nodes	10

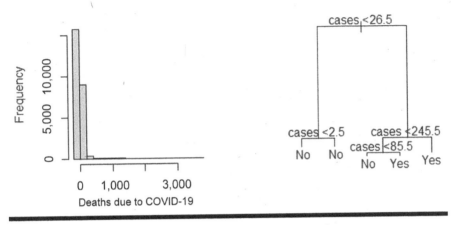

Figure 10.2   Histogram and tree classifier for COVID-19 dataset

Table 10.2   Model's Confusion Matrix, Accuracy, Precision, Specificity, Recall, and F1 Score Results

		True Class	
	N = 170	No	Yes
Predicted Class	No	58	20
	Yes	12	79
Accuracy		0.810650888	
Precision		0.797979798	
Specificity		0.743589744	
Recall		0.868131868	
F1 Score		0.831578947	

Table 10.1. The number of terminal nodes was 10. Figure 10.2 shows a histogram and tree classification.

The observations were divided into two: (1) test set; and (2) training set. Prediction accuracy of >80% was obtained. The confusion matrix given in Table 10.2 gives the performance of the classification model.

10.10.2 Fitting Regression Trees

A training set was created, and the tree was fitted to it. The cumulative number of cases every 14 d per 100,000 of the population was used as the dependent variable. The regression line is given as

$$Y = -733.7 - 0.000559X_1 + 0.03854X_2 + 0.3632X_3$$
$$+ 0.005738X_4 + 0.0292X_5 \tag{10.7}$$

The variables used when constructing the trees were the number of cases, months, population data, territories, and the number of deaths. The regression tree test set mean square error (MSE) was 0.1785 and the square root was around 0.4224, indicating a test prediction that was around 422.4 of the true median cumulative number of cases for COVID-19 in Nigeria.

10.10.3 Hybridization of Bag and Random Forest

Bag was performed on the data using the actual variables used in the regression trees to see how well the bagged model performed on the test set, as given in Table 10.3. From the residuals of the sum of squares, the MSE was calculated. Then, the sum of squares was divided by the number of observations (n), to obtain the mean of the squared residuals.

Growing a random forest showed a test set MSE of 0.234065, which yielded an improvement over Bag with a value of 0.2632. Then, the importance of each variable was reported in Table 10.4.

The higher the value of the mean decreased accuracy or mean decreased Gini score, the more important the variable was to the model.

The mean decrease accuracy (IncMSE), which was calculated from a reduction in the accuracy mean in predictions when the model excluded a variable and mean decrease Gini (IncNodePurity) measured the total decrease in node impurity that resulted from splits over those variables that were averaged over all trees, as shown in Figure 10.3.

For classification trees, the node impurity measurement arises from deviance, while in regression trees, it was measured by the training RSS. Plots of these important measures are shown in Figure 10.4.

Table 10.3 Summary of Bag Results

Variable	Value
Number of trees	500
Mean of squared residuals	0.0155
% Var explained	99.04

Table 10.4   Importance of each Variable for Hybridization

Variable	% IncMSE	IncNodePurity
Day	-0.3567	1.3696
Month	13.5567	37.2178
Year	0	0.1495
Cases	68.3093	215.6263
Deaths	9.1845	17.7558
popData	0	0.0000
continentExp	0	0.0000
%IncMSE = Mean decrease accuracy		
IncNodePurity = Mean decrease Gini		

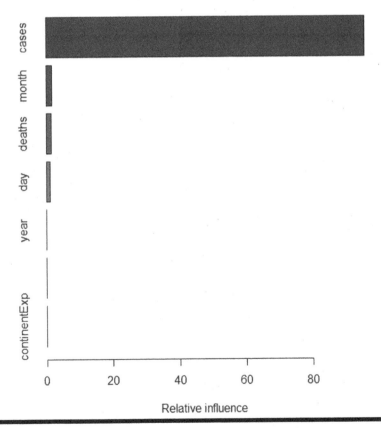

Figure 10.3   Importance measures plot for COVID-19 data

rf.covid

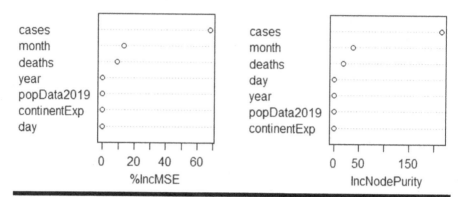

Figure 10.4 Plots of importance measured produced from the random forest

Table 10.5 Boosting Relative Influence Statistics Summary

Variable	Relative Influence
Cases	95.495
Month	1.830
Deaths	1.564
Day	1.111
Year	0.000
popData	0.000
continentExp	0.000

The results indicated that across all the trees considered in the random forest, the number of cases, months, and number of deaths were the most important variables.

10.10.4 Boosting

Boosting is a sequential process: each generated following model is added to improve on the previous model. Table 10.5 indicates that the number of cases, months, and number of deaths were the most important variables. The test MSE obtained was 0.02877, which was close to Bag.

Table 10.6   Comparison of MSE of the Algorithms

Tree Algorithm	MSE
Regression tree	0.1785
Bag	0.2632
Random forest	0.234065
Boosting	0.02877
BART	4.3678

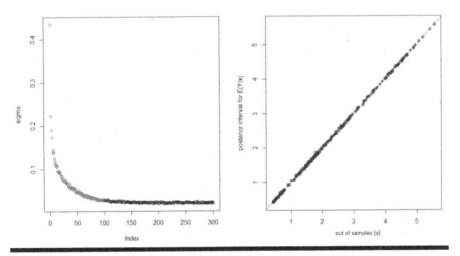

Figure 10.5   Plot of BARTS

10.10.5 BART

BART, which is a sum-of-trees, appears to be very robust to small changes in the previous and the choice of the number of trees. The MSE was 4.3678. The plot in blue has the input-dependent vectors of the response variable on the horizontal axis and posterior intervals for the corresponding function on the vertical axis (Figure 10.5). Table 10.6 shows a comparison of MSEs using the algorithms.

10.11 Limitations and Future Work

COVID-19 data is still being generated; therefore, DT models will fluctuate, because a change in data can lead to a structural change in the optimal DTs. Also, if the outcome of some variables are linked, the calculation becomes very complex. It is recommended for future studies to provide an EL method that can model continuous data in large volumes with several variables over time.

10.12 Conclusions

The outbreak of COVID-19 has questioned the world's readiness to handle an unexpected outbreak of a deadly disease(s). The need to improve the response time, accuracy of diagnosis, and efficiency of resource(s) distribution in the face of an epidemic or pandemic has brought about the use of computational techniques, especially ML techniques. DT, which is an ML technique can be applied to regression and classification problems. On their own, DTs perform poorly; however, when used as ensembles they showed improved performance. Selected DT ensembles were compared using the Nigerian COVID-19 data taken from the world COVID 19 data.

Finally, this chapter discussed the phylogenetics of coronavirus and the three main approaches to COVID-19 diagnosis. The contribution of this chapter was in the application of hybridized DT algorithms for fitting an optimal regression line for COVID-19 data. In addition, the implementation and comparison of different DT ensemble techniques were discussed. The COVID-19 model's result showed an accuracy of 81%, precision of approximately 80%, specificity of 74%, and recall had the highest rate of 86% and an F-score of 83%. The results showed that the DT-based model was reliable.

References

Adewole, M. O., Onifade, A. A., Abdullah, F. A., Kasali, F., & Ismail, A. I. M. (2021). Modeling the dynamics of COVID-19 in Nigeria. *International Journal of Applied and Computational Mathematics, 7*(67), 1–25. doi.10.1007/s40819-021-01014-5

Ahmad, A., Safi, O., Malebary, S., Alesawi, S., & Alkayal, E. (2021). Decision tree ensembles to predict coronavirus disease 2019 Infection: A comparative study. *Complexity, 2021,* 1–8. doi.10.1155/2021/5550344

Ai, T., Yang, Z., Hou, H., Zhan, C., Chen, C., Lv, W., ... Xia, L. (2019). Correlation of chest CT and RT-PCR testing in coronavirus disease 2019 (COVID-19) in China: A report of 1014 Cases. *Radiology, 29*(2),1–23.

Akinsola, J. E. T., Adeagbo, M. A., & Awoseyi, A. A. (2019). Breast cancer predictive analytics using supervised machine learning techniques. *International Journal of Advanced Trends in Computer Science and Engineering, 8*(6). doi.10.30534/ijatcse/2019/70862019

Akinsola, J. E. T., Akinseinde, S., Kalesanwo, O., Adeagbo, M., Oladapo, K., Awoseyi, A., & Kasali, F. (2021). Application of artificial intelligence in user interfaces design for cyber security threat modeling. In L. M. Castro, D. Cabero, & R. Heimgartner (Eds.) *Software Usability*. IntechOpen. 1–28. doi.10.5772/intechopen.9653

Akinsola, J. E. T., Awodele, O., Idowu, S. A., & Kuyoro, S. O. (2020). SQL injection attacks predictive analytics using supervised machine learning techniques. *International Journal of Computer Applications Technology and Research, 9*(4), 139–149. doi.10.7753/ijcatr0904.1004

Akinsola, J. E. T., Awodele, O., Kuyoro, S. O., & Kasali, F. A. (2019). Performance evaluation of supervised machine learning algorithms using multi-criteria decision making techniques. *International Conference on Information Technology in Education and Development (ITED)*, 17–34.

Akinsola, J. E. T., Kuyoro, A., Adeagbo, M. A., & Awoseyi, A. A. (2020). Performance Evaluation of Software using Formal Methods. *Global Journal of Computer Science and Technology: C Software & Data Engineering, 20*(1).

Ali, A., Qadir, J., Rasool, R. ur, Sathiaseelan, A., Zwitter, A., & Crowcroft, J. (2016). Big data for development: applications and techniques. *Big Data Analytics, 1*(1). doi.10.1186/ s41044-016-0002-4

Anirudh, V. K. (2019). What is machine learning: Definition, types, applications and examples. Potentia Analytics Inc. Retrieved from https://potentiaco.com/what-is-machine-learn ing-definition-types-applications-and-examples/#:~:text=As%20explained%2C%20 machine%20learning%20algorithms,unsupervised%20learning%2C%20and%20re inforcement%20learning.

Ardakani, A. A., Kanafi, A. R., Acharya, U. R., Khadem, N., & Mohammadi, A. (2020). Application of deep learning technique to manage COVID-19 in routine clinical practice using CT images: Results of 10 convolutional neural networks. *Computers in Biology and Medicine, 121*, 103795. doi.10.1016/j.compbiomed.2020.103795

Berekaa, M. M. (2021). Insights into the COVID-19 pandemic: Origin, pathogenesis, diagnosis, and therapeutic interventions. *Frontiers in Bioscience, 13*, 117–139.

Bharati, S., Podder, P., & Mondal, M. R. H. (2020). Hybrid deep learning for detecting lung diseases from X-ray images. *Informatics in Medicine Unlocked, 20*, 100391. doi.10.1016/j.imu.2020.100391

Bharati, S., Podder, P., Mondal, M. R. H., & Prasath, V. B. S. (2021a). CO-ResNet: optimized ResNet model for COVID-19 diagnosis from X-ray images. *International Journal of Hybrid Intelligent Systems, 17*(1–2), 71–85. doi.10.3233/his-210008

Bharati, S., Podder, P., Mondal, M. R. H., & Prasath, V. B. S. (2021b). Medical imaging with deep learning for COVID- 19 diagnosis: A comprehensive review. *International Journal of Computer Information Systems and Industrial Management Applications, 13*, 91–112. https://arxiv.org/abs/2107.09602v1

Brownlee, J. (2019). 14 Different types of learning in machine learning. Machine Learning Mastery. Retrieved from https://machinelearningmastery.com/types-of-learning-in-machine-learning/

Chauhan, N. S. (2021). Decision Tree Algorithm Explained. KDnuggets. Retrieved from https://kdnuggets.com/2020/01/decision-tree-algorithm-explained.html

Chipman, H. A., George, E. I., & McCulloch, R. E. (2012). BART: Bayesian additive regression trees. *Annals of Applied Statistics, 6*(1), 266–298. doi.10.1214/09-AOAS285

Chou, J.-S., Chiu, C.-K., Farfoura, M., & Al-Taharwa, I. (2010). Optimizing the prediction accuracy of concrete compressive strength based on a comparison of data-mining techniques. *Journal of Computing in Civil Engineering, 25*(3), 242–253. doi.10.1061/ (ASCE)CP.1943-5487.0000088

Ciotti, M., Ciccozzi, M., Terrinoni, A., Jiang, W. C., Wang, C. B., & Bernardini, S. (2020). The COVID-19 pandemic. *Critical Reviews in Clinical Laboratory Sciences, 57*(6), 365–388. doi.10.1080/10408363.2020.1783198

Colson, P., Lagier, J., Baudoin, J., Khalil, J., Scola, B. La, & Raoult, D. (2020). Ultrarapid diagnosis, microscope imaging, genome sequencing, and culture isolation of SARS-CoV-2. *European Journal of Clinical Microbiology and Infectious Disease, 39*(8), 1601–1603.

Davenport, T., & Kalakota, B. R. (2019). The potential for artificial intelligence in healthcare. *Future Healthcare Journal, 6*(2), 94–98. doi.10.7861/futurehosp.6-2-94

Dhiraj, K. (2019). Top 5 advantages and disadvantages of decision tree algorithm. Medium. Retrieved from https://dhirajkumarblog.medium.com/top-5-advantages-and-disadv antages-of-decision-tree-algorithm-428ebd199d9a

Erdal, H. I. (2013). Two-level and hybrid ensembles of decision trees for high perform- ance concrete compressive strength prediction. *Engineering Applications of Artificial Intelligence, 26*(7), 1689–1697. doi.10.1016/j.engappai.2013.03.014

Gorbalenya, A. E., Baker, S. C., Baric, R. S., de Groot, R. J., Drosten, C., Gulyaeva, A. A., and Ziebuhr, J. (2020). The species severe acute respiratory syndrome-related cor- onavirus: classifying 2019-nCoV and naming it SARS-CoV-2. *Nature Microbiology.* doi.10.1038/s41564-020-0695-z

Hani, C., Trieu, N. H., Saab, I., Dangeard, S., Bennani, S., Chassagnon, G., & Revel, M. P. (2020). COVID-19 pneumonia: A review of typical CT findings and differential diagnosis. *Diagnostic and Interventional Imaging, 101*(5), 263–268. doi.10.1016/ j.diii.2020.03.014

Hinmikaiye, J. O., Awodele, O., & Akinsola, J. E. T. (2021). Disruptive technology and regulatory response: The Nigerian perspective. *Computer Engineering and Intelligent Systems, 12*(1), 42–47. doi.10.7176/ceis/12-1-06

Ho, T. K. (1995). Random decision forest. In: Proceedings of the Third International Conference on Document Analysis and Recognition, 278– 282.

Ho, T. K. (1998). The random subspace method for constructing decision forests. *IEEE Transactions on Pattern Analysis and Machine Intelligence, 20*(8), 832–844. doi.10.1109/ 34.709601

Idowu, S. A., Awodele, O., Kuyoro, S. O., & Akinsola, J. E. T. (2020). Taxonomy and characterization of structured query language injection attacks for predictive analytics. *International Journal of Software & Hardware Research in Engineering, 8*(3), 15–25.

Krishna, M. V., & Prakash, J. (2020). Mathematical modelling on phase based transmis- sibility of Coronavirus. *Infectious Disease Modelling, 5*, 375–385. doi.10.1016/ j.idm.2020.06.005

Kumar, V., Singh, D., Kaur, M., & Damaševičius, R. (2021). Overview of current state of research on the application of artificial intelligence techniques for COVID-19. *Peer Journal of Computer Science, 7*, e564. doi.org10.7717/peerj-cs.564

Lalmuanawma, S., Hussain, J., & Chhakchhuak, L. (2020). Applications of machine learning and artificial intelligence for Covid-19 (SARS-CoV-2) pandemic: A review. *Chaos, Solitons and Fractals, 139.* doi.10.1016/j.chaos.2020.110059

Mondal, M. R. H., Bharati, S., & Podder, P. (2021). CO-IRv2: Optimized InceptionResNetV2 for COVID-19 detection from chest CT images. *PlosOne, 16*(10), e0259179. doi.10.1371/JOURNAL.PONE.0259179

Mondal, M. R. H., Bharati, S., Podder, P., & Podder, P. (2020). Data analytics for novel coronavirus disease. *Informatics in Medicine Unlocked, 20*, 100374. doi.10.1016/ j.imu.2020.100374

Osisanwo, F. Y., Akinsola, J. E. T., Awodele, O., Hinmikaiye, J. O., Olakanmi, O., & Akinjobi, J. (2017). Supervised machine learning algorithms: Classification and com- parison. *International Journal of Computer Trends and Technology (IJCTT), 48*(3), 128–138.

Phillips-Wren, G., Ichalkaranje, N., & Jain, L. C. (2008). *Intelligent Decision Making: An AI-Based Approach. Studies in Computational Intelligence* (97th ed.). Berlin Heidelberg: Springer-Verlag. doi.10.1007/978-3-540-76829-6

Podder, P., Khamparia, A., Rubaiyat Hossain Mondal, M., Rahman, M. A., & Bharati, S. (2021). Forecasting the spread of COVID-19 and ICU requirements. *International Journal of Online and Biomedical Engineering, 17*(5), 81–99. doi.10.3991/ijoe.v17i05.20009

Ribeiro, M. H. D. M., da Silva, R. G., Mariani, V. C., & Coelho, L. dos S. (2020). Short-term forecasting COVID-19 cumulative confirmed cases: Perspectives for Brazil. *Chaos, Solutions and Fractals: The Interdisciplinary Journal of Nonlinear Science, and Nonequilibrium and Complex Phenomena*, 109853. doi.10.1016/j.chaos.2020.109853

Rochmawati, N., Hidayati, H. B., Yamasari, Y., Yustanti, W., Rakhmawati, L., Tjahyaningtijas, H. P. A., & Anistyasari, Y. (2020). Narrative for COVID-19 decision tree for people in schools, youth, and child care programs introduction. Paper presented at the Third International Conference on Vocational Education and Electrical Engineering (ICVEE), IEEE Xplore, 8–12.

Samuel, A. L. (1959). Some studies in machine learning using the game of checkers. *IBM Journal of Research and Development, 3*(3), 210–229. doi.10.1147/rd.441.0206

Shahid, O., Nasajpour, M., Pouriyeh, S., Parizi, R. M., Han, M., Valero, M., Li, F., ... Sheng, Q. Z. (2021). Machine learning research towards combating COVID-19: Virus detection, spread prevention, and medical assistance. *Journal of Biomedical Informatics, 117*. doi.10.1016/J.JBI.2021.103751

Shin, J. (2020). Random subspace ensemble learning for functional near-infrared spectroscopy brain-computer interfaces. *Frontiers in Human Neuroscience, 14*(July), 1–9. doi.10.3389/fnhum.2020.00236

Slowik, A., & Kwasnicka, H. (2020). Evolutionary algorithms and their applications to engineering problems. *Neural Computing and Applications, 32*(16), 12363–12379. doi.10.1007/s00521-020-04832-8

Vaishya, R., Javaid, M., Haleem, I., & Haleem, A. (2020). Artificial intelligence (AI) applications for COVID-19 pandemic. *Diabetes & Metabolic Syndrome: Clinical Research & Reviews, 14*(4), 337–339. doi.10.1016/j.dsx.2020.04.012

Vikhar, P. A. (2016). Evolutionary algorithms: A critical review and its future prospects. Paper presented at the IEEE 2016 International Conference on Global Trends in Signal Processing, Information Computing and Communication (ICGTSPICC) (pp. 261–265). Jalagon, India.

WHO. (2021). WHO Coronavirus (COVID-19) Dashboard with Vaccination Data. Retrieved from https://covid19.who.int/

Yoo, S. H., Geng, H., Chiu, T. L., Yu, S. K., Cho, D. C., Heo, J., Choi, M. S., ... Lee, H. (2020). Deep learning-based decision-tree classifier for COVID-19 diagnosis from chest X-ray imaging. *Frontiers in Medicine, 7*(427), 1–8. doi.10.3389/FMED.2020.00427

Zhou, Z.-H., Yu, Y., & Qian, C. (2019). *Evolutionary learning: Advances in theories and algorithms*. Singapore: Springer. doi.10.1007/978-981-13-5956-9_1

Chapter 11

CoVICU: A Smart Model for Predicting the Intensive Care Unit Stay of COVID-19 Patients Using Machine Learning Techniques

Sakthi Jaya Sundar Rajasekar

Melmaruvathur Adhiparasakthi Institute of Medical Sciences and Research, Melmaruvathur, Tamil Nadu, India

V. Aruna Devi and Varalakshmi Perumal

MIT Campus, Anna University, Chennai, India

Contents

DOI: 10.1201/9781003324447-11

11.1 Introduction

Coronavirus has affected people throughout the world. This has been noted as one of the greatest disasters in the world's record. According to the World Health Organization (WHO), more than 18 million confirmed cases were recorded. Meanwhile, above 40 lakhs death cases were recorded (WHO, 2021). The prediction of COVID positive is important because early detection of diseases will always help to the necessary actions to be taken earlier. Therefore, many medical and research organizations have released datasets to help forecast COVID-19. The significant features from the datasets need to be selected. Some of the attributes might show significant performance improvements. Some may not give a significant improvement in the results. Most of the features have missing values; therefore, the missing values need to be filled or remove the attribute that has many missing values. All these things need to be sorted out before performing the classification. Once all the data was preprocessed, the model was chosen for classification purposes. The model could be any machine learning (ML) model or mathematical model. As usual, ML has an impact on the medical field. Most of the papers discussed the significance of ML algorithms when forecasting COVID-19 cases.

The main contributions of this chapter are as follows.

1. This work was proposed mainly for predicting whether COVID patients need to stay in ICUs or not
2. The dataset preprocessing was carried out by considering the missing value replacement and balancing the dataset
3. A variety of ML algorithms were used for predicting whether the patient needed to stay in the ICU or not and the results were compared to choose the best algorithm
4. The results were also compared to determine during which period of testing results the algorithms provided superior results

This chapter is organized as follows. Section 11.2 describes the existing methods for the prognosis of COVID-19 cases. The proposed method is explained in Section 11.3. The implementation and the results of all the models are described in Section 11.4. Conclusions are drawn in Section 11.5 and some of the future scopes are given in Section 11.6.

11.2 Related Works

From the chest X-ray images of patients, the features were extracted using histograms of oriented gradients (Eljamassi, 2020). The classification was carried out using a few ML algorithms, which include K-nearest neighbors (KNN), support vector machine (SVM), and random forest (RF) algorithms. Their work results were compared with other existing works. Consequently, they got better results when classifying the images with an SVM classifier. When considering the prediction of COVID-19, the COVID-19 cases were divided into death, infected, and recovered cases. In Saudi Arabia and Bahrain, the ML models, such as SVM, long short-term memory, linear regression (LR), and polynomial regression (PR) were employed for the forecasting of the previously mentioned cases. Finally, for the prediction of COVID-19 confirmed cases, SVM and LR showed better results for Saudi Arabia and Bahrain, respectively (Khaloofi, 2021). ML algorithms, such as least absolute shrinkage and selection operator (LASSO), decision tree (DT) regressor, LR, SVM, and RF algorithms were compared for the prediction of COVID-19 in India. As a result, they got better results with polynomial LASSO and polynomial LR algorithms (Bhadana, 2020). The forecasting of COVID-19 infection can also be carried out using research on the genome (Wang, 2020). RF classifiers and neural networks (NN) were used for classifying the COVID cases.

Contact tracing is the main contribution to control the spread of COVID-19. The infectious people were identified using Wi-Fi signals from their mobile phones (Narzullaev, 2020). Among the SVM, KNN, LR, and DT algorithms, which have been deployed for classification, SVM outperformed the other algorithms. The PR algorithm was used and compared against the SVM algorithm for the prediction of COVID-19 patients utilizing the dataset released by the Indian Government (Gambhir, 2020). LR, LASSO, SVM, and exponential smoothing (ES) were employed for the prediction of COVID-19 in three cases, such as the number of people recovered, number of newly affected people, and number of deaths (Rustam, 2020). The best results were achieved with the ES algorithm while SVM showed poor performance. Some of the supervised ML algorithms like SVM, NNs, and DT were employed (Yusuf, 2020) and the performance of the models was evaluated by an ANOVA test. They performed four-fold cross-validation after some of the standard preprocessing techniques were used like mutual information and Chi-squared statistical methods.

To determine whether the patient was infected by COVID-19, it might take some time within which the patient's status will become critical. To identify the corona-affected people, ahead of the actual virus test, the relationship between the blood and virus tests was examined (Almansoor, 2020). But unfortunately, they could not find any significant correlation between them. A novel algorithm voting classifier ensemble based on logistic regression, RF and AdaBoost classifier

(SV-LAR) was proposed for the prediction of COVID-19 cases using blood samples from the patient (Darapaneni, 2021). Using their novel algorithm, they proved that analyzing the blood samples of a patient helps to predict if a person was infected by COVID-19 or not. Various ML models to forecast COVID-19 were discussed that could identify COVID-19 easily and quickly; therefore, crowds in hospitals when identifying COVID cases could be avoided. Another approach was proposed to predict COVID-19, which was based on the patient's cough sounds (Anupam, 2021). The ML models like LR, SVM, KNN, and DT classifiers were employed to categorize it into a normal cough, COVID cough, or healthy cough. Using the same supervised ML algorithms with standard feature extracting methods, the predominant features were selected and trained for cough sounds (Vrindavanam, 2021). Ensemble approaches will also enhance the prediction of COVID-19 patients. The ensemble of XGBoost (XGB), RF, and LR algorithms was utilized for forecasting COVID-19 (Podder, 2020). Supervised ML algorithms were used for the prediction of COVID cases based on the laboratory data of the patients. They have also classified the need for ICU if the patient is identified as COVID positive. Both these tasks were completed with the help of supervised ML algorithms (Darapaneni, 2020).

To predict the number of confirmed cases in Xinjiang, China, a mathematical method was built (Liu, 2020). They got better accuracy with PR. So far, numerous ML algorithms to forecast COVID-19 positive cases have been discussed. The number of recovering cases has also been predicted using ML models (Hossen, 2020). COVID-19 is one of the greatest pandemics of the twentieth century. However, there is a chance to recover from this disease if a patient has a healthy immune system. The immune system of a patient will depend on the diet followed by them. They have experimented with some ML algorithms including SVM, RF, and KNN to predict the possibility of COVID-19 patients recovering based on their dietary intake. Computed tomography (CT) images of a patient help to determine the presence of COVID-19 cases. But for classification and segmentation, a number of image samples are required. To increase the number of CT images, the generative adversarial network was used (Jiang, 2020). Like ML models, mathematical models could also be used for the identification of COVID-19 cases. The mathematical, logistic model, susceptible exposed infective removed, susceptible infective removed, and autoregressive integrated moving average mathematical methods were employed (Zhou, 2020) and compared. Based on the literature survey, various ML models were proposed in this chapter to predict whether there is a need to admit COVID patients to ICU or not. The model, which showcased a better performance, would be suggested for deployment in the healthcare sector. Understanding the spatial spread of COVID-19 is important in this pandemic situation (Jenila, 2020). The Internet of Things also has its impact to predict COVID cases. The possible contact tracing was carried out using radio-frequency identification tags and the individual's mobile phone, which was cost-effective (Rajasekar, 2021). When using mobile phones, the security and privacy of the user need to be considered. Following this, the security and privacy issues in contract tracing methods were also discussed (Sowmiya, 2021). It is also possible that the criticality of COVID-19 can be determined using the hybrid regression models with clinical and CT images (Perumal, 2021a). Hybrid learning techniques can also be used for the classification of COVID-19 CT images (Perumal, 2021b). The detection of COVID-19 was carried out by classifying the clinical images using transfer learning, and haralick features were used for feature extraction (Perumal, 2021c). Through data visualization, people could easily understand the impact of COVID-19 cases. The authors collected the data from Johns Hopkins University, Baltimore, MD, US which has been used for data visualization to show the impact on people and the data from Israelita Albert Einstein Hospital, Sao Paulo, Brazil was used for classification (Podder, 2021). The analysis of the factors of COVID-19 will help to expose the widespread disease across the world. So, the authors analyzed and gave a visualization of the agents that majorly influenced the COVID-19 cases (Mondal, 2020). The novel deep learning algorithm known as an optimized residual network was developed and used on the novel dataset, which was created by the combination of two publicly available datasets (Bharati, 2021b). A convoluted neural network might have a drawback because of imperfect staging at rotation, flipping, and blurring. Considering this, the authors presented a hybrid network, which is an amalgamation of the visual geometry group and a spatial transformer network for the classification of lung diseases using X-ray images (Bharati, 2020). The assistance of deep learning in medical imaging is important today. The authors utilized this feature for imaging activities as well as classification and accomplished a great result but with limited data (Bharati, 2021c). As mentioned previously, predicting whether the patient needs to stay in ICU or not is also important. The categorization of confirmed and death cases for COVID-19 is carried out using regression analysis and to classify whether the patient needs to stay in ICU or not is also analyzed (Podder, 2021). The authors also made a review of the significance of artificial intelligence (AI) in the prognosis of COVID-19 using the residual NN and DenseNet (Mondal, 2021a). The Internet of Health Things (IoHT) can also be used for the prognosis of COVID-19 disease by continuously monitoring the patient (Bharati, 2021a). Clinical data is always sensitive. Handling this data is very critical. To maintain the security and confidentiality of the dataset, the Internet of Medical Things (IoMT) was used. The authors used servers and data acquisition systems in the IoMT to avoid security threats (Pinto Kumar Paul, 2021). Furthermore, the diagnosis of COVID-19 has been explored using an optimized InceptionResNetV2 algorithm with a different type of optimizer known as RMSProp, Nadam, and Adam. CT images were preprocessed and used as the input dataset. The combination of an InceptionResNetV2 and Nadam algorithms gave better results for the CT images (Mondal, 2021b).

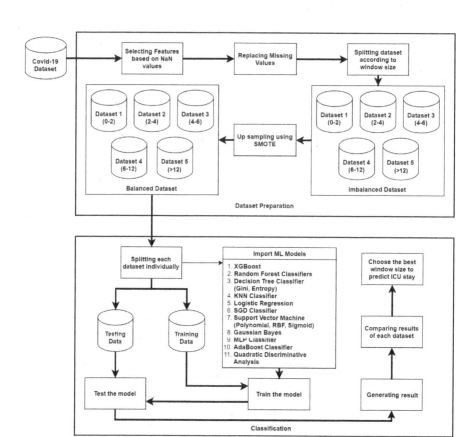

Figure 11.1   Architecture of the proposed system

11.3 Proposed System

Based on the literature survey, the proposed system could be divided into two sections. The architecture of the proposed diagram is shown in Figure 11.1. First, prepare the dataset for categorizing whether the patient needs to stay in ICU or not. The dataset has many missing values where it has 231 attributes and 1,925 records. In the first section, the methods and strategies used to preprocess the dataset will be discussed. To fill out the missing values, the median function was used, and to balance the dataset, the numerical up sampling method was used [synthetic minority oversampling technique (SMOTE)]. In the second section, the employed ML algorithms were discussed. The ML algorithms were evaluated for all five datasets. The results among all five datasets were compared to determine at which period the prediction of ICU stay exhibited better results.

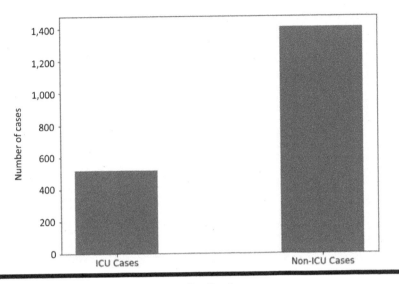

Figure 11.2   ICU and non-ICU cases distribution

11.3.1 Data Preprocessing

The dataset was taken from Kaggle (Kaggle Repository, 2021). It has a total of 231 attributes and 1,925 records. This was binary classification, where the target variable ICU had values of zero or one indicating whether the patient needed to stay in ICU or not, respectively. The distribution of ICU and non-ICU cases are shown in Figure 11.2.

This shows that the COVID-19 dataset was an imbalanced one. The patient group's previous diseases were represented with nine features, vital signs were represented with six features, patient demographic information was given three features, and 36 features were used to represent blood test results; therefore, a total of 54 basic attributes were considered in this work. The dataset also consisted of blood gas statistics. Most of the attributes were expanded into at least four columns, which included mean, median, minimum, and maximum values for the corresponding attributes.

However, from the 231 attributes, most of the attributes didn't have proper values. So, these features were removed, which had <10% of the overall instances. No significant improvement in the results was achieved with these features. After removing the unwanted attributes from the attribute list, there were 51 features in the list including the patient visit identifier and the target that was ICU stay (e.g., 0 = no need to stay in ICU and 1= need to stay in ICU). In addition, categorical attribute AGE_PERCENTIL was used, where the values of age were the 10th, 20th, 30th, 40th, 50th, 60th, 70th, 80th, 90th, and above the 90th percentile. The distribution of the values in the AGE_PERCENTIL attribute is shown in Figure 11.3.

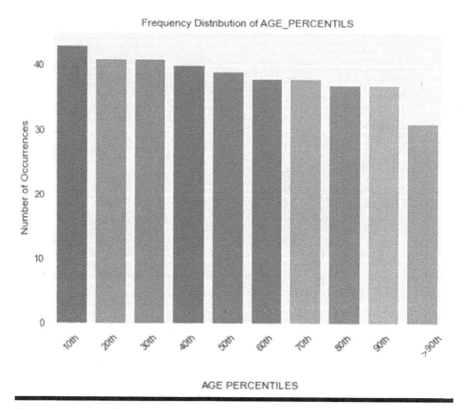

Figure 11.3 **Distribution of AGE_PERCENTIL attribute in COVID-19 dataset**

Since it had categorical values, it could not be prepared for the training ML models. Hence, one-hot encoding was used to make it a purely numerical dataset. After using one-hot encoding, this single attribute was divided into 10 attributes using AGE_ as the prefix. The dataset was composed of 385 patient instances, where each patient's record was taken for five different durations. These durations were indicated by periods, such as 0–2, 2–4, 4–6, 6, and >12 h from the time of admission. Since there were 385 patient instances, a total of 385 × 5 = 1,925 instances were present in the dataset. Then, the dataset was split into five different datasets, according to the period. Then, there were five individual datasets, each with 60 features. Among the five, four were biased datasets since non-ICU instances had more records than ICU instances. All five datasets were balanced using the SMOTE algorithm to make them a balanced dataset. The distribution of the ICU and non-ICU instances for all five datasets is shown in Figure 11.4.

Figure 11.5 shows the relationship between age and the need for an ICU stay.

From these figures, the patient >65 years old had more probability of staying in ICU. Figure 11.5(left), shows the age statistics for not staying in ICU (ICU = 0) and Figure 11.5(right) shows the age statistics for staying in ICU (ICU = 1). As shown in

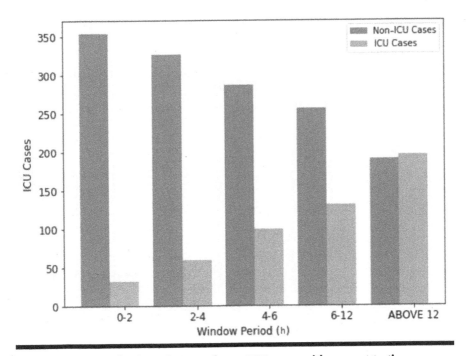

Figure 11.4   Distribution of ICU and non-ICU cases with respect to time

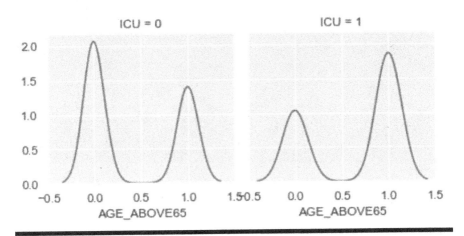

Figure 11.5   Relationship between age and ICU stay of COVID patients (left) age distribution for ICU = 0; and (right) age distribution for ICU = 1

Figure 11.5(left), if the person was <65 years old (i.e., AGE_ABOVE65 = 0), then the probability of not staying in ICU was high (i.e., the high peak at AGE_ABOVE65=0), and for a person >65 years old (AGE_ABOVE65=1), the probability for not staying in ICU was low (i.e., comparatively low peak at AGE_ABOVE65=1). As shown in Figure 11.5(right), if the person was <65 years old (AGE_BELOW65=0), then the probability of staying in ICU was less (i.e., the low peak at AGE_ABOVE65=0), whereas, for a person >65 years old (AGE_ABOVE65=1), the probability for staying in ICU is high (comparatively low peak at AGE_ABOVE65=1). Hence, Figures 11.5(left and right) depict the same meaning with slightly different representations. Similarly, the correlation between the attribute hypertension (HTN) and the probability of an ICU stay is shown in Figure 11.6. From Figure 11.6, it can be seen that a person without HTN has a much lower probability of a stay in the ICU.

Similar to the previous figures, as shown in Figure 11.7, the relationship between the attributes IMMUNOCOMPROMISED and ICU stay is shown.

Other than these attributes, some of the significant notable attributes like heart rate, respiratory rate, temperature, and oxygen saturation are also in the dataset. The correlation between these attributes with the probability of ICU stay is shown in Figure 11.8. For this pair–plot, the mean attributes of the previously mentioned variables were used. As shown in Figure 11.8, the diagonal elements show the correlation between the same attributes (i.e., the histogram of the same attribute). The first diagonal image (X= HEART_RATE_MEAN, y=HEART_RATE_MEAN) describes the frequency of occurrence of the attribute HEART_RATE_MEAN with respect to an ICU stay. The next one (i.e., first row and second column) (X= HEART_RATE_MEAN, y= RESPIRATORY_RATE_MEAN) correlates both variables HEART_RATE_MEAN and RESPIRATORY_RATE_MEAN with respect to an ICU stay. Similarly, all other subplots are shown in Figure 11.8.

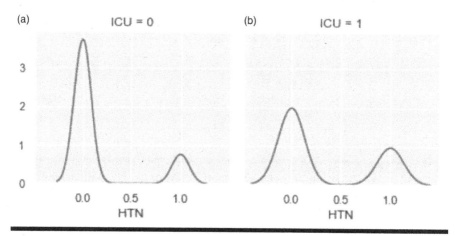

Figure 11.6 Relationship between HTN and ICU stay of COVID patients: (a) HTN distribution for ICU = 0; and (b) HTN distribution for ICU = 1

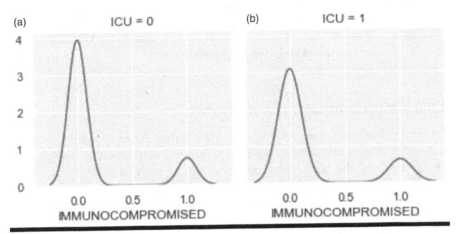

Figure 11.7 Relationship between IMMUNOCOMPROMISED and ICU stay: (a) distribution of IMMUNOCOMPROMISED for ICU = 0; and (b) distribution of IMMUNOCOMPROMISED for ICU = 1

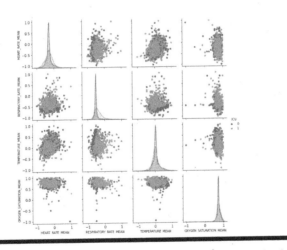

Figure 11.8 Interrelationship between heart rate, respiratory rate, temperature, and oxygen saturation

11.3.2 Classification

Most of the ML algorithms were used on the preprocessed dataset. The ML algorithms like SVM (Kernel = Polynomial, Sigmoid, RBF), DT (criteria= gini, entropy), KNN, XGB, LR, RF, multilayer perceptron (MLP), quadratic discriminative analysis, stochastic gradient descent (SGD), AdaBoost, and Gaussian naive Bayes were used for classification. There were five different datasets, each one representing one window size. The results were evaluated for all five datasets, and better results were achieved for the first dataset, which had the records collected during the first 2 h. The records also described that the XGB algorithm showed better results for most of the datasets, especially for the first 2 h of collected information.

11.4 Implementation and Results

The Jupiter notebook from Anaconda installed in the system was used. It has a backend of Python 3.8. Loading the dataset, manipulating data, checking the null values, dropping the unwanted attributes, selecting the significant features, and replacing the null values of attributes were carried out using the utilities of the Numpy and Pandas modules. Following that, the imbalanced datasets were balanced by the data augmentation technique SMOTE, which is intended for numerical data augmentation, imported from Python's imblearn module. After the preprocessing of the dataset, splitting the dataset into training and testing datasets, importing the selected ML model, fitting the attribute values for training, evaluating the model using the testing dataset, and generating classification results for the model were carried out with the functionalities of Python's sci-kit-learn library. The distribution of attributes in the dataset and the comparison of ML algorithms were visualized with the help of methodologies imported from the matplotlib and seaborn modules. Notably, the interrelationship between the significant attributes was drawn from the pair–plot function, which is available in the seaborn module. The dataset was split based on the window size, which described the period within which the samples were collected. Every dataset was modeled and trained using most of the ML algorithms. The results of all the algorithms were compared for each dataset. The algorithms were evaluated in terms of most of the essential ML evaluation metrics including F1-score, precision, sensitivity (recall), specificity, and accuracy. All these evaluation metrics could provide more significant details for better results. Table 11.1 gives the results for the dataset, collected from 0–2 h from the admission time.

From Table 11.1, the XGB algorithm performed well compared with all other algorithms. Table 11.2 shows the results for the dataset collected from 2–4 h from the admission time.

From Table 11.2, the RF algorithm performed well compared with all other algorithms. Table 11.3 shows the results for the dataset collected from 4–6 h from the admission time.

From Table 11.3, for the dataset collected for 4–6 h, the RF algorithm provided better results. From Table 11.4, for the dataset collected for 6–12 h from the admission, the XGB algorithm showed a better performance. Table 11.5 gives the results for the dataset collected >12 h from the admission time.

From Table 11.5, in the dataset collected >12 h of admission, the XGB algorithm shows better performance. From the results given in the tables, Table 11.1 provided better results compared with all other datasets, which indicated the first 0–2 h of samples provided significant results. Also, the XGB algorithm showed

Table 11.1 Results for the Dataset Collected for 0–2 h

ML Algorithms	Accuracy	Sensitivity (Recall)	Specificity	Precision	F1-Score
XGB	**95.07**	**93.75**	**96.15**	**95**	**94**
RF classifier	93.66	93.75	93.58	92	93
DT (entropy)	92.25	89.06	94.87	93	91
DT (gini)	90.14	85.93	93.58	92	89
K-Neighbors classifier	88.73	93.75	84.61	83	88
Logistic regression	85.91	85.93	85.89	83	85
SGD classifier	85.91	71.87	97.43	96	82
SVM (kernel = linear)	87.32	84.37	89.74	87	86
SVM (kernel = poly)	88.73	89.06	88.46	86	88
SVM (kernel = RBF)	87.32	85.93	88.46	86	86
SVM (kernel = sigmoid)	77.46	85.93	70.51	71	77
Gaussian naive Bayes	80.98	95.31	69.23	72	82
MLP classifier	93.66	93.75	93.58	92	93
AdaBoost classifier	92.25	87.5	96.15	95	91
Quadratic discriminant analysis	81.69	98.43	67.94	72	83

Table 11.2 Results for the Dataset Collected for 2–4 h

ML Algorithms	Accuracy	Sensitivity (Recall)	Specificity	Precision	F1-Score
XGB	85.21	87.87	81.63	87	87
RF classifier	86.08	90.90	79.59	86	88
DT (entropy)	78.26	82.08	72.91	81	81
DT (gini)	73.91	79.10	66.66	77	78
K-Neighbors classifier	72.17	80.59	60.41	74	77
Logistic regression	73.04	77.61	66.66	76	77
SGD classifier	62.60	100	10.41	61	76
SVM (kernel = linear)	75.65	79.10	70.83	79	79
SVM (kernel = poly)	73.04	77.61	66.66	76	77
SVM (kernel = RBF)	71.30	74.62	66.66	76	75
SVM (kernel = sigmoid)	66.95	67.16	66.66	74	70
Gaussian naive Bayes	60	56.71	64.58	69	62
MLP classifier	80.86	86.56	72.91	82	84
AdaBoost classifier	81.73	82.08	81.25	86	84
Quadratic discriminant analysis	71.30	52.23	97.91	97	68

Table 11.3 Results for the Dataset Collected for the Window Period of 4–6 h

ML Algorithms	Accuracy	Sensitivity /(Recall)	Specificity	Precision	F1-Score
XGB	93.58	88.88	97.61	97	93
RF classifier	94.87	88.88	100	100	**94**
DT (entropy)	89.74	88.88	77.77	89	89
DT (gini)	84.61	83.33	85.71	83	83
K-Neighbors classifier	87.17	80.55	92.85	91	85
Logistic regression	92.30	83.33	100	100	91
SGD classifier	91.02	80.55	100	100	89
SVM (kernel = linear)	93.58	86.11	100	100	93
SVM (kernel = poly)	92.30	83.33	100	100	91
SVM (kernel = RBF)	91.02	80.55	100	100	89
SVM (kernel = sigmoid)	89.74	77.77	100	100	88
Gaussian naive Bayes	82.05	69.44	92.85	89	78
MLP classifier	92.30	83.33	100	100	91
AdaBoost classifier	87.17	83.33	90.47	88	86
Quadratic discriminant Analysis	67.94	94.44	45.23	60	73

Table 11.4 Results for the Dataset Collected for the Window Period of 6–12 h

ML Algorithms	Accuracy	Sensitivity (Recall,	Specificity	Precision	F1-Score
XGB	**90.07**	**85.96**	**93.24**	**91**	**88**
RF classifier	89.31	91.22	87.83	85	88
DT (entropy)	80.15	80.70	79.72	75	78
DT (Gini)	82.44	84.21	81.08	77	81
K-Neighbors classifier	76.33	85.96	68.91	68	76
Logistic regression	78.62	73.68	82.43	76	75
SGD classifier	77.86	92.98	66.21	68	79
SVM (kernel = linear)	80.91	68.42	90.54	85	76
SVM (kernel = poly)	84.73	80.70	87.83	84	82
SVM (kernel = RBF)	82.44	85.96	79.72	77	81
SVM (kernel = sigmoid)	74.80	85.96	66.21	66	75
Gaussian naive Bayes	72.51	94.73	55.40	62	75
MLP classifier	83.20	75.43	89.18	84	80
AdaBoost classifier	88.54	87.71	89.18	86	87
Quadratic discriminant analysis	80.15	64.91	91.89	86	74

Table 11.5   Results for the Dataset Collected for >12 h

ML Algorithms	Accuracy	Sensitivity (Recall)	Specificity	Precision	F1-Score
XGB	**86.27**	**84.61**	**88**	**88**	**86**
RF classifier	84.31	84.61	84	85	85
DT (entropy)	80.39	82.69	78	80	81
DT (Gini)	82.35	84.61	80	81	83
K-Neighbors classifier	79.41	86.53	72	76	81
Logistic regression	79.41	75	84	83	79
SGD classifier	71.56	98.07	44	65	78
SVM (kernel = linear)	77.45	75	80	80	77
SVM (kernel = poly)	76.47	69.23	84	82	75
SVM (kernel = RBF)	77.45	73.07	82	81	77
SVM (kernel = sigmoid)	77.45	73.07	82	81	77
Gaussian naive Bayes	74.50	65.38	84	81	72
MLP classifier	82.35	76.92	88	87	82
AdaBoost classifier	80.39	80.76	80	81	81
Quadratic discriminant analysis	78.43	69.23	88	86	77

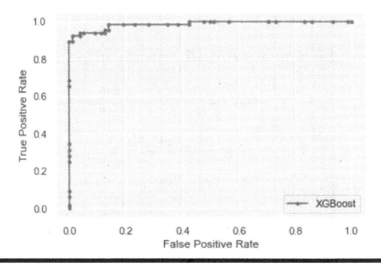

Figure 11.9 AUC Curve for XGB algorithm using 0–2 h

better results for most of the datasets. The AUC curve for the same model is shown in Figure 11.9. The AUC value for the XGB algorithm was 98.6.

The confusion matrix for the same model is shown in Figure 11.10.

11.5 Conclusions

The need for ICU is the most emerging topic in the current COVID situation. It is essential to check whether the COVID patient needs to stay in ICU based on their medical reports taken as window periods (0–2, 2–4, 4–6, 6–12, and >12 h from the admission time). The datasets that were taken were compared at all window periods individually. The first 2 h of patient records from the admission time provided better results. The data acquired from the patients during the first 2 h from admission proved to be the best indicator of the patient outcome in terms of ICU stay in this study. The data set was preprocessed, and the data set was turned into a balanced data set. Different ML models were tried with the balanced data set to choose the best one of the various ML models. The XGB algorithm performed well compared with all other algorithms for 0–2 h. This model could be suggested for clinical deployment. This would provide key insights to physicians and decision makers to better combat the pandemic. Finally, the XGB algorithm outperformed all the other algorithms that were used in this experiment with an accuracy of 95.07%, specificity of 96.15%, sensitivity of 93.75%, precision of 0.95, and F1-score of 0.94 and the test results taken during the first 2 h provide a better outcome for all the ML algorithms.

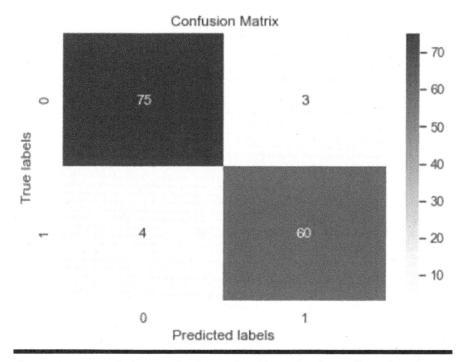

Figure 11.10   Confusion matrix of XGB algorithm using data collected 0–2 h from admission

11.6 Future Work

In data preprocessing, most of the records were ignored because of the missing values. Hence, the number of instances decreased. In further research, an attempt will be made to resolve this problem. Moreover, ML algorithms were used for this experiment. In future, deep learning algorithms could be used to further improve performance.

References

Almansoor, M., & Hewahi, N. M. (2020). Exploring the relation between blood tests and Covid-19 using machine learning. Paper presented at the 2020 IEEE International Conference on Data Analytics for Business and Industry: Way Towards a Sustainable Economy (ICDABI) (pp. 1–6).

Anupam, A., Mohan, N. J., Sahoo, S., & Chakraborty, S. (2021). Preliminary diagnosis of COVID-19 based on cough sounds using machine learning algorithms. Paper presented at the 2021 IEEE 5th International Conference on Intelligent Computing and Control Systems (ICICCS) (pp. 1391–1397). Madurai, India.

Bhadana, V., Jalal, A. S., & Pathak, P. (2020, December). A comparative study of machine learning models for COVID-19 prediction in India. Paper presented at 2020 IEEE 4th Conference on Information & Communication Technology (CICT) (pp. 1–7). Chennai, India.

Bharati, S., & Mondal, M., R., H. (2021a). 12 Applications and challenges of AI-driven IoHT for combating pandemics: A review. In A. Khamparia, R. Hossain Mondal, P. Podder, B. Bhushan, V. Albuquerque, & S. Kumar (Eds.) *Computational Intelligence for Managing Pandemics* (pp. 213–230). Berlin, Boston: De Gruyter.

Bharati, S., Podder, P., & Mondal, M., R., H. (2020). Hybrid deep learning for detecting lung diseases from X-ray images. *Informatics in Medicine Unlocked, 20,* 100391.

Bharati, S., Podder, P., Mondal, M., & Prasath, V., B., (2021a). CO-ResNet: Optimized ResNet model for COVID-19 diagnosis from X-ray images. *International Journal of Hybrid Intelligent Systems,* 17(1–2) (pp. 71–85).

Bharati, S., Podder, P., Mondal, M., & Prasath, V., B. (2021c). Medical imaging with deep learning for COVID-19 diagnosis: A comprehensive review. *arXiv 2107.09602.*

Darapaneni, N., Gupta, M., Paduri, A. R., Agrawal, R., Padasali, S., Kumari, A., & Purushothaman, P. (2021)). A novel machine learning based screening method for high-risk Covid-19 patients based on simple blood exams. Paper presented at the 2021 IEEE International IOT, Electronics and Mechatronics Conference (IEMTRONICS) (pp. 1–6).

Darapaneni, N., Singh, A., Paduri, A., Ranjith, A., Kumar, A., Dixit, D., & Khan, S. (2020). A machine learning approach to predicting covid-19 cases amongst suspected cases and their category of admission. Paper presented at the 2020 IEEE 15th International Conference on Industrial and Information Systems (ICIIS) (pp. 375–380).

Eljamassi, D. F., & Maghari, A. Y. (2020). COVID-19 detection from chest X-ray scans using machine learning. Paper presented at the 2020 IEEE International Conference on Promising Electronic Technologies (ICPET), (pp. 1–4).

Gambhir, E., Jain, R., Gupta, A., & Tomer, U. (2020). Regression analysis of COVID-19 using machine learning algorithms. Paper presented at the 2020 IEEE International conference on smart electronics and communication (ICOSEC) (pp. 65–71).

Hossen, M. S., & Karmoker, D. (2020). Predicting the probability of Covid-19 recovered in South Asian countries based on healthy diet pattern using a machine learning approach. Paper presented at the 2020 IEEE 2nd International Conference on Sustainable Technologies for Industry 4.0 (STI) (pp. 1–6).

Jenila, V. M., Varalakshmi, P., & Rajasekar, S., J., S. (2020). Geospatial mapping, epidemiological modelling, statistical correlation and analysis of COVID-19 with forest cover and population in the districts of Tamil Nadu, India. Paper presented at the 2020 IEEE International Conference on Advent Trends in Multidisciplinary Research and Innovation (ICATMRI) (pp. 1–7).

Jiang, Y., Chen, H., Loew, M., & Ko, H. (2020). Covid-19 CT image synthesis with a conditional generative adversarial network. *IEEE Journal of Biomedical and Health Informatics, 25*(2) (pp. 441–452).

Kaggle repository. (2021) COVID-19 – Clinical Data to assess diagnosis. Retrieved from www.kaggle.com/S%C3%ADrioLibanes/covid19

Khaloofi, H., Hussain, J., Azhar, Z., & Ahmad, H. F. (2021). Performance evaluation of machine learning approaches for COVID-19 forecasting by infectious disease modeling. Paper presented at the 2021 IEEE International Conference of Women in Data Science at Taif University (WiDSTaif) (pp. 1–6).

Liu, Y., & Xiao, Y. (2020). Analysis and prediction of COVID-19 in Xinjiang based on machine learning. Paper presented at the 2020 IEEE 5th International Conference on Information Science, Computer Technology and Transportation (ISCTT) (pp. 382–385).

Mondal, M. R. H., Bharati, S., & Podder, P. (2021a). *Diagnosis of COVID-19 using machine learning and deep learning: A review.* Current Medical Imaging.

Mondal, M. R.H., Bharati, S., & Podder, P. (2021b). CO-Irv2: Optimized InceptionResNetV2 for COVID-19 detection from chest CT images. *PLoS One, 16(*10), e0259179.

Mondal, M. R. H., Bharati, S., Podder, P., & Podder, P. (2020). Data analytics for novel coronavirus disease. *Informatics in Medicine Unlocked, 20,* 100374.

Narzullaev, A., Muminov, Z., & Narzullaev, M. (2020). Contact tracing of infectious diseases using Wi-Fi signals and machine learning classification. Paper presented at the 2020 IEEE 2nd International Conference on Artificial Intelligence in Engineering and Technology (IICAIET) (pp. 1–5).

Perumal, V., Narayanan, V., & Rajasekar, S. J. S. (2021a). Prediction of COVID criticality score with laboratory, clinical and CT images using hybrid regression models. *Computer Methods and Programs in Biomedicine, 209,* 106336.

Perumal, V., Narayanan, V., & Rajasekar, S. J. S. (2021b). Prediction of COVID-19 with computed tomography images using hybrid learning techniques. *Disease Markers.*

Perumal, V., Narayanan, V., & Rajasekar, S. J. S. (2021c). Detection of COVID-19 using CXR and CT images using transfer learning and Haralick features. *Applied Intelligence, 51(*1) (pp. 341–358).

Pinto Kumar Paul, S. B., Podder, P., & Mondal, M. R. H. 10 the role of IoMT during pandemics. *Intelligence for Managing Pandemics, 169.*

Podder, P., Bharati, S., Mondal, M. R. H., & Kose, U. (2021). Application of machine learning for the diagnosis of COVID-19. *Data Science for COVID-19* (pp. 175–194). Academic Press.

Podder, P., Khamparia, A., Mondal, M. R. H., Rahman, M. A., & Bharati, S. (2021). *Forecasting the Spread of COVID-19 and ICU Requirements.*

Podder, P., & Mondal, M. R. H. (2020). Machine learning to predict COVID-19 and ICU requirement. Paper presented at the 2020 IEEE 11th International Conference on Electrical and Computer Engineering (ICECE*)* (pp. 483–486).

Rajasekar, S. J. S. (2021). An enhanced IoT based tracing and tracking model for COVID-19 cases. *SN Computer Science, 2(*1) (pp. 1–4).

Rustam, F., Reshi, A. A., Mehmood, A., Ullah, S., On, B. W., Aslam, W., & Choi, G. S. (2020). COVID-19 future forecasting using supervised ML models. *IEEE Access, 8,* 101489–101499.

Sowmiya, B., Abhijith, V. S., Sudersan, S., Sundar, R. S. J., Thangavel, M., & Varalakshmi, P. (2021). A survey on security and privacy issues in contact tracing application of Covid-19. *SN computer science, 2(*3) (pp. 1–11).

Vrindavanam, J., Srinath, R., Shankar, H. H., & Nagesh, G. (2021). Machine learning based COVID-19 cough classification models: A comparative analysis. Paper presented at the 2021 IEEE 5th International Conference on Computing Methodologies and Communication (ICCMC) (pp. 420–426).

Wang, R. Y., Guo, T. Q., Li, L. G., Jiao, J. Y., & Wang, L. Y. (2020). Predictions of COVID-19 infection severity based on co-associations between the SNPs of co-morbid diseases and COVID-19 through machine learning of genetic data. Paper presented at the 2020 IEEE 8th International Conference on Computer Science and Network Technology (ICCSNT) (pp. 92–96).

WHO. (2021) WHO Coronavirus (COVID-19) Dashboard. Retrieved from https://covid19.who.int/

Yusuf, R. (2020). Comparing different supervised machine learning accuracy on analyzing COVID-19 data using ANOVA test. Paper presented at the 2020 IEEE 6th International Conference on Interactive Digital Media (ICIDM) (pp. 1–6).

Zhou, Q., Tao, W., Jiang, Y., & Cui, B. (2020). A comparative study on the prediction model of COVID-19. Paper presented at the 2020 IEEE 9th Joint International Information Technology and AI Conference (ITAIC) 9(pp. 1348–1352).

Chapter 12

Long Short-Term Memory-Based Recurrent Neural Network Model for COVID-19 Prediction in Different States of India

Mredulraj S. Pandianchery, V. Sowmya,
E. A. Gopalakrishnan, and K. P. Soman

Center for Computational Engineering and Networking, Amrita School of Engineering, Coimbatore, Amrita Vishwa Vidyapeetham, India

Contents

DOI: 10.1201/9781003324447-12

12.1 Introduction

In December 2019, an outbreak of pneumonia with an unknown cause was found in Wuhan, Hubei, China. On January 12, 2020, it was named 2019-nCoV and the whole genome sequence was shared with the World Health Organization (WHO) (Dhar Chowdhury & Oommen, 2020). To detect infections by the COVID-19 virus, a real time reverse transcriptase-polymerase chain reaction (RT-PCR) diagnostic test was developed (Wang et al., 2020). The major symptoms found in COVID-19 infected patients were fever, illness, and dry cough. The COVID-19 virus has a bad effect on the respiratory system of infected people. The chest radiography images can help to detect the damage that has been done to the lungs of infected people (Anand et al., 2021; Garlapati et al., 2021). Many researchers have carried out medical imaging for COVID-19 diagnosis with machine learning and deep learning algorithms (Bharati et al., 2021; Mondal et al., 2021a; Mondal et al., 2021b).

In India, the first case of COVID-19 infection was reported in the Thrissur district of Kerala on January 27, 2020. On January 30, 2020, the COVID-19 outbreak was declared a public health emergency of international concern by WHO (Andrews et al., 2020). WHO declared the COVID-19 outbreak a global pandemic on March 11, 2020 (Dhar Chowdhury & Oommen, 2020). The transmission of the COVID-19 virus takes place when an infected person sneezes or breathes heavily in the open atmosphere. In order to mitigate transmission among the population, it was made mandatory to wear face masks, use sanitizers, and maintain social distancing in public areas. The Indian government imposed a lockdown in India on March 24, 2020. In the initial phase, there were no vaccines for COVID-19, and the measures to control the transmission of COVID-19 were social distancing and wearing personal protective equipment (Suresh et al., 2021). There was a strong requirement for good health infrastructures, which included frontline workers, the number of hospital beds and ventilators, and testing services to overcome this pandemic. Since 65%–68% of the population of India lives in rural areas, it was a particularly high threat to the country to maintain strict measures (Kumar et al., 2020). It was proposed that about 98% of the entire country would be affected by the COVID-19 virus until July 2020 (Acharya & Porwal, 2020).

The forecasting for the transmission of COVID-19 and the requirements for ICU helped the government to overcome the different phases of the pandemic

(Podder et al., 2021). The dynamics in the transmission of the COVID-19 virus can be traced using mathematical models and deep learning algorithms. Deep learning offers many tools to build data-driven models. Deep learning algorithms, which include simple recurrent neural networks (RNN), long short-term memory (LSTM), and gated recurrent neural networks (GRU), play a key role to capture the patterns that are present in the time series data. Forecasting the time series plays a key role in epidemics and finance (Selvin et al., 2017). LSTM performs better when forecasting time series data compared with other traditional techniques, such as moving average, simple exponential smoothing, and autoregressive integrated moving average (Siami-Namini et al., 2018).

The primary aspect of the research carried out in this chapter are mentioned below.

1. The LSTM-based RNN model is proposed for the prediction of active cases per day, confirmed cases per day, and cumulative confirmed cases for each province in India
2. In India, 36 provinces include the state and union territories. India is one of the countries that was badly affected by COVID-19 during the first and second waves of the pandemic. The proposed LSTM-based RNN model is trained on the first wave of the pandemic and tested for the second wave of the pandemic for each province in India

Despite the prediction for the whole country (India), the prediction of active cases per day, confirmed cases per day, and cumulative confirmed cases for each province helped to capture the dynamics more effectively. In India, provinces including Maharashtra, Karnataka, Kerala, Andhra Pradesh, Uttar Pradesh, and West Bengal were badly affected compared with other states during the first and second waves of the pandemic. Some provinces including Arunachal Pradesh, Manipur, Meghalaya, Mizoram, Nagaland, Sikkim, and Tripura were comparatively less affected. The reason behind the undistributed dynamics of COVID-19 in each province was due to the geographical areas of the provinces and the population density. The spread of COVID-19 also depended on the geographical area and population density. The prediction for each province helped the state governments to make better decisions and impose restrictions at the state level. So, the state-level prediction gives better insights into the future dynamics of COVID-19 compared with the country-level prediction. The proposed model with the same hyperparameters is used for the prediction of COVID-19 cases in each province of India. So, this chapter focuses on the effectiveness and robustness of the proposed model to capture the different dynamics of COVID-19, which were seen during the first and second waves of the pandemic in different provinces of India.

12.2 Related Work

Bahri et al. (2020) proposed an LSTM model to predict the number of deceased cases due to COVID-19 in three countries, such as India, Italy, and the US. Their study focused on the training data from January 22, 2020, to June 22, 2020, and testing data from June 23, 2020, to June 29, 2020, which was extracted from Johns Hopkins University Centre's publicly available dataset (Johns Hopkins, 2020). The proposed model carried out the prediction for deceased cases about 7 days ahead with error rates of 1.37%, 1.99%, and 2.69% for the US, India, and Italy, respectively.

Iqbal et al. (2021) proposed an LSTM model for the prediction of daily patient count from the percentage of positive patients. The percentage of positive patients is the ratio of the number of daily positive tests to the total tests conducted per day. This study used the dataset from the Ministry of Health, Pakistan from March 11, 2020, to May 31, 2020, (Government of Pakistan, 2020) and carried out the prediction for the first 24 days of June 2020. The study considered the effect of LSTM units, epochs, and batches on the results obtained. It was concluded that with an increase in the LSTM units, epochs, and batches, the mean absolute percentage error (MAPE) was reduced in the model. The prediction was carried out with a MAPE value of 0.049 with 20 LSTM nodes, 100 epochs, and a batch size configuration of 15 for daily positive patients.

Cruz-Mendoza et al. (2020) proposed an LSTM model to predict the infected cases per day in Peru using two different simulation environments including MATLAB and Google Colab. The study stated that the model was trained on the infected cases from March to April 2020 and the test data consisted of data collected in May 2020. The computational cost is high in MATLAB as it requires 250 LSTM units, while in Google Colab it requires 30 LSTM units. But in MATLAB, the predicted results have a root mean square error (RMSE) of 678, which was less compared with Google Colab with an RMSE of 813. Even though MATLAB requires a high computational cost, it performed well with the test data compared with Google Colab.

Bodapati et al. (2020) proposed an LSTM model to predict the infected cases in different cities in China. The study was carried out on the dataset extracted from Johns Hopkins University's publicly available datasets (Johns Hopkins, 2020). LSTM model considered 104 days for training and carried out the prediction for 12 days ahead. The accuracy of the proposed LSTM model is 77.895%.

Ghany et al. (2021) proposed an LSTM model to predict the confirmed and death cases in different Gulf Cooperation Council (GCC) countries, such as Saudi Arabia (KSA), United Arab Emirates (UAE), Kuwait, Bahrain, Oman, and Qatar. Their study involved the dataset extracted from Johns Hopkins University Centre from January 22, 2020, to January 25, 2021. In the proposed model, there was an input step equal to seven, an LSTM layer with 10 hidden units, and relu as an activation function. The RMSEs for confirmed cases in KSA, Qatar, Oman, Kuwait, UAE, and Bahrain were 1768.35, 735.21, 730.53, 456.90, 446.44, and 320.79, respectively. The RMSEs for death cases in KSA, Qatar, Oman, Kuwait, UAE, and Bahrain were 21.78, 2.09, 9.99, 3.75, 3.27, and 1.84, respectively.

From this literature review, it is observed that there was a scope for the prediction of COVID-19 cases for entire provinces in India. The implementation of deep learning algorithms for the prediction of COVID-19 in each province in India shows the robustness of the model behavior to capture the different dynamics. The deep learning model with the same hyperparameter helped to detect the biased decisions taken under different circumstances. So, this chapter involved an LSTM-based RNN model for the prediction of active cases per day, confirmed cases per day, and cumulative confirmed cases for every province in India.

12.3 Methodology

12.3.1 Dataset Description

The dataset (Dong et al., 2020) for the entire states and union territory in India was extracted from Johns Hopkins University Centre's publicly available dataset (Johns Hopkins, 2020) and preprocessed in Python. The dataset consisted of active cases per day, case fatality, cumulative confirmed cases, cumulative death cases, incident rate, and cumulative recovered cases for all the provinces in India. The dataset was collected from June 10, 2020, to August 4, 2021. Due to discrepancies in the cumulative confirmed cases for five different states including Telangana, Tripura, Uttar Pradesh, Uttarakhand, and West Bengal, the cumulative confirmed cases from July 29, 2020, to August 4, 2021, were considered. The active cases per day were calculated based on confirmed cases, death cases, and recovered cases per day. The confirmed cases per day were calculated from the cumulative confirmed cases present in the dataset. The dataset consisted of the first and second waves of the pandemic that hit the different provinces of India. The total confirmed cases and recovered cases for each state and union territory are shown in Figures 12.1 and 12.2, respectively. Maharashtra, Karnataka, Kerala, Andhra Pradesh, Uttar Pradesh, and West Bengal had a total of confirmed cases and recovered cases of >10,00,000 up to August 4, 2021. Maharashtra reported the highest number of total confirmed cases among the other provinces in India. Arunachal Pradesh, Meghalaya, Mizoram, Nagaland, Sikkim, and Tripura reported a total of confirmed cases <1,00,000 cases up to August 4, 2021. Among the union territories, Delhi had a total of confirmed cases and recovered cases of >10,00,000 cases up to August 4, 2021, while the other union territory had comparatively fewer cases. The first case of COVID-19 was reported on January 18, 2021, in Lakshadweep. The total death cases in the states and union territories are shown in Figure 12.3.

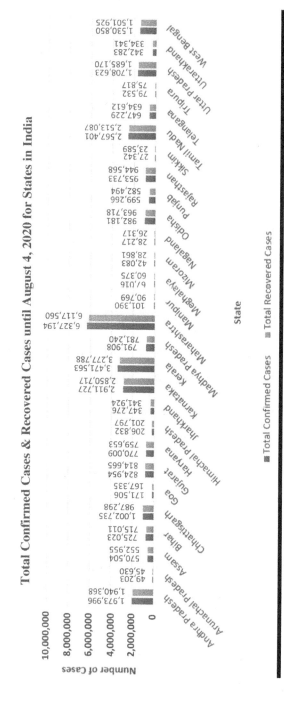

Figure 12.1 Total confirmed cases and recovered cases for states in India (up to August 4, 2021)

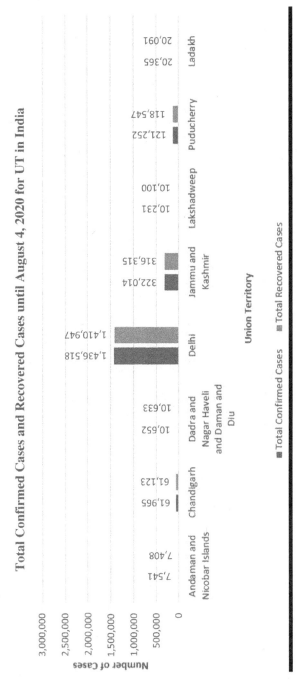

Figure 12.2   Total confirmed cases and recovered cases for union territories in India (up to August 4, 2021)

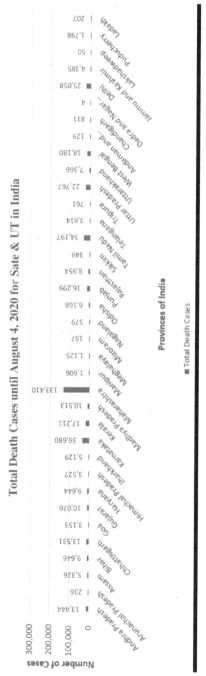

Figure 12.3   Total death cases for states and union territories in India (up to August 4, 2021)

12.3.2 Proposed Methodology

LSTM consists of a gating mechanism, which helps to sustain the long-term dependencies. An LSTM cell consists of an input and forget gates, cell state, and output gate. By the input gate, the LSTM decides which information should be retained in the current cell state. The forget gate decides which information must be removed from the previous LSTM cell. The output gate calculates the value of the output by a combination of the current input, and the output and cell value from the previous iteration (Van Houdt, 2020).

LSTM was implemented for the prediction of COVID-19 cases for different provinces in India as follows.

1. Active cases per day
2. Confirmed cases per day
3. Cumulative confirmed cases

The layout of the proposed LSTM model is shown in Figure 12.4. In the LSTM model, for the prediction of active cases per day and confirmed cases per day, an LSTM was incorporated with 10 hidden units. The total learnable parameters in the LSTM model for the prediction of active cases per day and confirmed cases per day was 531. In the prediction of the cumulative confirmed cases, an LSTM was incorporated with 100 hidden units. As in the prediction of cumulative confirmed cases, the number of hidden units was increased for a better prediction. The total learnable parameters in the LSTM model to predict the cumulative confirmed cases was 41,301.

The quantitative parameter for error calculation between actual and predicted data was carried out by the following metrics (Khair et al., 2017).

$$MAE\ (Mean\ Absolute\ Error) = \frac{\sum_{i=1}^{n}|p_i - a_i|}{n} \qquad (12.1)$$

$$MAPE\ (Mean\ Absolute\ Percentage\ Error) = \frac{\sum_{i=1}^{n}\left\{\frac{|p_i - a_i|}{a_i}\right\}}{n} * 100 \qquad (12.2)$$

where:
n = total number of days for prediction
p_i and a_i = predicted and actual cases for ith day in Equations 12.1 and 12.2.

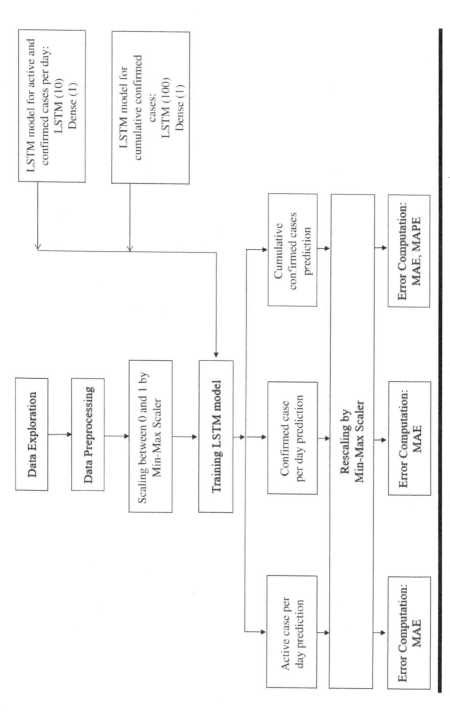

Figure 12.4   Layout of LSTM model (proposed LSTM model)

12.4 Experimental Results and Discussion

In the proposed LSTM model, the input step size was two and the prediction was carried out for 1 day ahead in the prediction of active cases per day, confirmed cases per day, and cumulative confirmed cases. About 200 days were used to train the model and the prediction was carried out for 219 days. Due to the data discrepancy in the cases in states including Telangana, Tripura, Uttar Pradesh, Uttarakhand, and West Bengal, 200 days were taken to train and 169 days to test the model for the prediction of cumulative confirmed cases. As the first case of COVID-19 was reported on January 18, 2021, in Lakshadweep, 300 days were used to train the model and the remaining days to test the model. The proposed LSTM model was trained for 100 epochs. In the LSTM model, the hard sigmoid function was used as the gate activation function and the tanh function was used as the block input and output activation function. For the prediction, the loss was measured in mean squared error and the optimizer was the root mean square propagation (rmsprop) The metrics for the LSTM model were measured in mean absolute error (MAE).

12.4.1 Prediction for Active Cases per Day

Based on the experiments in the proposed model in this chapter, the prediction for active cases was carried out with single variable input. The MAE was calculated between actual and predicted active cases per day as given later in Table 12.1. The MAPE was not used for active cases per day, as many states have reported zero cases for some days. For states including Andhra Pradesh, Arunachal Pradesh, Assam, Bihar, Chhattisgarh, Goa, Gujarat, Haryana, Kerala, Karnataka, Madhya Pradesh, Manipur, Meghalaya, Rajasthan, Odisha, and Punjab, the proposed LSTM model carried out the prediction with the exact trend as in the actual active cases. The active case prediction for Kerala is shown in Figure 12.5. For the rest of the states in India, the proposed LSTM model carried out the prediction with some deviations from the actual trend at the peak of the second wave of the pandemic. The large deviation at the peak of the second wave of the pandemic was seen in Mizoram and Tamil Nadu with MAEs of 103.52 and 4767.05, respectively. The active case prediction for Tamil Nadu is shown in Figure 12.5. The model was trained with fewer dynamics for Mizoram. For Tamil Nadu, the model did not capture the dynamics properly. The number of hidden units in the LSTM model had to be increased to reduce the deviation from the actual trend. The MAEs for Maharashtra and Karnataka were 9454.41 and 9357.41, respectively, because the active cases per day reported at the peak of the second wave of the pandemic were >6,00,000 and 5,00,000 cases. The active case prediction for Maharashtra and Karnataka is shown in Figure 12.5. For the union territories, except for Lakshadweep, the proposed LSTM model carried out the prediction as per the actual trend. For Lakshadweep, the model was trained with fewer dynamics compared with the other union territories.

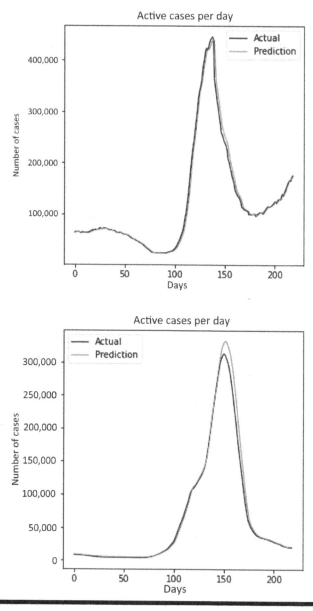

Figure 12.5 Active cases per day prediction (prediction by proposed LSTM model) (Continued)

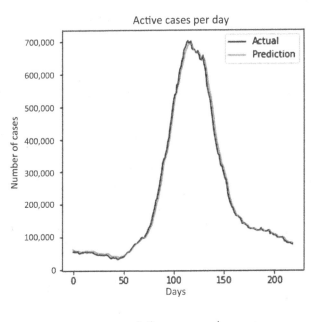

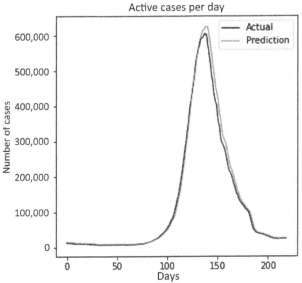

Figure 12.5 (Continued) Active cases per day prediction (prediction by proposed LSTM model)

12.4.2 Prediction for Confirmed Cases per Day

The prediction of confirmed cases per day followed the same procedure as the active cases per day. The MAE was calculated between the actual and predicted confirmed cases per day as given later in Table 12.1. The MAPE was not used for confirmed cases per day, as many states have reported zero cases for some days. The MAEs for Maharashtra and Karnataka were 2259.44 and 1217.57, respectively, as they had reported confirmed cases per day at the peak of the second wave of the pandemic >45,000. The MAEs for Kerala and Uttar Pradesh were 2593.3 and 924.66, respectively, as both states reported confirmed cases per day at the peak of the second wave of the pandemic >35,000. The confirmed case per day prediction for Maharashtra, Karnataka, Kerala, Uttar Pradesh, and Gujarat is shown in Figure 12.6. For the rest of the states, the proposed LSTM model carried out predictions similar to the actual trend with MAEs <1,000. Among the union territories, the proposed LSTM model carried out the prediction as per the actual trend, except for Lakshadweep because it reported confirmed cases per day <400. The MAE for Delhi was 725.86, as they reported confirmed cases per day at the peak of the second wave of the pandemic >25,000. The confirmed case per day prediction for Delhi is shown in Figure 12.6. For union territories including Andaman and Nicobar Islands, Dadra and Nagar Haveli and Daman and Diu, Chandigarh, Jammu and Kashmir, Puducherry and Ladakh, the proposed LSTM model carried out better prediction with lower MAEs.

12.4.3 Prediction for Cumulative Confirmed Cases

The prediction was carried out for the cumulative confirmed cases for different provinces with it as a single variable input and the error between the actual and predicted data was formulated with MAE and MAPE. As seen later in Figure 12.10, the MAPE for all the states was <4%. For states including Andhra Pradesh, Bihar, Jharkhand, Karnataka, Kerala, Maharashtra, and Tamil Nadu, the prediction for cumulative confirmed cases with a single variable input was carried out with MAPEs of 0.99%, 1.07%, 1.15%, 1.18%, 1.24%, 1.35%, and 1.29% respectively. This result showed that the proposed LSTM model carried out better predictions and captured the dynamics in the data. For states including Himachal Pradesh, Nagaland, and Uttarakhand, the MAPEs for the prediction of cumulative confirmed cases were 3.25%, 3.31%, and 3.32% respectively. For all union territories, except for Lakshadweep, the prediction for cumulative confirmed cases was carried out with MAPEs <3%. For Lakshadweep, the prediction for cumulative confirmed cases was carried out MAPE of 4.32%. The prediction for cumulative confirmed cases with a single variable input for Andhra Pradesh, Jharkhand, Tamil Nadu, and Uttarakhand is shown in Figure 12.7. Figures 12.8–12.11 show the quantitative analysis of the prediction for cumulative confirmed cases.

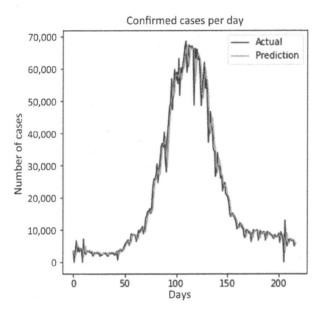

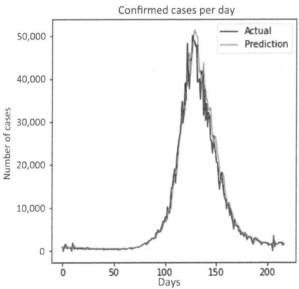

Figure 12.6 Confirmed cases per day prediction (prediction by proposed LSTM model) (Continued)

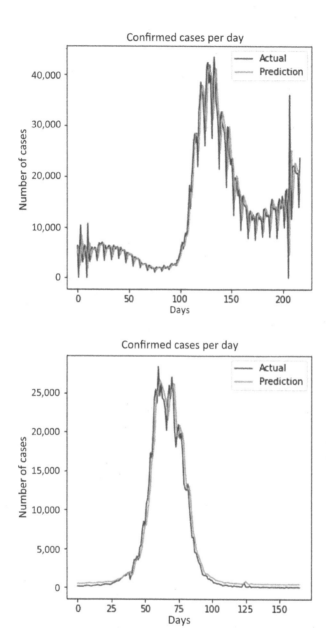

Figure 12.6 (Continued)   Confirmed cases per day prediction (prediction by proposed LSTM model) (Continued)

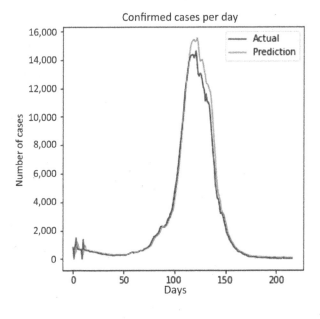

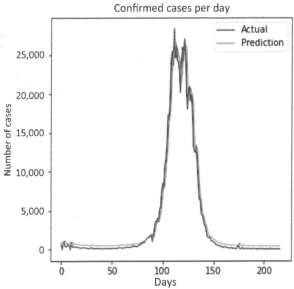

Figure 12.6 (Continued) **Confirmed cases per day prediction (prediction by proposed LSTM model)**

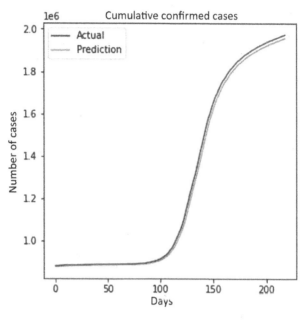

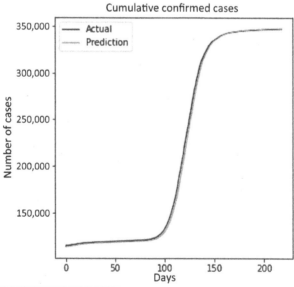

Figure 12.7 Cumulative confirmed cases prediction (prediction by proposed LSTM model) (Continued)

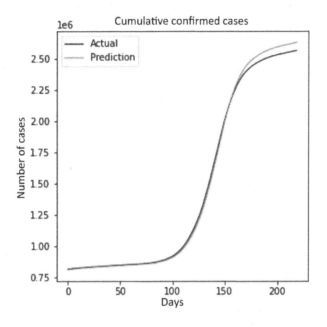

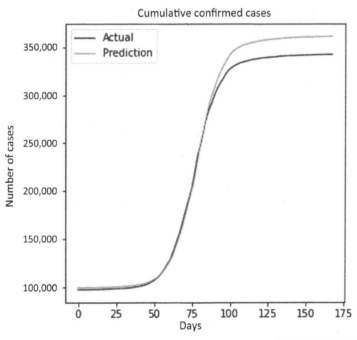

Figure 12.7 (Continued) Cumulative confirmed cases prediction (prediction by proposed LSTM model)

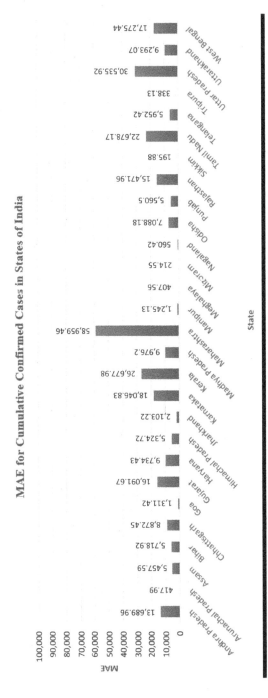

Figure 12.8 MAEs for cumulative confirmed cases in the states of India (quantitative analysis of proposed LSTM model)

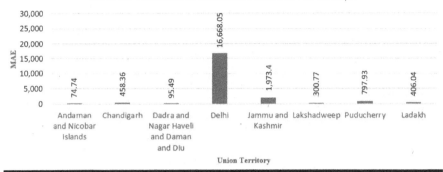

Figure 12.9 MAEs for cumulative confirmed cases in union territories of India (quantitative analysis of proposed LSTM model)

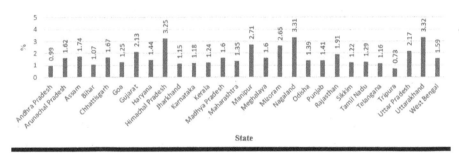

Figure 12.10 MAPEs for cumulative confirmed cases in states of India (quantitative analysis of proposed LSTM model)

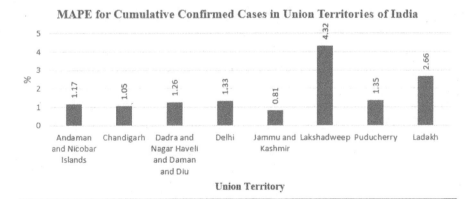

Figure 12.11 MAPE for cumulative confirmed cases in union territories of India (quantitative analysis of proposed LSTM model)

The data-driven deep learning model performed better for the prediction of COVID-19 cases for different provinces in India. The proposed LSTM model with an input step size of two captured the trend in COVID-19 for different provinces. The model worked with a lower input size and learnable parameters, which reduced the computational cost compared with the LSTM model proposed by Ghany et al. (2021) for the prediction of confirmed and death cases in GCC countries. The state-wise prediction of COVID-19 cases for India efficiently captured the dynamics compared with the deceased cases prediction for whole countries including the US, India, and Italy (Bahri et al., 2020). The LSTM model successfully predicted the trend during the second wave of the pandemic with long-term dependency. The effectiveness and robustness of the LSTM model to capture the dynamics for different provinces with the same hyperparameters were achieved.

12.5 Conclusions

In this chapter, the proposed LSTM model was implemented for the prediction of active cases per day, confirmed cases per day, and cumulative confirmed cases for different provinces in India. The different transmission dynamics of COVID-19 were shown in the provinces of India. The proposed LSTM model with the same hyperparameters captured the dynamics during the first and second waves of the pandemic efficiently. The proposed LSTM model resulted in better predictions for the majority of provinces in India. The data-driven model provided by deep learning help to achieve the early prediction of COVID-19 cases efficiently. Based on the understanding of the predictions achieved by the model, the state governments could take the necessary precautions and impose restrictions or lockdowns to overcome the pandemic.

12.6 Limitation and Future Scope

The proposed LSTM model was used to predict the active cases per day, confirmed cases per day, and cumulative confirmed cases for each province in India as shown in Table 12.1. The LSTM model must be trained and tested for each province. This increases the time complexity when training and testing the model. For some of the provinces, the proposed LSTM model could not capture the dynamics in the data. The biased behavior of the proposed LSTM model was noted in the experiments. For a better understanding of the model behavior, the proposed LSTM model should be integrated with explainable artificial intelligence to give robustness to the model and enhance its performance (Adadi & Berrada, 2018). The LSTM model must be trained with favorable dynamics once and should carry out the predictions for all the provinces. This approach could help to understand the biased behavior of the model, leverage the prediction with lower error, and reduce the time complexity.

Table 12.1 MAE for Active Cases per Day and Confirmed Cases per Day for Each Province in India (Quantitative Analysis of Proposed LSTM Model)

Number	Province	Active Cases per Day	Confirmed Cases per Day	Number	Province	Active Cases per Day	Confirmed Cases per Day
		MAE	*MAE*			*MAE*	*MAE*
1	Andhra Pradesh	3,177.42	785.21	19	Odisha	13,68.2	348.32
2	Arunachal Pradesh	79.56	44.03	20	Punjab	1,057.63	202.65
3	Assam	749.14	296.06	21	Rajasthan	3,467.41	345.78
4	Bihar	1,845.52	346.52	22	Sikkim	81.49	37.53
5	Chhattisgarh	1,855.88	511.77	23	Tamil Nadu	4,767.05	690.45
6	Goa	447.93	103.42	24	Telangana	1,098.38	285.63
7	Gujarat	2,768.78	303.81	25	Tripura	198.2	76.91
8	Haryana	1,615.61	272.45	26	Uttar Pradesh	5,417.55	924.66
9	Himachal Pradesh	524.42	1,46.41	27	Uttarakhand	1,610.14	498.41
10	Jharkhand	879.71	202.18	28	West Bengal	1,909.76	399.98
11	Karnataka	9,357.41	1,217.57	29	Andaman and Nicobar Islands	13.82	5.08
12	Kerala	5,995.79	2,593.3	30	Chandigarh	121.67	22.7
13	Madhya Pradesh	1,665.64	251.83	31	Dadra and Nagar Haveli and Daman and Diu	32.35	11.21

(continued)

Table 12.1 (Continued) MAE for Active Cases per Day and Confirmed Cases per Day for Each Province in India (Quantitative Analysis of Proposed LSTM Model)

Number	Province	Active Cases per Day	Confirmed Cases per Day	Number	Province	Active Cases per Day	Confirmed Cases per Day
		MAE	MAE			MAE	MAE
14	Maharashtra	9,454.41	2,259.44	32	Delhi	2,093.45	725.86
15	Manipur	192.49	83.56	33	Jammu and Kashmir	758.27	125.3
16	Meghalaya	121.91	53.36	34	Lakshadweep	72.99	41.1
17	Mizoram	103.52	77.41	35	Puducherry	241.62	64.96
18	Nagaland	82.86	48.77	36	Ladakh	55.22	22.63

References

Acharya, R., & Porwal, A. (2020). A vulnerability index for the management of and response to the COVID-19 epidemic in India: an ecological study. *The Lancet. Global Health, 8*(9), e1142–e1151. doi.10.1016/S2214-109X(20)30300-4

Adadi, A., & Berrada, M. (2018). Peeking inside the black box: A survey on explainable artificial intelligence (XAI). *IEEE Access, 6,* 52138–52160. doi.10.1109/ACCESS.2018.2870052

Anand, R., Sowmya, V., Gopalakrishnan, E. A. & Soman, K.P. (2021). Modified Vgg deep learning architecture for Covid-19 classification using bio-medical images. *IOP Conference Series: Materials Science and Engineering, 1084*(1), 12001. doi.10.1088/1757-899x/1084/1/012001.

Andrews, M. A., Areekal, B., Rajesh, K. R., Krishnan, J., Suryakala, R., Krishnan, B., ... Santhosh, P. V. (2020). First confirmed case of COVID-19 infection in India: A case report. *The Indian Journal of Medical Research, 151*(5), 490–492. doi.10.4103/ijmr.IJMR_2131_20

Bahri, S., Kdayem, M. & Zoghlami, N. (2020). *Deep learning for COVID-19 prediction.* Paper presented at the 4th International Conference on Advanced Systems and Emergent Technologies, Hammamet, Tunisia. (pp. 406–411). doi.10.1109/IC_ASET49463.2020.9318297

Bharati, S., Podder, P., Mondal, M., & Prasath, V. B. (2021). Medical imaging with deep learning for COVID-19 Diagnosis: A comprehensive review. *arXiv* preprint arXiv:2107.09602.

Bodapati, S., Bandarupally, H., & Trupthi, M. (2020). *COVID-19 time series forecasting of daily cases, deaths caused and recovered cases using long short term memory networks.* Paper presented at 2020 IEEE 5th International Conference on Computing Communication and Automation (ICCCA). doi.10.1109/ICCCA49541.2020.9250863

Cruz-Mendoza, I., Quevedo-Pulido, J., & Adanaque-Infante, L. (2020). *LSTM performance analysis for predictive models based on Covid-19 dataset.* Paper presented at the 2020 IEEE XXVII International Conference on Electronics, Electrical Engineering and Computing (INTERCON), pp. 1–4. doi.10.1109/INTERCON50315.2020.9220248

Dhar Chowdhury, S., & Oommen, A. M. (2020). Epidemiology of COVID-19. *Journal of Digestive Endoscopy, 11*(1), 3–7. doi.10.1055/s-0040-1712187.

Dong, E., Du, H., & Gardner, L., (2020). An interactive web-based dashboard to track COVID-19 in real time. *Lancet Infectious Diseases, 20*(5):533–534. doi.10.1016/S1473-3099(20)30120-1

Garlapati, K., Kota, N., Mondreti, Y. S., Gutha, P. & Nair, A. K. (2021). Detection of COVID-19 using X-ray image classification. Paper presented at the 5th International Conference on Trends in Electronics and Informatics (ICOEI), (pp. 745–750) doi.10.1109/ICOEI51242.2021.9452745

Ghany, K., Zawbaa, H. M., & Sabri, H. M. (2021). COVID-19 prediction using LSTM algorithm: GCC case study. *Informatics in Medicine Unlocked, 23,* 100566doi.10.1016/j.imu.2021.100566.

Government of Pakistan (2020) Health Advisory Platform. Retrieved from https://covid.gov.pk/

Iqbal, M., Al-Obeidat, F., Maqbool, F., Razzaq, S., Anwar, S., Tubaishat, A. … Shah, B. (2021). COVID-19 patient count prediction using LSTM. *IEEE Transactions on Computational Social Systems, 8*(4), 974–981. doi.10.1109/TCSS.2021.3056769

Johns Hopkins. (2020). Coronavirus Resource Center. Retrieved from https://coronavirus. jhu.edu/about/how-to-use-our-data

Khair, U., Fahmi, H., Hakim, S., & Rahim, R. (2017). Forecasting error calculation with mean absolute deviation and mean absolute percentage error. *Journal of Physics: Conference Series, 930.* doi.10.1088/1742-6596/930/1/012002

Kumar, A., Rajasekharan Nayar, K., & Koya, S. F. (2020). COVID-19: Challenges and its consequences for rural health care in India. *Public Health in Practice, 1,* 100009. doi.10.1016/j.puhip.2020.100009

Mondal, M. R. H., Bharati, S., & Podder, P. (2021a). Diagnosis of COVID-19 using machine learning and deep learning: A review. *Current Medical Imaging,* 17(12), 1403–1418

Mondal, M. R. H., Bharati, S., & Podder, P. (2021b). CO-IRv2: Optimized InceptionResNetV2 for COVID-19 detection from chest CT images. *PLoS One, 16*(10), e0259179.

Podder, P., Khamparia, A., Mondal, M. R. H., Mohammad, A. R., & Subrato, B. (2021). Forecasting the spread of COVID-19 and ICU requirements. *International Journal of Online and Biomedical Engineering, 17*(5), 81–99. doi.10.20944/preprints202103. 0447.v1

Selvin, S., Vinayakumar, R., Gopalakrishnan, E. A., Menon, V. K. & Soman, K. P. (2017) *Stock price prediction using LSTM, RNN and CNN-sliding window model.* Paper presented at the International Conference on Advances in Computing, Communications and Informatics (ICACCI), pp. 1643–1647. doi.10.1109/ICACCI.2017.8126078.

Siami-Namini, S., Tavakoli, N., & Siami Namin, A. (2018). *A comparison of ARIMA and LSTM in forecasting time series.* Paper presented at the 17th IEEE International Conference on Machine Learning and Applications (ICMLA), (pp. 1394–1401). doi.10.1109/ICMLA.2018.00227

Suresh, K., Palangappa, M., & Bhuvan, S. (2021). *Face mask detection by using optimistic convolutional neural network.* Paper presented at the 6th International Conference on Inventive Computation Technologies (ICICT), (pp. 1084–1089). doi.10.1109/ ICICT50816.2021.9358653

Van Houdt, G., Mosquera, C., & Nápoles, G. (2020). A review on the long short-term memory model. *Artificial Intelligence Review, 53,* 5929–5955. doi.10.1007/ s10462-020-09838-1

Wang, W., Xu, Y., Gao, R., Lu, R., Han, K., Wu, G., & Tan, W. (2020). Detection of SARS-CoV-2 in different types of clinical specimens. *Journal of American Medical Association, 323*(18), 1843–1844. doi.10.1001/jama.2020.3786

Chapter 13

Dengue in the Presence of COVID-19: Evaluation of Tree-Based Classifiers Using Stratified K-Fold on Dengue Dataset

Supreet Kaur and Sandeep Sharma

*Department of Computer Engineering and Technology,
Guru Nanak Dev University, Amritsar, India*

Contents

DOI: 10.1201/9781003324447-13

13.1 Introduction

Machine learning decreases the analysis burden on humans from the automatic learning patterns hidden in humongous data to ease decision-making with iterative aspects. With each iteration, experience is gained that enables computers to independently adapt and give reliable decisions when new data is introduced. This allows us to build systems that can study a broad range of variables (factors) with a disease (e.g., understanding the biological mechanism and risk factors involved) rapidly; therefore, allowing medical practitioners to diagnose diseases early and effectively. A global pandemic of dengue began after World War II (in Southeast Asia) and intensified over the next 15 years making it a rapidly emerging pandemic disease in tropical and subtropical regions of the globe. Scientists have also found traces of dengue infection disease in the parts of the world that experience the coldest climatic conditions throughout, hence highlighting the threat of the adaptability of this infection-carrying mosquito and negating the previous claims that dengue is the disease of tropical and subtropical countries. Each year, dengue claims >390 million infections and recent estimations put half of the world's population at risk (1). The current COVID pandemic has already told the whole world how insufficient human efforts have become to curb the issue when a disease escalates to a pandemic level. The research teams around the globe came together in a race against the COVID pandemic and many machines and deep learning algorithms were trained using any available data to help medical staff when saving lives (2). Dengue virus and the COVID-19 causing virus exhibit similar symptomatic scenarios in their onset period even though their mode of spread is completely different. As stated previously, the dengue virus is spread through the bite of female Aedes mosquitoes whereas COVID-19 is thought to be caused primarily by respiratory droplets that are produced by the infected person. However, in India, the medical sector in addition to numerous obstacles when fighting against COVID-19 faced the danger of a worsening dengue epidemiological profile. Experts believed one of the reasons was the main allocation of the country's entire resources to fight against COVID-19, which resulted in major setbacks in the treatment and diagnosis of other diseases, mainly dengue. Another reason was the under-diagnosis due to the somewhat similar clinical profile of COVID-19 with dengue because the complexity of a diagnosis between both is a very challenging task for healthcare professionals. The initial symptoms of both are common, such as fever, body pain, headache, and abdominal pain and both disease-causing viruses share similar biochemical and hematological characteristics (3).

Similarly, in various other parts of Asia, as in Brazil, a spike in severe dengue cases was observed with COVID-19, where experts believed lockdown was the primary cause that let mosquito population increase due to the absence of vector control programs during the pandemic situation (4). Medication used for COVID-19 treatment could worsen dengue patients, which leads to an increased risk of bleeding, hence making the situation quite alarming (3). In countries in Asia, to reduce the burden of the dengue epidemic it's necessary to implement methods that allow early and accurate detection of dengue cases, in particular, the severe cases to reduce the overall disease burden (4). A supervised machine learning algorithm could allow the learning program to learn from hidden patterns in the input dengue dataset; therefore, it could use this experience when classifying a new observation. Various popular classifiers are available in machine learning, such as logistic regression, naive Bayes (NB), K-nearest neighbor, support vector machine (SVM), random forest (RF), and decision tree (DT). A typical classifier after receiving the preprocessed data splits it into two parts: training data (learning is achieved from this part) and testing data (this is used to identify the experience's efficiency in the previous part) (5). The algorithm used in this chapter was a tree-based classifier that included DTs and various algorithms associated with them that come under this classification. To ensure the best working of the model, various conditions are performed to improve predictions, such as eliminating duplicate data and missing value data, using label encoders, and applying stratified sampling to conserve the percentage of sample for each resultant class.

The process of data mining is performed using the Jupyter Notebook in Python 3 and the Scikit-learn machine learning libraries. The dengue dataset is imported as a CSV file and the results are predicted and the best among them are chosen as classifiers based on the accuracy. The dengue dataset consists of various attributes, such as fever, nausea, retro-orbital headache, and fatigue. As the physical file-sourced data were manually collected from government hospitals over 2 years, first a soft copy of the dengue dataset was constructed in Excel and preprocessed to eliminate any missing or incorrect values. To improvise the selection of attributes combination for learning, duplicate data is also dropped and stratified K-fold cross-validation is implemented to ensure the proportion of the feature of interest remains the same across original data (training as well as testing). In this chapter, the performance of classification algorithms like DT, classification and regression tree (CART), ID3, C4.5, CHAID, and RF on the dengue dataset was evaluated and compared based on the accuracy and error rate obtained. The main objective of this chapter is to improvise the efficiency of machine learning methods when forecasting the classification of dengue patients accurately, which is further compared by plotting the confusion matrix for each classifier. So, the stratified K-fold cross-validation technique was used to improve the goodness of each iteration by ensuring that each data split was as good as the entire data along with removing duplicate rows, which might result in a smaller dataset than the original but improve the learning ability of the classification algorithm.

Machine learning is widely popular due to its capabilities and various software packages are available that give inbuilt working libraries, such as Python, which is the most commonly used tool among data scientists.

The main contribution of this chapter can be broadly categorized as follows.

■ A comparative approach is termed to evaluate various tree-based classifiers in machine learning
■ The symptomatic dataset is formulated by combining data accumulated from various cities in India
■ A K-fold stratified approach is followed to ensure quality training and testing dataset
■ The infected person is diagnosed and based on the risk factor; a target class is assigned
■ The infected person is advised to get medical aid on an emergency basis if their input symptoms (either alone or in combination) indicate a possible internal hemorrhagic manifestation
■ Comparative evaluation is carried out, and the best tree-based classifier is selected

The rest of this chapter is structured as follows; Section 13.2 summarizes the existing related work. The model to predict dengue-infected patients is proposed in Section 13.3. The experimental results and performance analysis of the proposed model are discussed in the "Results and Discussions". The "Conclusion" gives the conclusions derived from the proposed model in this chapter.

13.2 Related Works

Based on physical symptoms alone, a dengue infection prediction model can be achieved by a machine learning algorithm, which acts as an early patient diagnosis system (1). This work emphasized the importance of the inclusion of the medical test parameters alongside the physical symptoms to properly find which stage of dengue the person is affected by. During this study, the author incorporated some symptoms, for example, fever, gastrointestinal findings, headache, pain, skin rash, eyeball pain, and clinical factors, such as white blood cell (WBC), aspartate aminotransferase (AST), alanine aminotransferase, C-reactive protein, partial thromboplastin time, and platelet (PLT) to offer results composed for three possible diagnoses; no dengue, probable dengue, and dengue confirmed (1). The technique used was the fuzzy toolbox in MATLAB, which generated 860 rules for 11 input parameters that were effective if not the best in predicting a dengue-infected person and representing the seriousness of this disease based on physical signs along with medical tests results. However, this system cannot evaluate the risk level classification, for example, dengue fever (DF), dengue hemorrhagic fever (DHF), and dengue shock syndrome (DSS). Similarly, (2) a study on 60 dengue patients' data was conducted in which predictors like systolic and diastolic blood pressure (BP), pulse rate, heart rate (HR), bleeding and clotting times, hematocrit, WBC, and PLT to classify patients based on the severity of dengue disease. The researcher used different models like DT, discriminant analysis, SVM, nearest neighbor classifier, and ensemble classifiers provided in MATLAB to perform the prediction, which showed that linear discriminant analysis performed the best for accuracy and median error rate. But when the confusion matrix results were generated it showed that the accuracy was only 50% for the testing for which the author believed missing data and an unbalanced distribution between the severity groups were the key reasons. Early detection of dengue disease can help not only in saving lives but also serves as a preventive step in its progress to the epidemic level. Focusing on its importance, a dengue diagnostic model was proposed that applies K-fold cross-validation on the three machine learning techniques, for example, artificial neural network (ANN), DT, and NB to detect dengue-infected cases embedded in the data set of 110 samples (3). There are nonclinical as well as clinical attributes in this dataset, such as age, gender, vomiting, abdominal pain, chills, body ache, headache, weakness, fever, PLT, temperature, HR, dengue virus antigen detection (NS1), Immunoglobulins G and M (IgG and IgM), and Elisa. It was observed that ANN had the best accuracy of 76.35% but suffered from larger computational time compared with the remaining techniques. One more point to emphasize, while generating a confusion matrix NB worked much better than others in true negative and positive values. A prognostic multivariate prediction system for children using seven warning signs highlighted by a revised World Health Organisation (WHO) classification was proposed, which took independent variables such as abdominal pain, persistent vomiting, lethargy, fluid accumulation, low platelet count, and mucosal bleed. It was observed that hematocrit with concurrent low platelet count were key indicators when predicting severe dengue in children (4). In other research (5, 6) an autoregressive integrated moving average (ARIMA) technique was proposed for modeling and forecasting DHF cases and it was seen that the number of cases tended to be high at the beginning as well as the end of the year, which indicates the development of the mosquito population during this period.

The author used a particle swarm optimization to optimize an ANN (PSO-ANN)-based model for the early prediction of dengue disease by taking physical signs as well as clinical test parameters as input and claimed to get higher accuracy, specificity, and sensitivity rate along with the highest AUC curve; however, it suffered from a long computational time (7). Two easily applicable dengue diagnostic models using early clinical signs using classification and regression tree analysis achieved a 97% sensitivity when identifying patients correctly that progressed to the fatal state of DSS using WBC count, AST, platelet count, and age (8). In this study, dengue confirmed cases were used to train RF algorithms using self-organizing maps to identify patient clusters with similar patterns and the author suggested that age should be considered as the first characteristic when dealing with the clinical profile of patients with dengue. The observations also emphasized the close monitoring of children who showed warning signs after acquiring this disease (9). The authors used an RF algorithm as a classification technique for their proposed dengue prediction system, which maintained the best accuracy compared with others when a prediction was made on input symptoms taken from the user or patient (10). From the literature survey, the existing models for potential dengue prediction have achieved promising accuracy. Although high accuracy was achieved, many dengue physical symptoms weren't considered during these studies. In addition, until an individual thinks they might have dengue disease, the chances of them undergoing lab tests are very minimal. If they did get a lab test, the idea of constructing an early diagnosis system collapse, because a lab test alone is insufficient to work out the infection status, for example, dengue-infected or not. This motivated the construction of a dengue detection model. In this model, input about a person's signs or symptoms could predict if the person was suffering from dengue disease. In addition, if any warning sign was present, the system would classify that person with DF with a warning (DFW). In the second category, people need to consult a doctor if they are showing dangerous complications of this disease, which might become fatal or life-threatening if left untreated.

13.3 Proposed Model

The proposed dengue prediction model was further classified into subsections to gain a better understanding of every stage's operation by starting with an overall working idea, which could eventually progress into more detailed information. Therefore, dengue predictions could be analyzed in a better and easier way, which could further help when designing tools for help in pandemics. In the following section, the proposed model's architecture is discussed to offer a generalized view and in the following sections, each stage is discussed highlighting the functionality and main features.

13.3.1 Model Architecture

The working design of the proposed model is divided into major three phases.

1. Data collection: information was screened and retrieved from dengue patients that were admitted or referred to the Government Medical College (GMC), Amritsar, India for dengue monitoring as well for those who were dengue positive, but hospitalization was not required. The positive patients were confirmed to have dengue infection through NS1 antigen test or IgM/IgG tests. The vital signs, as well as clinical test parameters, were then recorded in a spreadsheet for further preprocessing in which missing values records were deleted.

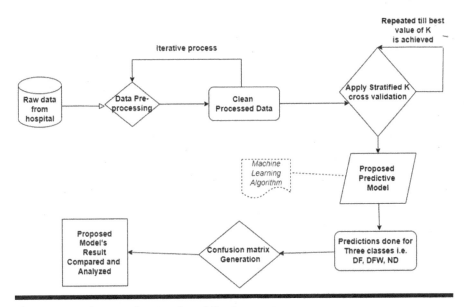

Figure 13.1 Proposed system's architecture

2. Prediction model: the tree algorithms in the machine learning library of Python were trained using training data. The stratified K-fold cross-validation for the value of k = 6 was applied to the dataset generated in the previous phase to get a quality training and testing data set. The predicting algorithms are saved in Jupyter Notebook for further work.
3. Validation and improvement: the predictive models were tested using a testing dataset (generated in Phase 2) and accuracy for each was calculated. The confusion matrix was then generated to verify the models' performance and on the comparison, the best algorithm was selected.

The architecture followed in the proposed system is shown in Figure 13.1.

13.4 Data Collection

The population for this study was composed of subjects with dengue infection which was collected manually from the GMC, Amritsar, India ensuring all legal and ethical formalities were followed during this study. The physical signs/symptoms along with clinical tests result were collected from the dengue patient's file records that are managed and stored in the dengue ward, at the GMC. An Excel spreadsheet was used for data entry, in which further data were grouped into two main classes, for example, DF and DFW. The dataset attributes were age, gender, address (city), fever, loss of appetite, nausea, rash, extreme weakness, retro-orbital headache, joint/muscle pain, mucosal bleed, blood in stool, abdomen pain, unusually heavy menstrual bleeding, loose motion, large BP drop along with result classed as DF and DFW. To ensure there was no violation of the privacy rights of patients, their personal information like postal address and phone number were not extracted from the hospital records for this study. In total, there were 16 data attributes in the input class and two data attributes in the output class of the data file with extension.CSV having values of either zero or one indicating NO and Yes respectively. Only the label class used letters as values, for example, DF and DFW, which will be converted into numeric values in further processing for operational ease.

13.5 Train the Test Dataset

The proposed model was trained using the dengue patient dataset, which was discussed in the previous section. During training the testing dataset generated some attributes like age, gender, and address, which are important from an analysis point of view but are of no help in the prediction models; therefore, the result was dropped. Moreover, for ease of classification the resulting class that had letter values was coded as 0 (DF) and 1(DFW) before processing it further in the Jupyter Notebook. The 13 attributes that composed the physical signs/symptoms experienced by a person infected with dengue disease were used as the predictors for which classification was carried out to get the response against the new data entry. The stratified K-fold cross-validation was applied to the data repeatedly for different values of k, to ensure that any subset acquired at a given time for the value of selected k, was a qualitative equivalent of the entire data representation. This ensure not only better accuracy but also unbalanced distribution was avoided. From the iterative process, k = 6 gave the best possible performance, and the method is shown in Figure 13.2.

13.6 Results

Dengue data containing vital signs/symptoms from patients suffering from dengue were trained using machine learning classifiers. In this study, >1 tree classifiers were selected and compared based on the accuracy achieved. The results given in Table 13.1 show each model type along with the accuracy, precision, and recall achieved by it. Among the selected models: C4.5, ID3, and RF showed high accuracy compared with DT and CHAID. The RF model prediction revealed the highest accuracy of 96.14% with 0.86 precision and 1.00 recall. Figure 13.3 shows the confusion matrix for the RF analysis in which the diagonal box's value indicated the predicted class was equal to the true class and the off-diagonal values specified the misclassification predictions.

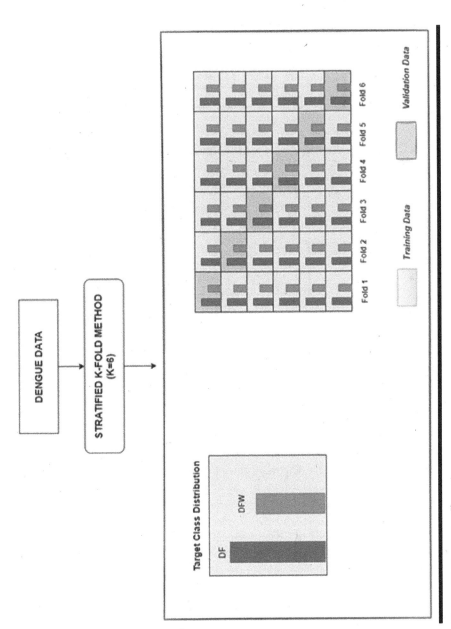

Figure 13.2 Data allocation

Table 13.1   Trained Model Accuracy, Precision, and Recall

Model Types	Accuracy (%)	Precision	Recall
DT	83.33	0.67	0.70
C4.5	94.83	0.95	0.92
ID3	93.75	0.93	0.91
CHAID	80	0.70	0.88
RF	**96.14**	**0.86**	**1.00**

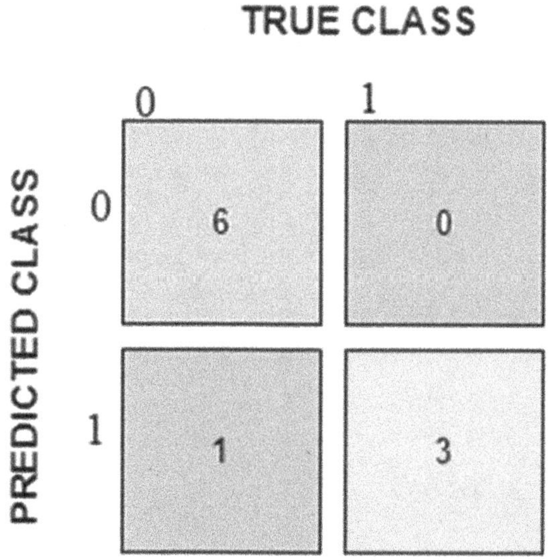

Figure 13.3   Confusion matrix for RF model

The higher value of the diagonal values in the matrix specified the prediction precision and the column on the right shows the accuracy for each predicted category. From Figure 13.3 there are two predicted categories: category 0 and category 1. Out of 10 dengue patients whose data were used as the test, the trained classifier predicted that six patients had DF (category 0) and three patients had DFW (category 1). For category 0, it was observed that the classifier could avoid any false-positive predictions but for category 1, only one patient was falsely predicted

Figure 13.4 shows the testing resulting tree for the model. The accuracy of the testing data was >90 %, which successfully classified 9 patients out of 10 test dengue patients. After the vital signs input, a classification would be provided depicting one of two classes, for example, DF or DFW. The selected classifier was visualized using a tree structure generation and tree (0) was selected among the others because it gave a more detailed idea of the workability of the RF model.

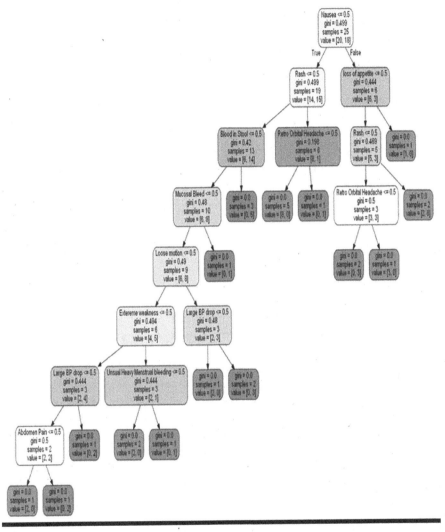

Figure 13.4   RF tree

13.7 Discussion

Although recall and F-1 scores for category 1 were relatively lower than category 0 it still gave promising results when predicting patients showing warning signs. The patients in category1 carried more risk than category 0, because the warning signs indicated the possibility of internal bleeding, which is usually the manifestation of a low platelet count. Thrombocytopenia is a condition in which an abnormally low platelet count causes nosebleeds, blood in the urine, heavy menstrual periods, bruising, and bleeding gums. Although it is easily treated, if left unattended it can easily escalate into a life-threatening situation, especially in tropical/subtropical areas where dengue is viewed as a rapidly emerging pandemic disease. Moreover, some obstacles were faced when carrying out this study, such as finding a large public dataset that was based on symptoms related to dengue disease for the implementation of this proposed model. Deep learning is preferred over machine learning for better accuracy compared with the latter when trained using a huge volume of data in this study as discussed previously, the data volume was not adequate. Also, the problem of handling old physical file records that have missing or unreadable values/pages is one of the important challenges in the construction of the dengue patient prediction model. This includes time constraints, manual work, and legal formalities (hospitals, laboratories), which are required when acquiring the resources required for the proposed system. However, these shortcomings can be addressed in future work.

The dataset for this study targeted patients who were suffering from signs/symptoms and after confirmation, they were labeled as dengue positive. The majority of training and testing data were from patients classified as category 0, for instance, DF whereas the patients classified under category 1, for instance, DFW need to be managed, which requires them to be admitted for hospital management. The RF algorithm was selected as the best classifier among the other selected machine learning tree algorithms based on its accuracy. One of the reasons for this higher accuracy could be the use of 13 predictors to train the model; however, its precision power was not the highest among the other classifiers. The C4.5 and ID3 models showed 0.95 and 0.93 precision scores, respectively, which was relatively higher than the precision of 0.86 that was achieved by the RF model for category 0. So, selecting the model based on the accuracy percentage alone is not a reliable option to a certain extent, the sensitivity/specificity are also important parameters that need to be taken into consideration in the prediction model development. Specificity gives the ability of the model to correctly classify those patients without disease and sensitivity gives the ability to correctly classify the dengue patients' levels. For this study, the sensitivity (recall) of RF was calculated as 1.00, which further explained how this model had a very low false-positive ratio in the confusion matrix results. It was also observed that parameters, such as precision, recall, and F-1 score had values for category 0 of 0.86, 1.00, and 0.92, respectively; and for category 1 of 1.00, 0.75, and 0.86, respectively.

13.8 Conclusions

The purpose of this chapter was to choose a suitable prediction model for DF that could further assist in improving the current dengue disease management practice, especially in areas that have minimal or no medical facilities or in current pandemics-like scenarios. Moreover, in the COVID-19 pandemic, all medical resources were concentrated on fighting against it, which resulted in the neglect of other diseases like dengue, which raised alarms in already burdened dengue-prone countries. This study showed that the trained RF classifier model gave the highest accuracy among all other tree-based machine learning classifiers. Overall, promising results were observed from the proposed model to classify the level of dengue patients, with an emphasis on patients showing warning signs that needed to consult a doctor for timely treatment. The proposed model was able to achieve good classification parameters, such as 96.14% accuracy, 0.86 precision, and 1.0 recall, which gave promising results among the selected pool of classifiers. The proposed model's novelty was not only in effectively diagnosing infected people based on risk but also in alerting them against the warning signs based on observed symptoms, which could stand alone or in combination with hemorrhagic manifestations. In dengue disease, internal hemorrhagic manifestations are the primary cause of mortality in patients as they are indicators of thrombocytopenia, which has been proven by researchers over time to be the main cause of the deadly effects in dengue. This study mimicked the usual way a doctor investigates patients suspected of being infected, which is why, unlike previous studies, this could pinpoint the cases that require medical help even before undergoing clinical tests. Due to similar symptomatic periods in dengue and COVID-19, the proposed method could be more useful in the early detection of severe cases of dengue and will lessen the burden on healthcare professionals with a decrease in fatal cases to curb dengue, which is a rapidly growing epidemic, on a timely basis.

However, a graphical user interface (GUI)-based front end could facilitate the workability of this proposed model on a large scale, and the addition of more data in category 1 and from patients who claimed to be dengue negative (although suffering from ≥1 symptoms, like dengue disease) could add to the diversity of symptomatic investigations. Deep learning can also enhance the overall disease prediction efficiency if sufficient data can be collected and then experimented with, which usually is one of the limitations in the study of this disease. Although the aims stated in the Introduction have been achieved, the effectiveness of the proposed system should be evaluated for larger databases on dengue disease. Future work will try to correctly calculate the severity index of dengue patients based on the classification provided by WHO and classify patients into three levels, for example, DF, DHF, and DSS to further enhance the disease prediction systems to withstand the current epidemic pressure and to help the medical sector to fight pandemic-like situations (COVID-19) in the future.

References

1. Anggraeni W, Abdillah A, Pujiadi, Trikoratno, L. T., Wibowo RP, Purnomo MH, Sudiarti, Y. Modelling and forecasting the dengue hemorrhagic fever cases number using hybrid fuzzy- ARIMA. 7th International Conference on Serious Games and Applications for Health; 2019 1–8. Available from: doi.10.1109/SeGAH.2019.8882433

2. Mondal MRH, Bharati S, Podder P. CO-IRv2: Optimized InceptionResNetV2 for COVID-19 detection from chest CT images. *PLoS One.* 2021; 16(10): e0259179.
3. Phadke R, Mohan A, Cavdaroglu S, Dapke K, Costa ACDS, Riaz MMA, et al. Dengue amidst COVID-19 in India: The mystery of plummeting cases. *J Med Virol.* 2021; 93(7):4120–1. doi: 10.1002/jmv.26987.
4. Lu X, Bambrick H, Pongsumpun P, Dhewantara PW, Toan DTT, Hu W. Dengue outbreaks in the COVID-19 era: Alarm raised for Asia. *PLoS Negl Trop Dis.* 2021; 15(10):e0009778.
5. Binti Mohd Zainee N, Chellappan K. A preliminary dengue fever prediction model based on a vital signs and blood profile. IECBES 2016 – IEEE-EMBS Conference on Biomedical Engineering and Sciences; 2016, Dec 4–8; Kuala Lumpur, Malaysia. doi.10.1109/IECBES.2016.7843530
6. Gambhir S, Malik SK, Kumar Y. PSO-ANN based diagnostic model for the early detection of dengue disease. *New Horiz Translational Med.* 2017, 4(1–4):1–8. doi.org/10.1016/j.nhtm.2017.10.001
7. Gambhir S, Malik SK, Kumar Y. The diagnosis of dengue disease: An evaluation of three machine learning approaches. *Int J Healthc Inf Syst Inform.* 2018; 13(3):1–19. doi.10.4018/IJHISI.2018070101
8. Hair GME, Nobre FF, Brasil P. Characterization of clinical patterns of dengue patients using an unsupervised machine learning approach. *BMC Infect Dis.* 2019; 19(1):1 11. doi.10.1186/s12879-019-4282-y
9. Centres for Disease Control and Prevention [Internet]. Available from https://cdc.gov/dengue/index.html. (n.d.). Dengue.
10. WHO [Internet] Available from: https://who.int/news-room/fact-sheets/detail/dengue-and-severe-dengue.
11. Nayak SDP, Narayan KA. Forecasting dengue fever incidence using ARIMA analysis. *Int J Collab Res Internal Med Pub Health.* 2019; 11(3):924–32. Available from: www.iomcworld.org/abstract/forecasting-dengue-fever-incidence-using-arima-analysis-44475.html
12. Pandiyarajan P, Thangairulappan K. Classification of dengue serotypes using protein sequence based on rule extraction from neural network. LNCS (LNAI LNBI). 2018; 11308 LNAI:127–37. doi.10.1007/978-3-030-05918-7_12
13. Potts JA, Gibbons RV, Rothman AL, Srikiatkhachorn A, Thomas SJ, Supradish P, et al . Prediction of dengue disease severity among pediatric Thai patients using early clinical laboratory indicators. *PLoS Negl Trop Dis.* 2010; 4(8):2–8. doi.10.1371/journal.pntd.0000769
14. Saikia D, Dutta JC. Early diagnosis of dengue disease using fuzzy inference system. 2016 International Conference on Microelectronics, Computing and Communications (MicroCom); 2016; Jan 23–25; Durgapur, India.. doi.10.1109/MicroCom.2016.7522513
15. Sreenivasan P, Geetha S, Sasikala K. Development of a prognostic prediction model to determine severe dengue in children. *Indian J Pediatr.* 2018; 85(6):433–9. doi.10.1007/s12098-017-2591-y
16. Idris MFIM, Abdullah A, Fauzi SSM. Prediction of dengue outbreak in Selangor using fuzzy logic. Proceedings of the Second International Conference on the Future of ASEAN (ICoFA). 2017; 2: p. 593–603. Singapore: Springer.

17. Divya A, Lavanya S. Real time dengue prediction using machine learning. *Indian J Public Health Res Dev*. 2020; 11(2).

18. Chakraborty A, Chandru V. A robust and non-parametric model for prediction of dengue incidence. *J Indian Inst Sci*. 2020; 100(4):1–7.

19. Pravin A, Jacob TP, Nagarajan G. An intelligent and secure healthcare framework for the prediction and prevention of Dengue virus outbreak using fog computing. *Health Technol*. 2019; 1–9.

20. Mohapatra C, Rautray SS, Pandey M. Prevention of infectious disease based on big data analytics and map-reduce. ICECCT. 2017 (1–4). IEEE.

21. Gambhir S, Malik SK, Kumar Y. The diagnosis of dengue disease: An evaluation of three machine learning approaches. *I J Healthc Inf Syst Inform*. 2018; 13(3):1–19.

22. Ooi JYL, Thomas JJ. DengueViz: A knowledge-based expert system integrated with parallel coordinates visualization in the dengue diagnosis. Advances in Visual Informatics International Visual Informatics Conference; 2017; 10645:50–61. Cham: Springer. doi.10.1007/978-3-319-70010-6_5.

23. Chellappan K. A preliminary dengue fever prediction model based on vital signs and blood profile. Conference on Biomedical Engineering and Sciences; 2016; Dec 4–8; Kuala Lumpur, Malaysia. IEEE.

24. Saikia D, Dutta JC. Early diagnosis of Dengue disease using fuzzy inference system. Microelectronics, Computing and Communications. 2016; Jan 23–25; Durgapur, India. IEEE.

25. Mondal MRH, Bharati S, Podder P, Podder, P. Data analytics for novel coronavirus disease. *Inform Med Unlocked*. 2020; 20:100374.

26. Bharati S, Podder P, Mondal M, Prasath VB. CO-ResNet: Optimized ResNet model for COVID-19 diagnosis from X-ray images. *Int J Hybrid Intell Syst*. 2021; 17(1–2):71–85

27. Bharati S, Podder P, Mondal MRH. Hybrid deep learning for detecting lung diseases from X-ray images. *Inform Med Unlocked*. 2020; 20:100391.

28. Bharati S, Mondal MRH. 12 Applications and challenges of AI-driven IoHT for combating pandemics: a review. In: Khamparia A , Mondal MRH , Podder P , Bhushan B , Albuquerque V , Kumar S, editors. *Computational Intelligence for Managing Pandemics*. Berlin, Boston: De Gruyter. pp. 213–30.

29. Paul P, Bharati S, Podder P, Mondal MRH. 10 The role of IoMT during pandemics. In: Khamparia A, Mondal RHM, Podder P, Bhushan B, Albuquerque V, Kumar S. *Computational Intelligence for Managing Pandemics*. Berlin, Boston: De Gruyter; 2021. pp. 169–86.

30. Mondal MRH, Bharati S, Podder P. Diagnosis of COVID-19 using machine learning and deep learning: A review. *Curr Med Imaging*. 2021;17(12):1403–18

31. Bharati S, Podder P, Mondal M, Prasath VB. Medical imaging with deep learning for COVID-19 diagnosis: A comprehensive review. *arXiv*: 2107.09602. 2021; Available from: https://arxiv.org/abs/2107.09602

32. Podder P, Khamparia A, Mondal MRH, Rahman MA, Bharati S. Forecasting the spread of COVID-19 and ICU requirements. *Int J online Biomed Eng*. 2021; 17(5):81

33. Podder P, Bharati S, Mondal MRH, Kose U. Application of machine learning for the diagnosis of COVID-19. In: Kose U , Gupta D , Albuquerque V , Khanna A. *Data Science for COVID-19*. Academic Press; 2021. pp. 175–94.

Index

287

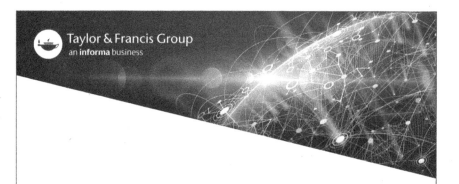